Molecular Imaging of
Neurodegenerative Disorders

Donna J. Cross · Karina Mosci
Satoshi Minoshima
Editors

Molecular Imaging of Neurodegenerative Disorders

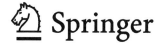

Springer

Editors
Donna J. Cross
Department of Radiology and Imaging
Sciences
University of Utah
Salt Lake City, UT, USA

Karina Mosci
Department of Nuclear Medicine
Hospital das Forças Armadas (HFA)
Brasilia, Distrito Federal, Brazil

Satoshi Minoshima
Department of Radiology and Imaging
Sciences
University of Utah
Salt Lake City, UT, USA

ISBN 978-3-031-35097-9   ISBN 978-3-031-35098-6   (eBook)
https://doi.org/10.1007/978-3-031-35098-6

This Springer imprint is published by the registered company Springer Nature Switzerland AG
The registered company address is: Gewerbestrasse 11, 6330 Cham, Switzerland

We would like to dedicate this book to the memory of Dr. David E Kuhl and Dr. Henry N. Wagner, Jr. who made unparalleled contributions to the field and inspired us to be molecular brain imagers.

Preface

It is with great pleasure that we present this textbook on *Molecular Imaging of Neurodegenerative Disorders*. Neurodegenerative disorders represent a significant burden on both individuals and society, and their prevalence is expected to increase as the population ages. Molecular imaging techniques provide a powerful tool for investigations, early diagnosis, tracking disease progression, and evaluating the effectiveness of therapeutic interventions.

The goal of this textbook is to provide a comprehensive and accessible resource for trainees, researchers, clinicians, and other professionals interested in the field of molecular imaging of neurodegenerative disorders. Leading experts in the field have contributed chapters on diverse topics ranging from the biology of neurodegeneration to the latest imaging modalities and techniques.

The textbook begins with an introduction to neurodegenerative disorders, common molecular imaging modalities and radiotracers used for diagnosis including Alzheimer's disease, and Parkinson's disease. The chapters also cover emerging techniques in molecular imaging, such as imaging of protein aggregates, neuroinflammation, and AI-based image analysis. The final chapter is a comprehensive tutorial with practice cases for how to read clinical brain images.

We hope that this textbook will serve as a valuable resource for all those interested in helping patients suffering from neurodegenerative disorders. We would like to express our gratitude to all the authors who have contributed to this textbook, and to the editorial team for their hard work and dedication in bringing this project to fruition.

Salt Lake City, UT, USA   Donna J. Cross
Brasilia, Distrito Federal, Brazil   Karina Mosci
Salt Lake City, UT, USA   Satoshi Minoshima

Acknowledgments

We would like to thank all of the authors who contributed to this book despite their extremely busy schedules as well as all of our colleagues collaborating across the globe. We would like to recognize the Society of Nuclear Medicine and Molecular Imaging (SNMMI) Brain Imaging Council and the International Atomic Energy Agency (IAEA) for their support and efforts to promote brain molecular imaging. We also would like to thank our family members who supported our efforts in this publication. Lastly, we would like to remember those patients who taught us every day how to be better molecular imaging scientists and physicians.

Contents

Contributors

Javier Arbizu Department of Nuclear Medicine, Clínica Universidad de Navarra, Pamplona, Navarra, Spain

Jaimie Barr The Division of Nuclear Medicine, Department of Radiology, University of Michigan, Ann Arbor, MI, USA

Morris K. Udall Center of Excellence for Parkinson's Disease Research, University of Michigan, Ann Arbor, MI, USA

University of Michigan Parkinson's Foundation Research Center of Excellence, Ann Arbor, MI, USA

Tammie L. S. Benzinger Neuroradiology Section, Department of Radiology, Mallinckrodt Institute of Radiology, Washington University in St. Louis, Saint Louis, MO, USA

Gérard N. Bischof Department of Nuclear Medicine, University Hospital Cologne, Cologne, Germany

Molecular Organization of the Brain, Institute for Neuroscience and Medicine (INM-2), Jülich, Germany

Nico Bohnen The Division of Nuclear Medicine, Department of Radiology, University of Michigan, Ann Arbor, MI, USA

Morris K. Udall Center of Excellence for Parkinson's Disease Research, University of Michigan, Ann Arbor, MI, USA

Department of Neurology, University of Michigan, Ann Arbor, MI, USA

GRECC and Neurology Service, VAAAHS, Ann Arbor, MI, USA

Per Borghammer Department of Nuclear Medicine and PET, Aarhus University Hospital, Aarhus, Denmark

Pierrick Bourgeat CSIRO The Australian e-Health Research Centre, Brisbane, Australia

David J. Brooks Department of Nuclear Medicine and PET, Aarhus University Hospital, Aarhus, Denmark

Positron Emission Tomography Centre, Newcastle University, Newcastle upon Tyne, UK

Richard E. Carson Department of Radiology and Biomedical Imaging, Yale University School of Medicine, New Haven, CT, USA

Department of Biomedical Engineering, Yale University, New Haven, CT, USA

Department of Radiology and Biomedical Imaging, Yale PET Center, Yale University, New Haven, CT, USA

Ciprian Catana Department of Radiology, Athinoula A. Martinos Center for Biomedical Imaging, Massachusetts General Hospital and Harvard Medical School, Charlestown, MA, USA

Ming-Kai Chen Department of Radiology and Biomedical Imaging, Yale University School of Medicine, New Haven, CT, USA

Harry T. Chugani Department of Neurology, NYU School of Medicine, New York, NY, USA

Ann D. Cohen Department of Psychiatry, University of Pittsburgh, Pittsburgh, PA, USA

Donna J. Cross Department of Radiology and Imaging Sciences, University of Utah, Salt Lake City, UT, USA

Vincent Doré Department of Molecular Imaging and Therapy, Austin Health, Melbourne, VIC, Australia

CSIRO Health and Biosecurity Flagship: The Australian e-Health Research Centre, Melbourne, VIC, Australia

Alexander Drzezga Department of Nuclear Medicine, Faculty of Medicine and University Hospital Cologne, University of Cologne, Cologne, Germany

German Center for Neurodegenerative Diseases (DZNE), Bonn-Cologne, Germany

Institute of Neuroscience and Medicine (INM-2), Molecular Organization of the Brain, Jülich, Germany

Sjoerd J. Finnema Neuroscience Discovery Research, Translational Imaging, AbbVie, North Chicago, IL, USA

Norman L. Foster Department of Neurology, University of Utah, Salt Lake City, UT, USA

Jean-Dominique Gallezot Department of Radiology and Biomedical Imaging, Yale PET Center, Yale University, New Haven, CT, USA

Kathrin Giehl Department of Nuclear Medicine, Faculty of Medicine and University Hospital Cologne, University of Cologne, Cologne, Germany

Institute of Neuroscience and Medicine (INM-2), Molecular Organization of the Brain, Jülich, Germany

Alexandra Gogola Department of Radiology, University of Pittsburgh, Pittsburgh, PA, USA

Dima A. Hammoud Radiology and Imaging Sciences, National Institutes of Health/Clinical Center, Bethesda, MD, USA

Peter Herscovitch Positron Emission Tomography Department, National Institutes of Health/Clinical Center, Bethesda, MD, USA

Jacob Horsager Department of Nuclear Medicine and PET, Aarhus University Hospital, Aarhus, Denmark

Department of Clinical Medicine, Aarhus University, Aarhus, Denmark

Milos D. Ikonomovic Geriatric Research Education and Clinical Center, VA Pittsburgh Healthcare System, Pittsburgh, PA, USA

Kazunari Ishii Department of Radiology, Kindai University Faculty of Medicine, Osakasayama, Osaka, Japan

Saurabh Jindal Neuroimaging Laboratories-Research Center, Mallinckrodt Institute of Radiology, Washington University in St. Louis, Saint Louis, MO, USA

Prabesh Kanel The Division of Nuclear Medicine, Department of Radiology, University of Michigan, Ann Arbor, MI, USA

Morris K. Udall Center of Excellence for Parkinson's Disease Research, University of Michigan, Ann Arbor, MI, USA

University of Michigan Parkinson's Foundation Research Center of Excellence, Ann Arbor, MI, USA

Kejal Kantarci Department of Radiology, Mayo Clinic, Rochester, MN, USA

Guillaume Lamotte Department of Neurology, University of Utah, Salt Lake City, UT, USA

Oscar Lopez Department of Neurology, University of Pittsburgh, Pittsburgh, PA, USA

Brian J. Lopresti Department of Radiology, University of Pittsburgh, Pittsburgh, PA, USA

N. Scott Mason Department of Radiology, University of Pittsburgh, Pittsburgh, PA, USA

David Matuskey Department of Radiology and Biomedical Imaging, Yale University School of Medicine, New Haven, CT, USA

Department of Psychiatry, Yale University School of Medicine, New Haven, CT, USA

Department of Neurology, Yale University School of Medicine, New Haven, CT, USA

Davneet Minhas Department of Radiology, University of Pittsburgh, Pittsburgh, PA, USA

Satoshi Minoshima Department of Radiology and Imaging Sciences, University of Utah, Salt Lake City, UT, USA

Karina Mosci Department of Nuclear Medicine, Hospital das Forças Armadas (HFA), Brasilia, Distrito Federal, Brazil

Neelesh Nadkarni Department of Geriatric Medicine, University of Pittsburgh, Pittsburgh, PA, USA

Mika Naganawa Department of Radiology and Biomedical Imaging, Yale PET Center, Yale University, New Haven, CT, USA

Niels Okkels Department of Nuclear Medicine and PET, Aarhus University Hospital, Aarhus, Denmark

Department of Clinical Medicine, Aarhus University, Aarhus, Denmark

Department of Neurology, Aarhus University Hospital, Aarhus, Denmark

Yoshiaki Ota The Division of Neuroradiology, Department of Radiology, University of Michigan, Ann Arbor, MI, USA

The Division of Nuclear Medicine, Department of Radiology, University of Michigan, Ann Arbor, MI, USA

Nicola Pavese Department of Nuclear Medicine and PET, Aarhus University Hospital, Aarhus, Denmark

Clinical Ageing Research Unit, Newcastle University, Newcastle upon Tyne, UK

Victor W. Pike Molecular Imaging Branch, National Institute of Mental Health, Bethesda, MD, USA

C. Chauncey Spears Morris K. Udall Center of Excellence for Parkinson's Disease Research, University of Michigan, Ann Arbor, MI, USA

Department of Neurology, University of Michigan, Ann Arbor, MI, USA

Tanyaluck Thientunyakit Division of Nuclear Medicine, Department of Radiology, Faculty of Medicine Siriraj Hospital, Mahidol University, Bangkok, Thailand

Victor L. Villemagne Department of Psychiatry, University of Pittsburgh, Pittsburgh, PA, USA

Department of Molecular Imaging and Therapy, Austin Health, Melbourne, VIC, Australia

Greg Zaharchuk Stanford University, Stanford, CA, USA

Burcu Zeydan Department of Radiology, Mayo Clinic, Rochester, MN, USA

Department of Neurology, Mayo Clinic, Rochester, MN, USA

1

Burcu Zeydan and Kejal Kantarci

Key Points

1. Neurodegeneration is defined as the process of structural and/or functional loss in neuronal cells.
2. The primary mechanisms underlying neurodegeneration include protein misfolding, protein aggregation, autophagy, lysosomal dysfunction, oxidative injury, mitochondrial dysfunction, and neuroinflammation.
3. The neurovascular unit comprises the multidimensional relationship between brain cells and their microvasculature.
4. Among the main imaging modalities of neurodegeneration are structural MRI, diffusion MRI, arterial spin labeling, MR spectroscopy, FDG, SV2A, beta-amyloid, and tau PET.
5. The neurotransmitter systems in neurodegenerative diseases can be investigated by dopaminergic and cholinergic imaging techniques.

6. Emerging imaging techniques of neurodegeneration include ultra-field MRI, functional MRI, quantitative susceptibility imaging, and TSPO PET.

Pathophysiology of Neurodegeneration

Neurodegeneration is defined as the process of structural and/or functional loss in neuronal cells. Neurodegenerative diseases such as Alzheimer's disease (AD) and Parkinson's disease (PD) comprise a progressive, irreversible, and often slow process affecting specific vulnerable subsets of cells in certain anatomic regions of the brain, which determine the clinical presentation and disease course [1]. Neurodegenerative diseases stand out with their high prevalence and cost as well as the challenge in discovery of mechanism-targeted effective treatments [2].

The concept of neurovascular unit includes the multi-dimensional relationship between brain cells and their microvasculature as well as the organized reaction of brain cells and vessels to injury [3]. Neurons, microglia, astrocytes, basal membrane, pericytes, and endothelial cells are the main components of the neurovascular unit [4]. The developmental, structural, and functional interactions of brain cells and blood vessels in the neurovascular unit contribute to the maintenance and regulation of cerebral blood flow, blood–

B. Zeydan (✉)
Department of Radiology, Mayo Clinic, Rochester, MN, USA

Department of Neurology, Mayo Clinic, Rochester, MN, USA
e-mail: zeydan.burcu@mayo.edu

K. Kantarci
Department of Radiology, Mayo Clinic, Rochester, MN, USA
e-mail: kantarci.kejal@mayo.edu

brain barrier function, and brain homeostasis [5, 6]. Therefore, the changes in the neurovascular unit function may trigger neurodegeneration by the decrease in cerebral blood flow leading to hypoxia, the decrease in production of trophic factors resulting in increased cell vulnerability, irregularities in the blood–brain barrier causing dysfunction in homeostasis, and the decrease in the clearance of metabolites leading to accumulation of proteins such as beta-amyloid and tau [5].

The main risk factor for neurodegenerative diseases is aging. Neuronal loss and alterations in neurotransmitters happen both during aging and also with neurodegenerative diseases that lead to cognitive and motor dysfunction in older individuals [2]. The precise etiology of neurodegenerative diseases mostly remains unknown, but the main underlying mechanisms are usually shared among distinct neurodegenerative diseases [7] and are likely to be influenced or triggered by numerous metabolic, genetic, or environmental factors [2].

Some of the main mechanisms underlying neurodegenerative diseases that result in progressive neuronal cell dysfunction and ultimately cell death through common neuronal pathways are: (1) Protein misfolding, defective degradation, extra and intracellular aggregation of misfolded proteins, (2) autophagy and lysosomal dysfunction, (3) reactive oxidative species and free radical formation, mitochondrial deficits, excitotoxicity, and dysregulation of intracellular calcium, and (4) neuroinflammation [2, 7–9].

Protein Misfolding and Aggregation

Protein aggregation is one of the basic underlying mechanisms in neurodegenerative diseases. Based on their flexibility, proteins shift between a variety of conformational substrates. Newly synthesized proteins convert to functional molecules after folding. Abnormal interactions between highly soluble proteins lead to protein misfolding through alterations in protein conformation. The insoluble, improperly folded or misfolded proteins self-accumulate as a result of structural change of the normal, functional proteins [9, 10].

Defective intra and extracellular protein aggregation and accumulation leads to mitochondrial dysfunction, oxidative stress, and reactive oxygen species, defects in ubiquitin-proteasome system and abnormal alternative mRNA exon splicing [11]. AD and PD are main examples of neurodegenerative diseases with protein misfolding and aggregation.

Autophagy and Lysosomal Dysfunction

As a catabolic process, autophagy is the degradation of protein aggregates, excess or damaged organelles and cytosolic contents in lysosomes [12]. In case of abnormalities in autophagy and lysosomal dysfunction, the cell contents are not degraded properly and they start to accumulate [13]. CAG-polyglutamine repeat diseases such as Huntington disease is an example of aberrant degradation of autophagy pathway [14].

Oxidative Injury and Mitochondrial Dysfunction

Oxidative stress is a major contributor in the development of neurodegeneration. The formation of reactive oxidative species may be due to mechanisms such as metal-associated Fenton reactions, electrons that escape from respiratory chain reactions with oxygen and lipid peroxidation [15]. Once the free radical formation exceeds antioxidant mechanisms, oxidative injury takes place. Consequently, oxidative injury leads to mitochondrial deficits, excitotoxity and dysregulation of intracellular calcium resulting in neuronal cell dysfunction [9].

Damage to mitochondrial DNA and oxidative stress lead to mitochondrial impairment, which particularly increase with aging. Mitochondrial dysfunction is followed by the promotion of cell death as the cells become more vulnerable to degeneration and neurotoxic insults once the cell energy metabolism and ion homeostasis get compromised [9, 16].

Neuroinflammation

Chronic inflammatory reactions play an important role in the pathogenesis of neurodegenerative diseases. With aging, inflammatory pathways lead to neurodegeneration by either becoming hyperactivated (too much function) or inadequate to manage aging associated stress (too little function) [9, 17]. Microglia activation is a key component of neuroinflammatory reactions as it has both neuroprotective and neurotoxic features and is seen as a double-edged sword in neurodegeneration, especially in AD [18]. Microglia is a key factor in beta-amyloid clearance, but continued beta-amyloid production leads to reduction in the ability of microglial beta-amyloid clearance and increase in beta-amyloid deposition.

Multimodality Imaging of Neurodegeneration

Pathology is the current gold standard for definite diagnosis of neurodegenerative diseases [8]. However, multimodality imaging biomarkers of neurodegeneration have recently provided a more objective and in vivo understanding of the pathological changes. By enlightening the pathophysiology and detecting subtle structural and molecular changes, imaging biomarkers offer a complementary window of opportunity to help diagnose neurodegenerative diseases early and accurately, even in preclinical stages, to delay or avoid hospitalization, and to initiate early symptomatic management. It is also used for evaluating disease severity and disease course. Moreover, imaging biomarkers of neurodegeneration help develop disease-modifying treatments [19]. Some of these practical imaging biomarkers are already included in diagnostic criteria of neurodegenerative diseases for more accurate diagnosis.

Primary clinical symptoms, anatomical distribution of regions affected by neurodegeneration, or the main cellular/molecular abnormality may be used in classification of neurodegenerative diseases [8]. Often, the underlying pathology is complex with contribution from multiple etiologies such as AD, dementia with Lewy bodies (DLB), limbic pre-dominant age-related TDP-43 encephalopathy (LATE), and cerebrovascular disease [20]. This etiological heterogeneity tends to increase with age.

Structural MRI

Structural MRI is the main and most widely used imaging technique in neurodegenerative diseases. Structural MRI is also used to exclude other possible etiologies of cognitive dysfunction such as mass lesions and intracranial hemorrhage [21]. It is a common biomarker of progression in neurodegenerative diseases and have been used as an outcome measure in disease-modifying intervention trials.

In assessment of neurodegenerative diseases, structural MRI primarily targets atrophy and is able to detect even subtle morphological changes by utilizing volumetry and regional morphometry metrics, but also qualitative measures such as visual ratings [22]. Although it can assess changes in brain volume globally, it can also evaluate region-specific volume loss in brain and by identifying these atrophy patterns specific to the disease process, it can help differentiate neurodegenerative diseases from each other.

The anatomic changes in hippocampus and entorhinal cortex of the limbic system and precuneus, which is part of medial parietal lobe are essential in interpreting early neurodegenerative processes [23, 24]. Significant and disproportionate structural atrophy in medial and lateral temporal lobes and medial parietal cortex is a biomarker of neurodegeneration used for AD as a diagnostic criterion [25]. The lack of medial temporal lobe atrophy or minimal atrophy in medial temporal lobe is more consistent with DLB [26]. However, as AD and DLB may coexist quite commonly [26], medial temporal lobe atrophy is not an exclusion criterion for DLB.

The frontal or anterior temporal lobe atrophy with relatively preserved hippocampal and medial temporal lobe volume is suggestive for the behavioral variant of frontotemporal dementia [27], whereas putamen, pons, middle cerebellar peduncle, or cerebellum atrophy on MRI is suggestive of multiple system atrophy (MSA) [28]. Relative midbrain atrophy compared to pons is a characteristic imaging finding for progressive supranuclear palsy (PSP) [29]. Lacunar and cortical infarcts and moderate to severe white matter hyperintensities seen on the FLAIR MRI may suggest cognitive impairment due to vascular disease.

Diffusion MRI

Diffusion MRI evaluates the random and thermally induced displacement of water molecules as they diffuse within the tissue [30] and provides information about the microstructural integrity and complexity of the white matter. This data can be used to make inferences on membrane permeability, myelination, and axonal density. Among diffusion MRI techniques, diffusion tensor imaging (DTI) is the most commonly used technique to study neurodegenerative diseases, but other new techniques such as neurite orientation dispersion and density (NODDI) and free-water imaging (FWI) have also been developed, to improve the specificity of DTI for axonal integrity and free-water in the tissue [31].

Diffusion MRI facilitates interpreting pathophysiological and microstructural alterations underlying neurodegenerative diseases such as AD, PD, and amyotrophic lateral sclerosis (ALS). For example, in AD, in addition to gray matter injury, white matter injury and related changes also occur and can be measured through the DTI metrics [32]. In AD, DTI can particularly detect the microstructural changes in white matter tracts that link regions affected early in the disease course such as parahippocampus and fornix [33, 34]. These microstructural changes also associate with abnormal beta-amyloid and tau deposits in cognitively unimpaired individuals [35].

Because diffusion MRI is a quantitative imaging tool of cell pathophysiology, tissue microstructure, and structural connectivity, it is also a good candidate for detecting and monitoring early pathological changes and can be used as a biomarker in clinical trials [36, 37].

Arterial Spin Labeling (ASL) MRI

Arterial spin labeling (ASL) is an emerging MRI technique that measures cerebral blood flow quantitively and provides information about perfusion changes in neurodegenerative diseases. Classically, the metabolic changes in the brain are identified by FDG PET. However, especially in patients who are already undergoing an MRI scan, ASL MRI can be a good alternative for FDG PET, because hypoperfusion patterns on ASL MRI generally overlap with hypermetabolism patterns on FDG PET [38, 39]. For example, in DLB, ASL MRI can help detect the cingulate island sign [39]. Yet, in patients with mild cognitive impairment (MCI) and AD, apart from the typical hypoperfused regions, ASL also detects regions of hyperperfusion that reflects the functional response to neurodegeneration [40]. In addition to being more accessible, faster and cheaper in acquisition compared to FDG PET, ASL MRI can be used for evaluation of vascular factors that play a role in neurodegeneration as well [40].

MR Spectroscopy

Although conventional MRI is adequately utilized for morphological changes in neurodegenerative diseases, it does not particularly provide information on molecular changes. Conversely, MR spectroscopy can illustrate alterations in cell type, cell density, metabolite levels/biochemical composition using the proton [^{1}H] of water, and it helps enlighten underlying disease mechanisms. Hence, conventional MRI and MR spectroscopy complement each other at every stage of the disease course including diagnosis, follow-up, and therapy response [41].

MR spectroscopy is utilized in biomarker research in many diseases including brain tumors, epilepsy, multiple sclerosis, traumatic brain injury, and stroke. In neurodegenerative diseases including AD, PD, and ALS, a decrease in total N-acetlyaspartate (tNAA) in the regions that reflect the characteristic pattern of neurodegenerative process of each disease is typically detected by MR spectroscopy [42, 43]. As a prognostic biomarker, the decrease in tNAA associates with clinical metrics and pathological severity [44, 45].

Elevation in myoinositol is closely associated with microglial activation seen in neurodegeneration [46]. It precedes reduction of total NAA, neuronal loss, and cognitive impairment in dementia [47, 48]. Besides the decrease in the total NAA and elevation in myoinositol levels [49, 50], reduction in glutamate [50, 51] and elevation in total choline levels [42] are other changes in neurochemical profiles commonly seen in neurodegeneration that are detected by MR spectroscopy. Moreover, functional response to treatment in neurodegenerative diseases can be observed with MR spectroscopy monitoring [41]. Temporary increase in tNAA level [52] and decreased myoinositol/total creatinine level [53] were observed following donepezil treatment in AD.

Fluorodeoxyglucose (FDG) PET

Fluorodeoxyglucose (FDG) is the most common radionucleotide ligand used in clinical practice. FDG is taken up by the cells through regular glucose transporters and its uptake is higher by cells which are metabolically more active. The brain uses glucose as its main energy source and most of the glucose utilization occurs with synaptic activity. The detection of hypometabolism by FDG PET may be used for evaluation of neurodegenerative diseases as neuronal injury and synaptic inactivity leads to metabolic dysfunction [21].

FDG PET helps in identification of regional glucose metabolism patterns, which may be useful in differential diagnosis of dementias. On FDG PET, the parietotemporal hypometabolism including precuneus and posterior cingulate cortex is considered the neurodegeneration biomarker of AD [25]. Conversely, the FDG uptake is decreased in the occipital lobe in DLB along with the cingulate island sign, which is supportive of the DLB diagnosis [26]. The cingulate island sign is observed when the metabolism of midcingulate and posterior cingulate cortex is relatively preserved, while there is hypometabolism in the cuneus and precuneus [54, 55].

In line with structural MRI findings, hypometabolism in the frontal or anterior temporal lobe is characteristic of the FDG PET in behavioral variant of FTD [27]. In PSP, midbrain hypometabolism relative to pons is observed in FDG PET [29]. Putamen hypometabolism in MSA-Cerebellar (MSA-C) and decreased metabolism in putamen, brainstem, and cerebellum may be seen in MSA-Parkinsonian (MSA-P) [28].

Synaptic Vesicle Glycoprotein 2A (SV2A) PET

Synapses are one of the main components of neurotransmission, linking neurons to each other via neurotransmitters. Loss or dysfunction in synapses is associated with motor, sensory, and cognitive impairment and is a crucial mechanism in neurodegeneration. Particularly, synaptic loss is a key feature and one of the earliest hallmarks of AD. It precedes beta-amyloid and tau accumulation in the preclinical stage of AD [56] and is correlated with cognitive impairment and disease severity in AD [57]. Similarly, synaptic dysfunction and loss is a characteristic component of PD and DLB pathogenesis. Apart from the loss of dopaminergic neurons in the nigrostriatal system, synaptic loss is found outside the nigrostriatal system as well in the nondopaminergic neurons of the cortex in neurodegenerative diseases including PD [58, 59].

Synaptic vesicle glycoprotein 2A (SV2A) is a widely expressed component of the synaptic vesicle in neuronal cells. In the central nervous system, it is commonly found as a presynaptic protein in GABAergic and glutamatergic neurons [60]. SV2A PET is the first noninvasive and in vivo method to directly evaluate synaptic density [61] and evaluation of synaptic density by SV2A PET is important at every stage of the disease course from diagnosis to prognosis in neurodegenerative diseases. So far, as a candidate biomarker of synaptic density, SV2A PET seems to have its highest potential in AD and PD. However, the use of SV2A PET is also promising in other diseases with synaptic abnormalities such as Huntington's disease, epilepsy, stroke, multiple sclerosis, depression, and autism spectrum disorders [59].

Amyloid PET

One of the main pathological hallmarks of AD is postmortem beta-amyloid plaques. As a molecular imaging technique, amyloid PET offers an in vivo antemortem histopathological picture of the central nervous system by demonstrating a characteristic distribution of amyloid-affected areas of the brain, in line with the pathological distribution [62].

Amyloid PET tracers can reliably quantify cortical beta-amyloid deposition with high sensitivity and specificity by crossing the blood–brain barrier and binding to beta-amyloid plaques. Among amyloid tracers, C11-Pittsburgh compound-B (PiB) tracer is widely used and PiB was the first published human amyloid PET tracer [63]. However, newer tracers such as F18-Florbetapir, F18-Florbetaben, and F18-Flutemetamol have been developed, which have longer radioactive half-lives with commercial availability.

Using amyloid PET in addition to non-PET biomarkers improves diagnostic precision in neurodegenerative diseases [64]. Increased cortical C11-PiB uptake is observed on PET in patients with AD compared to controls, showing the deposition of beta-amyloid plaques in the cerebral cortex [63]. Amyloid PET is also found positive in about 10–44% of cognitively unimpaired individuals aged 50–90 years, but the clinical relevance is not known [65]. Moreover, amyloid PET alone is not sufficient in determining the clinical transition from prodromal stages and disease staging in AD [66]. However, the use of amyloid PET has been suggested in identification of individuals with MCI with clinical uncertainty, individuals with dementia suggestive of AD, but with a mixed or atypical presentation, and individuals who present with early-onset progressive cognitive decline [67].

Tau PET

Tau pathology plays an important role in the development of various neurodegenerative diseases such as AD. Tau function depends on phosphorylation; however, its physiology is modified if tau becomes hyperphosphorylated and hyperphosphorylation of tau leads to increase in intracellular aggregation of tau [68].

Tau PET enables quantification of tau deposition in the brain by using tau PET tracers that target tau deposits in vivo in the brain [69]. As tau PET visualizes and reflects the regional patterns of tau throughout the brain in different pathologies, it is a promising tool for diagnosis of neurodegenerative diseases [70]. Tau PET also correlates with cognitive impairment and neurodegeneration and therefore provides information on prognosis [70, 71].

Imaging of Neurotransmitter Systems

Dopaminergic Imaging (DatSCAN)

For evaluation of parkinsonian syndromes, dopamine transporter (DAT) can be measured with single-photon emission computed tomography (SPECT). DAT SPECT serves as the standard in vivo molecular imaging biomarker of presynaptic dopaminergic nigrostriatal neurons. It is a supportive diagnostic tool used in differentiation of PD and atypical parkinsonisms (such as PSP, MSA, corticobasal disease) from vascular or drug-induced parkinsonisms, avoiding misdiagnosis and unnecessary dopaminergic treatment [72, 73]. Although DAT imaging (DatSCAN) cannot differentiate PD from atypical parkinsonisms, it improves the accuracy of diagnosis and shortens the time to diagnosis in PD [72, 74]. A normal DatSCAN is one of the Movement Disorders Society PD exclusion criteria [75] because DatSCAN is considered as a very reliable biomarker of degenerative parkinsonism.

DAT decline appears to be non-linear in PD [76] and DAT imaging is helpful in both diagnosis and early stages of PD, but also in monitoring treatment response. As downregulation of DAT happens early in the disease course [77], DATSCaN can detect changes in DAT density before symptoms become evident showing early synaptic dysfunction. Once the dopaminergic neuronal terminal loss surpasses 50% at symptom onset later in the disease course, DATSCaN shows the decline in striatal DAT uptake reflecting the neurodegeneration of presynaptic dopaminergic nerve terminals [73].

F18-DOPA PET is another functional imaging technique of dopamine deficiency that is especially useful in differential diagnosis of patients with early age at onset, atypical presentations, or mild symptoms of parkinsonian syndrome [78]. F18 DOPA PET evaluates the integrity of presynaptic dopaminergic activity and dopamine terminal loss by quantifying dopamine precursor uptake [79, 80] and is a reliable in vivo diagnostic tool for PD with high sensitivity and specificity [78].

Cholinergic Imaging

The cholinergic system is crucial in cognitive function and is involved in the processing of numerous circuits associated with cognition [81]. Consequently, the dysfunction in the cholinergic system is closely related to mechanisms involved in neurodegenerative processes underlying cognitive impairment and dementia [82]. Thus, targeting the cholinergic (both pre- and post-synaptic) system using molecular imaging of PET or SPECT provides an opportunity to investigate the multiple elements of dementia pathophysiology.

PET studies using ligands targeting acetylcholine esterase (AChE) show decreased AChE activity in AD, which is associated with attention and working memory [83] and based on the age of onset, the binding patterns appear to vary [84]. Furthermore, cholinergic imaging can be used for evaluation of treatment response. In patients with AD treated with donepezil and rivastigmine, cholinergic PET studies detected inhibition of AChE activity [85]. Molecular imaging of the cholinergic system is also used in parkinsonian dementias

and depict significantly decreased cortical AChE activity in PD dementia and DLB [86].

Emerging Imaging Techniques

Ultra-High Field MRI

3 T and 1.5 T MRIs are widely used in clinic and research for investigation of neurodegenerative diseases. However, higher field 7T MRI has several benefits over lower field MRIs, given its increased sensitivity in early detection of neurodegenerative changes. With increase in magnetic field strength and associated higher signal-to-noise ratio, high field MRI provides significant improvement in image quality along with higher spatial resolution and reduced acquisition time [87]. Furthermore, iron depositions leading to neurotoxicity can be detected early on with high field imaging, because the sensitivity of image contrast increases to iron levels in the tissue. Similarly, image quality is increased, and background suppression is improved in high field MR angiography with longer T1 values of blood and tissue [87].

In comparison to MR spectroscopy at lower magnetic fields, higher field MR spectroscopy enables a more accurate in vivo quantification of brain metabolites as a result of better resolution, greater dispersion of chemical shifts, and increased signal-to-noise ratio [88]. With improved sensitivity [89], higher field MR spectroscopy can reliably quantify a greater range of metabolites, even from small structures of the brain, due to higher signal-to-noise ratio and associated higher anatomical consistency [88, 90]. The improvement in MR spectroscopy performance (including quantification and dispersion) becomes more relevant as the alterations in metabolite concentrations are often small and therefore may be harder to detect. With reliable quantification of metabolites, higher field MR spectroscopy helps clinical decisions regarding patient management including but not limited to early diagnosis, evaluation of treatment response, and longitudinal changes in metabolite levels in AD [88].

Functional Connectivity

Functional MRI specifically during the resting state is a noninvasive technique for evaluation of the strength and spatial topology of interactions between brain networks [91–93]. By utilizing the blood-oxygenation-level-dependent (BOLD) signals, functional MRI provides information on specific brain networks through quantification of temporal association of functional activation in different brain areas [92].

Functional MRI is helpful in investigating mechanisms underlying neurodegenerative diseases [93], because the connectivity of distinct large-scale distributed brain networks is impacted early on in neurodegenerative diseases [94]. Functional MRI studies reveal individual patterns of atrophy within functional networks [94] and detect alterations in the default mode network connectivity in neurodegenerative diseases [91].

Quantitative Susceptibility Mapping (QSM)

Iron is critical in metabolic pathways, but also is a key player in neurotransmitter and myelin synthesis [95]. Excess iron deposition plays an important role in pathology of neurodegenerative diseases such as AD and PD [96] as iron triggers oxidative injury and cell death [97]. However, iron also interacts with proteins such as beta-amyloid and tau leading to their aggregation and escalation in subsequent cell death.

Although it cannot quantify iron content directly, a recently developed MRI technique, QSM can offer a reliable evaluation of tissue magnetic susceptibility and changes in brain iron content [98, 99]. Quantitative Susceptibility Mapping (QSM) can provide a comprehensive investigation in vivo of the brain iron profile and related pathophysiology underlying neurodegenerative diseases [100]. Most importantly, it can help define patterns of iron distribution in the brain, which are disease-specific and reflect brain regions associated with pathology of each disease [100]. For example, QSM is sensitive to the increased magnetic susceptibility due to

higher iron content in the substantia nigra in DLB [101].

Translocator Protein (TSPO) PET

Chronic neuroinflammation is a common hallmark of many neurodegenerative diseases and is critical in pathogenesis and progression of neurodegeneration [102]. Hence, the evaluation of neuroinflammation is important in identification of underlying mechanisms and the disease spectrum [103].

The translocator protein 18 kDa (TSPO), which is a mitochondrial membrane protein, is upregulated in neuroinflammation and TSPO PET is an emerging imaging technique for evaluating neuroinflammation. In numerous diseases of the central nervous system including AD, PD, and multiple sclerosis, TSPO PET detects the fluctuations in TSPO expression [104–106], and it provides information on microglia activity, microglia phenotypes and temporal changes in microglia and astrocyte function during neuroinflammation [102]. Therefore, TSPO PET seems to be a promising molecular imaging biomarker in vivo in tracking neuroinflammation, treatment response in clinical trials, and disease progression.

Clinical Trials and Future Perspectives

Molecular imaging may provide much needed information on enrichment of clinical trials with individuals who may respond to disease-modifying treatments targeting a specific pathological process. A good example is the use of beta-amyloid PET for enrollment of participants to beta-amyloid modifying treatments as well as determining treatment efficacy. Overall, imaging biomarkers are becoming central to patient selection, assessment of target engagement, and treatment efficacy in disease-modifying clinical trials [107]. Furthermore, imaging biomarkers may be critical in determining multiple etiologies contributing to cognitive impairment for individualized approaches to patient care and potentially identifying new targets for drug development in neurodegenerative diseases.

References

1. Przedborski S, Vila M, Jackson-Lewis V. Neurodegeneration: what is it and where are we? J Clin Invest. 2003;111:3–10. https://doi.org/10.1172/JCI17522.
2. Relja M. Pathophysiology and classification of neurodegenerative diseases. EJIFCC. 2004;15:97–9.
3. Iadecola C. The pathobiology of vascular dementia. Neuron. 2013;80:844–66. https://doi.org/10.1016/j.neuron.2013.10.008.
4. Bell AH, Miller SL, Castillo-Melendez M, et al. The neurovascular unit: effects of brain insults during the perinatal period. Front Neurosci. 2019;13:1452. https://doi.org/10.3389/fnins.2019.01452.
5. Iadecola C. The neurovascular unit coming of age: a journey through neurovascular coupling in health and disease. Neuron. 2017;96:17–42. https://doi.org/10.1016/j.neuron.2017.07.030.
6. Schaeffer S, Iadecola C. Revisiting the neurovascular unit. Nat Neurosci. 2021;24:1198–209. https://doi.org/10.1038/s41593-021-00904-7.
7. Fan J, Dawson TM, Dawson VL. Cell death mechanisms of neurodegeneration. Adv Neurobiol. 2017;15:403–25. https://doi.org/10.1007/978-3-319-57193-5_16.
8. Dugger BN, Dickson DW. Pathology of neurodegenerative diseases. Cold Spring Harb Perspect Biol. 2017;9:a028035. https://doi.org/10.1101/cshperspect.a028035.
9. Jellinger KA. Basic mechanisms of neurodegeneration: a critical update. J Cell Mol Med. 2010;14:457–87. https://doi.org/10.1111/j.1582-4934.2010.01010.x.
10. Hartl FU, Hayer-Hartl M. Converging concepts of protein folding in vitro and in vivo. Nat Struct Mol Biol. 2009;16:574–81. https://doi.org/10.1038/nsmb.1591.
11. Tan SH, Karri V, Tay NWR, et al. Emerging pathways to neurodegeneration: dissecting the critical molecular mechanisms in Alzheimer's disease, Parkinson's disease. Biomed Pharmacother. 2019;111:765–77. https://doi.org/10.1016/j.biopha.2018.12.101.
12. Gan L, Cookson MR, Petrucelli L, et al. Converging pathways in neurodegeneration, from genetics to mechanisms. Nat Neurosci. 2018;21:1300–9. https://doi.org/10.1038/s41593-018-0237-7.
13. Menzies FM, Fleming A, Caricasole A, et al. Autophagy and neurodegeneration: pathogenic mechanisms and therapeutic opportunities. Neuron. 2017;93:1015–34. https://doi.org/10.1016/j.neuron.2017.01.022.
14. Ochaba J, Lukacsovich T, Csikos G, et al. Potential function for the Huntingtin protein as a scaffold for selective autophagy. Proc Natl Acad Sci U S A. 2014;111:16889–94. https://doi.org/10.1073/pnas.1420103111.
15. Halliwell B. Oxidative stress and neurodegeneration: where are we now? J Neurochem. 2006;97:1634–58. https://doi.org/10.1111/j.1471-4159.2006.03907.x.
16. Yang JL, Weissman L, Bohr VA, et al. Mitochondrial DNA damage and repair in neurodegenerative disorders. DNA Repair (Amst). 2008;7:1110–20. https://doi.org/10.1016/j.dnarep.2008.03.012.
17. Lucin KM, Wyss-Coray T. Immune activation in brain aging and neurodegeneration: too much or too little? Neuron. 2009;64:110–22. https://doi.org/10.1016/j.neuron.2009.08.039.
18. Hickman S, Izzy S, Sen P, et al. Microglia in neurodegeneration. Nat Neurosci. 2018;21:1359–69. https://doi.org/10.1038/s41593-018-0242-x.
19. Shimizu S, Hirose D, Hatanaka H, et al. Role of neuroimaging as a biomarker for neurodegenerative diseases. Front Neurol. 2018;9:265. https://doi.org/10.3389/fneur.2018.00265.
20. Schneider JA, Arvanitakis Z, Bang W, et al. Mixed brain pathologies account for most dementia cases in community-dwelling older persons. Neurology. 2007;69:2197–204. https://doi.org/10.1212/01.wnl.0000271090.28148.24.
21. Patel KP, Wymer DT, Bhatia VK, et al. Multimodality imaging of dementia: clinical importance and role of integrated anatomic and molecular imaging. Radiographics. 2020;40:200–22. https://doi.org/10.1148/rg.2020190070.
22. Koikkalainen J, Rhodius-Meester H, Tolonen A, et al. Differential diagnosis of neurodegenerative diseases using structural MRI data. Neuroimage Clin. 2016;11:435–49. https://doi.org/10.1016/j.nicl.2016.02.019.
23. Karas G, Scheltens P, Rombouts S, et al. Precuneus atrophy in early-onset Alzheimer's disease: a morphometric structural MRI study. Neuroradiology. 2007;49:967–76. https://doi.org/10.1007/s00234-007-0269-2.
24. Morris JC, Csernansky J, Price JL. MRI measures of entorhinal cortex versus hippocampus in preclinical AD. Neurology. 2002;59:1474; author reply 1474–5. https://doi.org/10.1212/wnl.59.9.1474.
25. Jack CR Jr, Albert MS, Knopman DS, et al. Introduction to the recommendations from the National Institute on Aging-Alzheimer's Association workgroups on diagnostic guidelines for Alzheimer's disease. Alzheimers Dement. 2011;7:257–62. https://doi.org/10.1016/j.jalz.2011.03.004.
26. McKeith IG, Boeve BF, Dickson DW, et al. Diagnosis and management of dementia with Lewy bodies: fourth consensus report of the DLB Consortium. Neurology. 2017;89:88–100. https://doi.org/10.1212/WNL.0000000000004058.
27. Rascovsky K, Hodges JR, Knopman D, et al. Sensitivity of revised diagnostic criteria for the

behavioural variant of frontotemporal dementia. Brain. 2011;134:2456–77. https://doi.org/10.1093/brain/awr179.

28. Gilman S, Wenning GK, Low PA, et al. Second consensus statement on the diagnosis of multiple system atrophy. Neurology. 2008;71:670–6. https://doi.org/10.1212/01.wnl.0000324625.00404.15.

29. Hoglinger GU, Respondek G, Stamelou M, et al. Clinical diagnosis of progressive supranuclear palsy: the movement disorder society criteria. Mov Disord. 2017;32:853–64. https://doi.org/10.1002/mds.26987.

30. Assaf Y, Pasternak O. Diffusion tensor imaging (DTI)-based white matter mapping in brain research: a review. J Mol Neurosci. 2008;34:51–61. https://doi.org/10.1007/s12031-007-0029-0.

31. Kamagata K, Andica C, Kato A, et al. Diffusion magnetic resonance imaging-based biomarkers for neurodegenerative diseases. Int J Mol Sci. 2021;22:5216. https://doi.org/10.3390/ijms22105216.

32. Brun A, Englund E. A white matter disorder in dementia of the Alzheimer type: a pathoanatomical study. Ann Neurol. 1986;19:253–62. https://doi.org/10.1002/ana.410190306.

33. Kantarci K, Murray ME, Schwarz CG, et al. White-matter integrity on DTI and the pathologic staging of Alzheimer's disease. Neurobiol Aging. 2017;56:172–9. https://doi.org/10.1016/j.neurobiolaging.2017.04.024.

34. Acosta-Cabronero J, Nestor PJ. Diffusion tensor imaging in Alzheimer's disease: insights into the limbic-diencephalic network and methodological considerations. Front Aging Neurosci. 2014;6:266. https://doi.org/10.3389/fnagi.2014.00266.

35. Jacobs HIL, Hedden T, Schultz AP, et al. Structural tract alterations predict downstream tau accumulation in amyloid-positive older individuals. Nat Neurosci. 2018;21:424–31. https://doi.org/10.1038/s41593-018-0070-z.

36. Kantarci K, Schwarz CG, Reid RI, et al. White matter integrity determined with diffusion tensor imaging in older adults without dementia: influence of amyloid load and neurodegeneration. JAMA Neurol. 2014;71:1547–54. https://doi.org/10.1001/jamaneurol.2014.1482.

37. Goveas J, O'Dwyer L, Mascalchi M, et al. Diffusion-MRI in neurodegenerative disorders. Magn Reson Imaging. 2015;33:853–76. https://doi.org/10.1016/j.mri.2015.04.006.

38. Young PNE, Estarellas M, Coomans E, et al. Imaging biomarkers in neurodegeneration: current and future practices. Alzheimers Res Ther. 2020;12:49. https://doi.org/10.1186/s13195-020-00612-7.

39. Nedelska Z, Senjem ML, Przybelski SA, et al. Regional cortical perfusion on arterial spin labeling MRI in dementia with Lewy bodies: associations with clinical severity, glucose metabolism and tau PET. Neuroimage Clin. 2018;19:939–47. https://doi.org/10.1016/j.nicl.2018.06.020.

40. Wolk DA, Detre JA. Arterial spin labeling MRI: an emerging biomarker for Alzheimer's disease and other neurodegenerative conditions. Curr Opin Neurol. 2012;25:421–8. https://doi.org/10.1097/WCO.0b013e328354ff0a.

41. Oz G, Alger JR, Barker PB, et al. Clinical proton MR spectroscopy in central nervous system disorders. Radiology. 2014;270:658–79. https://doi.org/10.1148/radiol.13130531.

42. Kantarci K, Jack CR Jr, Xu YC, et al. Regional metabolic patterns in mild cognitive impairment and Alzheimer's disease: a 1H MRS study. Neurology. 2000;55:210–7.

43. Sturrock A, Laule C, Decolongon J, et al. Magnetic resonance spectroscopy biomarkers in premanifest and early Huntington disease. Neurology. 2010;75:1702–10. https://doi.org/10.1212/WNL.0b013e3181fc27e4.

44. Kantarci K, Knopman DS, Dickson DW, et al. Alzheimer disease: postmortem neuropathologic correlates of antemortem 1H MR spectroscopy metabolite measurements. Radiology. 2008;248:210–20. https://doi.org/10.1148/radiol.2481071590.

45. Oz G, Hutter D, Tkac I, et al. Neurochemical alterations in spinocerebellar ataxia type 1 and their correlations with clinical status. Mov Disord. 2010;25:1253–61. https://doi.org/10.1002/mds.23067.

46. Ross BD, Bluml S, Cowan R, et al. In vivo MR spectroscopy of human dementia. Neuroimaging Clin N Am. 1998;8:809–22.

47. Godbolt AK, Waldman AD, MacManus DG, et al. MRS shows abnormalities before symptoms in familial Alzheimer disease. Neurology. 2006;66:718–22. https://doi.org/10.1212/01.wnl.0000201237.05869.df.

48. Kantarci K, Boeve BF, Wszolek ZK, et al. MRS in presymptomatic MAPT mutation carriers: a potential biomarker for tau-mediated pathology. Neurology. 2010;75:771–8. https://doi.org/10.1212/WNL.0b013e3181f073c7.

49. Miller BL, Moats RA, Shonk T, et al. Alzheimer disease: depiction of increased cerebral myoinositol with proton MR spectroscopy. Radiology. 1993;187:433–7. https://doi.org/10.1148/radiology.187.2.8475286.

50. Oz G, Iltis I, Hutter D, et al. Distinct neurochemical profiles of spinocerebellar ataxias 1, 2, 6, and cerebellar multiple system atrophy. Cerebellum. 2011;10:208–17. https://doi.org/10.1007/s12311-010-0213-6.

51. Rupsingh R, Borrie M, Smith M, et al. Reduced hippocampal glutamate in Alzheimer disease. Neurobiol Aging. 2011;32:802–10. https://doi.org/10.1016/j.neurobiolaging.2009.05.002.

52. Krishnan KR, Charles HC, Doraiswamy PM, et al. Randomized, placebo-controlled trial of the effects of donepezil on neuronal markers and hippocampal volumes in Alzheimer's disease. Am J Psychiatry.

2003;160:2003–11. https://doi.org/10.1176/appi.ajp.160.11.2003.

53. Bartha R, Smith M, Rupsingh R, et al. High field (1)H MRS of the hippocampus after donepezil treatment in Alzheimer disease. Prog Neuro-Psychopharmacol Biol Psychiatry. 2008;32:786–93. https://doi.org/10.1016/j.pnpbp.2007.12.011.

54. Lim SM, Katsifis A, Villemagne VL, et al. The 18F-FDG PET cingulate island sign and comparison to 123I-beta-CIT SPECT for diagnosis of dementia with Lewy bodies. J Nucl Med. 2009;50:1638–45. https://doi.org/10.2967/jnumed.109.065870.

55. Graff-Radford J, Murray ME, Lowe VJ, et al. Dementia with Lewy bodies: basis of cingulate island sign. Neurology. 2014;83:801–9. https://doi.org/10.1212/WNL.0000000000000734.

56. Shankar GM, Walsh DM. Alzheimer's disease: synaptic dysfunction and Abeta. Mol Neurodegener. 2009;4:48. https://doi.org/10.1186/1750-1326-4-48.

57. Scheff SW, Price DA, Schmitt FA, et al. Hippocampal synaptic loss in early Alzheimer's disease and mild cognitive impairment. Neurobiol Aging. 2006;27:1372–84. https://doi.org/10.1016/j.neurobiolaging.2005.09.012.

58. Hou Z, Lei H, Hong S, et al. Functional changes in the frontal cortex in Parkinson's disease using a rat model. J Clin Neurosci. 2010;17:628–33. https://doi.org/10.1016/j.jocn.2009.07.101.

59. Cai Z, Li S, Matuskey D, et al. PET imaging of synaptic density: a new tool for investigation of neuropsychiatric diseases. Neurosci Lett. 2019;691:44–50. https://doi.org/10.1016/j.neulet.2018.07.038.

60. Bajjalieh SM, Frantz GD, Weimann JM, et al. Differential expression of synaptic vesicle protein 2 (SV2) isoforms. J Neurosci. 1994;14:5223–35.

61. Finnema SJ, Nabulsi NB, Eid T, et al. Imaging synaptic density in the living human brain. Sci Transl Med. 2016;8:348–96. https://doi.org/10.1126/scitranslmed.aaf6667.

62. Jack CR Jr, Lowe VJ, Senjem ML, et al. 11C PiB and structural MRI provide complementary information in imaging of Alzheimer's disease and amnestic mild cognitive impairment. Brain. 2008;131:665–80. https://doi.org/10.1093/brain/awm336.

63. Klunk WE, Engler H, Nordberg A, et al. Imaging brain amyloid in Alzheimer's disease with Pittsburgh Compound-B. Ann Neurol. 2004;55:306–19. Comparative Study Research Support, Non-U.S. Gov't Research Support, U.S. Gov't, P.H.S. https://doi.org/10.1002/ana.20009.

64. Chetelat G, Arbizu J, Barthel H, et al. Amyloid-PET and (18)F-FDG-PET in the diagnostic investigation of Alzheimer's disease and other dementias. Lancet Neurol. 2020;19:951–62. https://doi.org/10.1016/S1474-4422(20)30314-8.

65. Jansen WJ, Ossenkoppele R, Knol DL, et al. Prevalence of cerebral amyloid pathology in persons without dementia: a meta-analysis. JAMA. 2015;313:1924–38. https://doi.org/10.1001/jama.2015.4668.

66. Mallik A, Drzezga A, Minoshima S. Clinical amyloid imaging. Semin Nucl Med. 2017;47:31–43. https://doi.org/10.1053/j.semnuclmed.2016.09.005.

67. Johnson KA, Minoshima S, Bohnen NI, et al. Appropriate use criteria for amyloid PET: a report of the Amyloid Imaging Task Force, the Society of Nuclear Medicine and Molecular Imaging, and the Alzheimer's Association. J Nucl Med. 2013;54:476–90. https://doi.org/10.2967/jnumed.113.120618.

68. Buee L, Bussiere T, Buee-Scherrer V, et al. Tau protein isoforms, phosphorylation and role in neurodegenerative disorders. Brain Res Brain Res Rev. 2000;33:95–130. https://doi.org/10.1016/s0165-0173(00)00019-9.

69. Chien DT, Bahri S, Szardenings AK, et al. Early clinical PET imaging results with the novel PHF-tau radioligand [F-18]-T807. J Alzheimers Dis. 2013;34:457–68. https://doi.org/10.3233/JAD-122059.

70. Groot C, Villeneuve S, Smith R, et al. Tau PET imaging in neurodegenerative disorders. J Nucl Med. 2022;63:20S–6S. https://doi.org/10.2967/jnumed.121.263196.

71. Nelson PT, Alafuzoff I, Bigio EH, et al. Correlation of Alzheimer disease neuropathologic changes with cognitive status: a review of the literature. J Neuropathol Exp Neurol. 2012;71:362–81. https://doi.org/10.1097/NEN.0b013e31825018f7.

72. Graebner AK, Tarsy D, Shih LC, et al. Clinical impact of 123I-Ioflupane SPECT (DaTscan) in a movement disorder center. Neurodegener Dis. 2017;17:38–43. https://doi.org/10.1159/000447561.

73. Palermo G, Ceravolo R. Molecular imaging of the dopamine transporter. Cells. 2019;8:872. https://doi.org/10.3390/cells8080872.

74. Kerstens VS, Fazio P, Sundgren M, et al. Reliability of dopamine transporter PET measurements with [(18)F]FE-PE2I in patients with Parkinson's disease. EJNMMI Res. 2020;10:95. https://doi.org/10.1186/s13550-020-00676-4.

75. Postuma RB, Berg D, Stern M, et al. MDS clinical diagnostic criteria for Parkinson's disease. Mov Disord. 2015;30:1591–601. https://doi.org/10.1002/mds.26424.

76. Sakakibara S, Hashimoto R, Katayama T, et al. Longitudinal change of DAT SPECT in Parkinson's disease and multiple system atrophy. J Parkinsons Dis. 2020;10:123–30. https://doi.org/10.3233/JPD-191710.

77. Nandhagopal R, Kuramoto L, Schulzer M, et al. Longitudinal evolution of compensatory changes in striatal dopamine processing in Parkinson's disease. Brain. 2011;134:3290–8. https://doi.org/10.1093/brain/awr233.

78. Ibrahim N, Kusmirek J, Struck AF, et al. The sensitivity and specificity of F-DOPA PET in a movement disorder clinic. Am J Nucl Med Mol Imaging. 2016;6:102–9.

79. Morrish PK, Sawle GV, Brooks DJ. Clinical and [18F] dopa PET findings in early Parkinson's disease.

J Neurol Neurosurg Psychiatry. 1995;59:597–600. https://doi.org/10.1136/jnnp.59.6.597.

80. Pavese N, Brooks DJ. Imaging neurodegeneration in Parkinson's disease. Biochim Biophys Acta. 2009;1792:722–9. https://doi.org/10.1016/j.bbadis.2008.10.003.

81. Berger-Sweeney J. The cholinergic basal forebrain system during development and its influence on cognitive processes: important questions and potential answers. Neurosci Biobehav Rev. 2003;27:401–11. https://doi.org/10.1016/s0149-7634(03)00070-8.

82. Roy R, Niccolini F, Pagano G, et al. Cholinergic imaging in dementia spectrum disorders. Eur J Nucl Med Mol Imaging. 2016;43:1376–86. https://doi.org/10.1007/s00259-016-3349-x.

83. Bohnen NI, Kaufer DI, Hendrickson R, et al. Cognitive correlates of alterations in acetylcholinesterase in Alzheimer's disease. Neurosci Lett. 2005;380:127–32. https://doi.org/10.1016/j.neulet.2005.01.031.

84. Kuhl DE, Minoshima S, Fessler JA, et al. In vivo mapping of cholinergic terminals in normal aging, Alzheimer's disease, and Parkinson's disease. Ann Neurol. 1996;40:399–410. https://doi.org/10.1002/ana.410400309.

85. Kaasinen V, Nagren K, Jarvenpaa T, et al. Regional effects of donepezil and rivastigmine on cortical acetylcholinesterase activity in Alzheimer's disease. J Clin Psychopharmacol. 2002;22:615–20. https://doi.org/10.1097/00004714-200212000-00012.

86. Klein JC, Eggers C, Kalbe E, et al. Neurotransmitter changes in dementia with Lewy bodies and Parkinson disease dementia in vivo. Neurology. 2010;74:885–92. https://doi.org/10.1212/WNL.0b013e3181d55f61.

87. Versluis MJ, van der Grond J, van Buchem MA, et al. High-field imaging of neurodegenerative diseases. Neuroimaging Clin N Am. 2012;22:159–71, ix. https://doi.org/10.1016/j.nic.2012.02.005.

88. Zhang N, Song X, Bartha R, et al. Advances in high-field magnetic resonance spectroscopy in Alzheimer's disease. Curr Alzheimer Res. 2014;11:367–88. https://doi.org/10.2174/1567205011666140302200312.

89. Barker PB, Hearshen DO, Boska MD. Single-voxel proton MRS of the human brain at 1.5T and 3.0T. Magn Reson Med. 2001;45:765–9. https://doi.org/10.1002/mrm.1104.

90. Tkac I, Andersen P, Adriany G, et al. In vivo 1H NMR spectroscopy of the human brain at 7 T. Magn Reson Med. 2001;46:451–6. https://doi.org/10.1002/mrm.1213.

91. Hohenfeld C, Werner CJ, Reetz K. Resting-state connectivity in neurodegenerative disorders: is there potential for an imaging biomarker? Neuroimage Clin. 2018;18:849–70. https://doi.org/10.1016/j.nicl.2018.03.013.

92. Smitha KA, Akhil Raja K, Arun KM, et al. Resting state fMRI: a review on methods in resting state connectivity analysis and resting state networks.

Neuroradiol J. 2017;30:305–17. https://doi.org/10.1177/1971400917697342.

93. Filippi M, Spinelli EG, Cividini C, et al. Resting state dynamic functional connectivity in neurodegenerative conditions: a review of magnetic resonance imaging findings. Front Neurosci. 2019;13:657. https://doi.org/10.3389/fnins.2019.00657.

94. Seeley WW, Crawford RK, Zhou J, et al. Neurodegenerative diseases target large-scale human brain networks. Neuron. 2009;62:42–52. https://doi.org/10.1016/j.neuron.2009.03.024.

95. Mills E, Dong XP, Wang F, et al. Mechanisms of brain iron transport: insight into neurodegeneration and CNS disorders. Future Med Chem. 2010;2:51–64. https://doi.org/10.4155/fmc.09.140.

96. Morris G, Berk M, Carvalho AF, et al. Why should neuroscientists worry about iron? The emerging role of ferroptosis in the pathophysiology of neuroprogressive diseases. Behav Brain Res. 2018;341:154–75. https://doi.org/10.1016/j.bbr.2017.12.036.

97. Ndayisaba A, Kaindlstorfer C, Wenning GK. Iron in neurodegeneration - cause or consequence? Front Neurosci. 2019;13:180. https://doi.org/10.3389/fnins.2019.00180.

98. Langkammer C, Schweser F, Krebs N, et al. Quantitative susceptibility mapping (QSM) as a means to measure brain iron? A post mortem validation study. Neuroimage. 2012;62:1593–9. https://doi.org/10.1016/j.neuroimage.2012.05.049.

99. Haacke EM, Liu S, Buch S, et al. Quantitative susceptibility mapping: current status and future directions. Magn Reson Imaging. 2015;33:1–25. https://doi.org/10.1016/j.mri.2014.09.004.

100. Ravanfar P, Loi SM, Syeda WT, et al. Systematic review: quantitative susceptibility mapping (QSM) of brain iron profile in neurodegenerative diseases. Front Neurosci. 2021;15:618435. https://doi.org/10.3389/fnins.2021.618435.

101. Chen Q, Boeve BF, Forghanian-Arani A, et al. MRI quantitative susceptibility mapping of the substantia nigra as an early biomarker for Lewy body disease. J Neuroimaging. 2021;31:1020–7. https://doi.org/10.1111/jon.12878.

102. Werry EL, Bright FM, Piguet O, et al. Recent developments in TSPO PET imaging as a biomarker of neuroinflammation in neurodegenerative disorders. Int J Mol Sci. 2019;20:3161. https://doi.org/10.3390/ijms20133161.

103. Tournier BB, Tsartsalis S, Ceyzeriat K, et al. In vivo TSPO signal and neuroinflammation in Alzheimer's disease. Cells. 2020;9:1941. https://doi.org/10.3390/cells9091941.

104. Hamelin L, Lagarde J, Dorothee G, et al. Early and protective microglial activation in Alzheimer's disease: a prospective study using 18F-DPA-714 PET imaging. Brain. 2016;139:1252–64. https://doi.org/10.1093/brain/aww017.

105. Lavisse S, Goutal S, Wimberley C, et al. Increased microglial activation in patients with Parkinson disease using [(18)F]-DPA714 TSPO PET imaging.

Parkinsonism Relat Disord. 2021;82:29–36. https://doi.org/10.1016/j.parkreldis.2020.11.011.

106. Sucksdorff M, Matilainen M, Tuisku J, et al. Brain TSPO-PET predicts later disease progression independent of relapses in multiple sclerosis. Brain. 2020;143:3318–30. https://doi.org/10.1093/brain/awaa275.

107. Kantarci K. 2021 marks a new era for Alzheimer's therapeutics. Lancet Neurol. 2022;21:3–4. https://doi.org/10.1016/S1474-4422(21)00412-9.

Appropriate Use of Biomarkers in Suspected Neurodegenerative Diseases

2

Guillaume Lamotte and Norman L. Foster

Abbreviations

A/T/N	Amyloid-tau-neurodegeneration
AD	Alzheimer's disease
ARIA	Amyloid-related imaging abnormalities
Aβ	abeta protein
CADASIL	Cerebral autosomal dominant arteriopathy with subcortical infarcts and leukoencephalopathy
CBD	Corticobasal degeneration
CJD	Creutzfeldt-Jakob disease
CLIA	Clinical Laboratory Improvement Amendments
CSF	Cerebrospinal fluid
DLB	Dementia with Lewy bodies
FDG	18F-fluorodeoxyglucose
FTD	Frontotemporal degeneration
GRE	Gradient echo MRI sequences
LATE	Limbic-predominant age-related TDP-43 encephalopathy
MCI	Mild cognitive impairment
MIBG	I-123 metaiodobenzylguanidine
MRI	Magnetic resonance imaging
MSA	Multiple system atrophy
MSA-C	Cerebellar subtype of multiple system atrophy
MSA-P	Parkinsonian subtype of multiple system atrophy
PART	Primary age-related tauopathy
PD	Parkinson's disease
PET	Positron emission tomography
p-tau	Phosphorylated tau protein
QIBA	Quantitative Imaging Biomarker Alliance
RBD	Rapid-eye-movement sleep behavior disorder
SPECT	Single-photon emission computerized tomography
SWI	Susceptibility-weighted imaging MRI sequences
α-syn	Alpha-synuclein

Key Points

- Imaging and fluid biomarkers are *measured* indicators of biological and disease processes or responses to an intervention.
- Biomarkers have clinical value if they increase the precision and accuracy of diagnosis and improve personalized drug treatment and disease management.
- Integrating clinical evidence obtained from a detailed history and focused examination is a

G. Lamotte · N. L. Foster (✉)
Department of Neurology, University of Utah,
Salt Lake City, UT, USA
e-mail: Guillaume.lamotte@hsc.utah.edu; Norman.
foster@hsc.utah.edu

© The Author(s), under exclusive license to Springer Nature Switzerland AG 2023
D. J. Cross et al. (eds.), *Molecular Imaging of Neurodegenerative Disorders*,
https://doi.org/10.1007/978-3-031-35098-6_2

precondition for selecting and interpreting biomarker results.

- The appropriate use of a biomarkers must be assessed independently for each intended purpose.
- Biomarkers should be used to answer pre-specified clinically relevant questions.
- Biomarker interpretation must consider patient factors, technical and statistical characteristics.
- Avoid overuse, underuse, overdependence errors, and misuses of biomarkers.

Introduction

A biomarker is "a defined characteristic that is *measured* as an indicator of normal biological processes, pathogenic processes or responses to an exposure or intervention" [1]. This broad definition includes quantitative clinical scales and psychometric tests, quantitative laboratory tests, genetic analyses, and quantitative imaging metrics when they are an accurate indicator of disease or biological outcomes. Demonstrating that a measure qualifies as a biomarker is a challenging and incremental process. Potential biomarkers are first identified by showing between group differences, but they often fail to meet the more stringent requirement of being useful in individuals. Biomarkers initially developed through research must be reliable and consistent in clinical settings. Finally, before becoming clinically useful, practical issues of regulatory approval, access, logistics, and reimbursement must be resolved.

We take for granted that oversight and quality standards required of Clinical Laboratory Improvement Amendments (CLIA) certification will assure the handling of biological fluid and tissue samples and assays meet biomarker standards. By contrast, most imaging is not "biomarker quality" and intended only for visual interpretation. The variability of visual interpretations is easily documented if standardized protocols and quantitative measurement are not used. In one study, a single patient receiving magnetic resonance imaging (MRI) scans at ten different centers over 3 weeks had 49 distinct findings reported, with 33 appearing in only 1 of the 10 reports [2]. In another study of 40 patients with behavioral variant frontotemporal degeneration (FTD), the characteristic atrophy pattern was described in 50%, but they were only reported as "consistent with atrophy" with no mention of FTD [3]. The Radiological Society of North America organized the Quantitative Imaging Biomarker Alliance (QIBA) to advance quantitative imaging and the use of imaging biomarkers [4]. With modest additional effort, radiology and nuclear medicine practices can implement QIBA profile quality standards. Biomarker measures then can be calculated with appropriate software using a supplemental billing code that insurers recognize for reimbursement of quantitative imaging.

Rapidly evolving research makes it impossible for us to consider all promising biomarker candidates. We will consider only well-validated biological (e.g., plasma, cerebrospinal fluid (CSF), and peripheral tissue biopsy) and imaging biomarkers used clinically in suspected neurodegenerative diseases, whether or not they are now practically available to all clinicians. We will not discuss the appropriate use of genetic biomarkers for disorders such as Huntington's disease, familial movement disorders and dementias, and genetic spinocerebellar ataxias. Genetic biomarkers require additional considerations including pre- and post-testing counseling, implications for other family members, issues of penetrance, variants of uncertain significance, managing unexpected mutations, and technical factors affecting the detection of repeat expansions, transpositions, and gene duplications. Fortunately, the principles for using non-genetic biomarkers are well established and can be applied broadly. We begin with the premise that biomarkers have clinical value if they increase the precision and accuracy of diagnosis and improve personalized drug treatment and disease management. We strongly believe integrating clinical evidence obtained from a detailed history and focused examination is a precondition for selecting and interpreting biomarker results that improve the diagnosis and care of individual patients.

Biomarker Classification Based on Intended Use

Indiscriminate use rapidly diminishes the value of biomarkers. First consider the purpose intended: diagnostic, disease monitoring, pharmacodynamic or drug response, predictive or prognostic, safety, and disease susceptibility or risk (Table 2.1). No single biomarker can be expected to be applicable for all purposes; the value for each intended use must be assessed independently. Fortunately, biomarkers may address more than one question. For example, amyloid positron emission tomography (PET) is a diagnostic biomarker of Alzheimer's disease (AD) dementia, a drug response biomarker in immunotherapy of AD, and a risk biomarker in mild cognitive impairment (MCI). Conversely, amyloid PET cannot be used as a predictive or prognostic biomarker to determine whether an individual will develop dementia in the future or how rapidly cognitive decline will occur.

Diagnostic biomarkers provide evidence that improves the accuracy and confidence in a specific disease. Few biomarkers are pathognomonic of a single disorder and they can be abnormal in more than one disease. Despite different disease mechanisms, CSF total tau is elevated in both AD and Creutzfeldt-Jakob disease (CJD), and in dementia with Lewy bodies (DLB) and vascular dementia [5] when AD is a co-pathology. Nevertheless, the potential confounds rarely lead to misdiagnosis if clinical context and the results of other biomarkers such as MRI, p-tau, and abeta (Aβ) are considered. Repeating biomarker measurements over time can sometimes be very helpful in clarifying uncertain diagnoses, such as repeating 18F-fluorodeoxyglucose (FDG) PET after symptoms have progressed [6]. Similarly, a

second dopamine scan can reduce diagnostic uncertainty in parkinsonian syndromes, even after a prolonged period of clinical observation [7]. Diagnostic biomarkers also refine and personalize diagnosis by identifying disease subtypes. Recognizing subtypes of AD and other neurodegenerative diseases can explain atypical presentations, distinctive clinical courses, treatment responses, and identify predictable complications [8]. Such biomarker-driven precision diagnosis offers the opportunity of individualizing care and tailoring management to different symptom trajectories and provide personalized education, support, and treatment [9, 10].

Disease monitoring biomarkers objectively track the course of a disease to guide treatment. They are commonly used in cardiology and oncology to decide on treatment, but their use in neurodegenerative diseases has lagged. Clinical cognitive and motor scales, neuropsychological tests, focal brain volume loss, FDG-PET, tau PET, and dopaminergic imaging correlate with disease pathology severity, providing a more realistic and objective assessment than categorical clinical "staging." To have clinical value, disease monitoring biomarkers must not fluctuate greatly in the same patient, so that changing levels can be accurately interpreted as a change in disease and acted on. Further research is needed to determine the minimal time needed to reliably detect that individual changes in disease; in the time frame of years, MRI and FDG-PET changes with disease progression are obvious.

Pharmacodynamic and drug response biomarkers measure the biochemical effects of treatment rather than the effects on disease. Pharmacodynamic biomarkers are not yet utilized clinically, but may be in the future. The potential for their use is illustrated by cholinergic PET ligands ability to measure dose-dependent inhibition of cholinesterase in the central nervous system before and after treatment [11]. Serial amyloid PET, tau PET, and dopaminergic imaging can be used as drug response biomarkers to demonstrate that drugs have successfully engaged pathological targets [12, 13].

Predictive and prognostic biomarkers track and predict disease progression and potential

Table 2.1 Classification of biomarkers based upon their intended use

- Diagnostic
- Disease monitoring
- Pharmacodynamic and drug response
- Predictive and prognostic
- Safety
- Susceptibility and risk

complications. For example, frontal hypometabolism measured with FDG-PET in AD is linked to apathy and behavior disturbance [14]. FDG-PET and amyloid PET are strong predictors of the future conversion of mild cognitive impairment to AD [15].

Safety biomarkers assess whether specific treatments should be given. Gradient echo sequences (GRE) and susceptibility-weighted imaging (SWI) MRIs identify whether multiple microhemorrhages are present to decide whether amyloid immunotherapies can be safely administered. MRI identifies amyloid-related imaging abnormalities (ARIA) that indicate amyloid immunotherapy should be suspended [16].

Susceptibility and risk biomarkers identify individual risks of developing the disease before symptom onset. The presence of an apolipoprotein APOE4 allele is an example of a genetic susceptibility biomarker because it increases the vulnerability to AD. However, APOE4 has low sensitivity (53%) and specificity (67%) for identifying individuals who eventually will develop AD. As a consequence, it is appropriate only in research [17]. Risk biomarkers allow identification of pathology before symptoms or full expression of disease develop. Even asymptomatic individuals with abnormal biomarkers can be at very high risk of developing progressive symptoms, which in some cases may justify beginning disease-modifying drug treatments.

Appropriate Use of Biomarkers in Clinical Care

A confident, accurate diagnosis is an important goal in clinical care. Misdiagnosis is especially common in neurodegenerative diseases that are by their nature complex and heterogeneous. Lack of provider diagnostic confidence is common, delaying treatment and inhibiting education and support for patients and families. Lack of patient diagnostic confidence, sometimes reflecting provider lack of confidence, contributes to poor follow-up and treatment adherence. Patients and their families too often are forced to endure a prolonged diagnostic odyssey and yet fail to get a

definitive evaluation. No wonder that outcomes are often less than ideal. Diagnosis is the basis of rational management and it is crucial in the doctor–patient relationship; without a clear diagnosis, both patient and physician feel disengaged. Without a clear and confident diagnosis, treatment may be misguided, and at worst, harmful. Accurate diagnosis also is important because it informs prognosis, which guides management and helps patients and families plan (e.g., financial management and end-of-life care). In the past, diagnostic testing was often performed to "rule-out" causes of dementia and movement disorders. Now, fully exploiting imaging data and using other biomarkers allows clinicians to "rule-in" disease.

Before using biomarkers, a clinical evaluation for a suspected neurodegenerative disease should include a comprehensive medical, family, and social history, review of medications, mental status, and neurological examination. Standardized cognitive scales, neuropsychological testing, and motor ratings are helpful. Blood tests should be performed including a complete blood count, comprehensive metabolic panel, thyroid-stimulating hormone, and vitamin B12 level. A review of the laboratory evaluation in atypical dementias and movement disorders (e.g., rapidly progressive dementia or ataxia, acute dystonia, myoclonus) is beyond the scope of this chapter but laboratory testing should be guided by the clinical presentation (e.g., paraneoplastic panel, ceruloplasmin, plasma and urine copper, EEG, etc.). The evaluation often includes structural brain imaging with a brain MRI or CT scan to detect occult brain lesions and focal abnormalities that cause or contribute to dementia and movement disorders. Images can be analyzed further with quantitative imaging software with little additional effort.

Biomarkers are not always needed. An accurate diagnosis without biomarkers can be made with high confidence if there is concordance between a typical medical history consistent from all sources and typical physical examination and laboratory findings. Conversely, biomarkers can be invaluable if there is diagnostic uncertainty even after a comprehensive evaluation or high diagnostic accuracy is needed before beginning high risk interventions. Neurodegenerative diseases are complex and often have co-pathologies, co-morbidities, complications, and variable presentations. Amyloid PET imaging may allow confident diagnosis of AD in a patient with cognitive impairment and depression but who did not respond to an appropriate trial of antidepressants. Dopaminergic imaging may identify DLB in a patient with dementia and behavior disturbance treated with antipsychotics. Biomarkers also are particularly important when high confidence in an accurate diagnosis is needed: before beginning antipsychotic treatment to avoid severe side effects when there is loss of striatal presynaptic dopamine transporters, deep brain stimulation, or anti-amyloid immunotherapy. Disease monitoring, drug response, predictive and safety biomarkers are applicable only in special circumstances. For example, a brain MRI may identify microhemorrhages or superficial siderosis, which would put a patient at higher risk of developing ARIA if treated with monoclonal antibodies targeting β-amyloid.

The use of one biomarker does not preclude the need for others. Several biomarkers can provide incremental evidence in support of a diagnosis or treatment plan if they provide complementary information. For example, dopaminergic imaging may identify central presynaptic dopaminergic denervation and differentiate parkinsonism from essential tremor, however, it does not differentiate PD from other parkinsonian syndromes. To confirm a diagnosis of PD, synuclein aggregates could be visualized on skin biopsy. Alternatively, the combined use of dopaminergic imaging and I-123 metaiodobenzylguanidine (MIBG) myocardial imaging showing denervation on both would also confirm a diagnosis of PD rather than MSA.

Clinical acceptance and feasibility of testing influence the choice of biomarker when alternatives are available. An individual with dementia may not be able to cooperate with a lumbar puncture or a brain MRI. Patients often prefer imaging biomarkers over more invasive procedures such as CSF studies or skin biopsies. A provider working in a busy clinical setting may not have the time, the staff support, or the capability to perform CSF studies or skin biopsies. Plasma biomarkers are easiest of all, but may not be an alternative until fully validated.

Insurance coverage and out-of-pocket costs are a significant factor in determining biomarker access and choice. In neurodegenerative diseases diagnostic costs, including the cost of biomarkers, represent only a small percentage of the economic burden of disease. Nevertheless, the cost-effectiveness of different diagnostic strategies should be taken into consideration. The National Institute on Aging—Alzheimer's Association (NIA-AA) clinical diagnostic criteria for MCI due to AD pathology requires evidence of amyloid or tau pathology with CSF or neuroimaging biomarkers [18]. However, this definition cannot be achieved if these biomarkers are not reimbursed by insurance or locally available. Wide access to biomarkers cannot be achieved without reimbursement. Alternatives that might indicate high likelihood of progressive dementia while still not meeting MCI due to AD pathology criteria include neuropsychological testing and brain MRI that may detect regional atrophy and cerebrovascular disease, which are associated with a higher risk of future dementia [19].

Relevant Clinical Questions Biomarkers Can Answer

The next step after determining the intended use of a biomarker is to identify the relevant clinical question the biomarker will answer. When diagnosis or management remains uncertain, biomarkers can answer relevant questions that address a differential diagnosis and treatment alternatives generated during the clinical assessment (Table 2.2). The expected results of clinically available biomarkers in common dementing diseases and movement disorders are summarized in Tables 2.3 and 2.4.

Table 2.2 Clinical questions relevant to biomarkers

1. Is there focal brain structural abnormality?
Uses: Diagnostic, disease monitoring, drug response (not yet), predictive (not yet), safety
2. Is there focal cerebral cortical or subcortical hypometabolism?
Uses: Diagnostic
3. Is there evidence of amyloid or tau pathology?
Uses: Diagnostic, drug response
4. Is there loss of presynaptic striatal dopaminergic innervation?
Uses: Diagnostic, drug response (not yet), safety, not prognostic, disease monitoring
5. Is cardiac postganglionic sympathetic innervation intact?
Uses: Diagnostic—MSA from PD, DLB from AD
6. Is there central or peripheral autonomic failure?
Uses: Diagnostic—MSA vs. PD
7. What is the neurophysiological characteristics of the tremor?
Uses: Diagnostic, drug response (not yet)—PD vs. ET vs. functional tremor
8. Is there evidence of alpha-synuclein pathology? (diagnostic)
Uses: Diagnostic PD and MSA vs. others

Is There a Focal Structural Brain Abnormality?

Many focal brain lesions cause or contribute to dementia including stroke, tumor, subdural hematoma, intracerebral hemorrhage, and abscess. Hyperintensities in the basal ganglia and cortical ribbon are characteristic of prion disease. Identification and quantification of microhemorrhages on brain MRI can identify cerebral amyloid angiopathy and may influence treatment (e.g., higher risk of intracranial hemorrhage with anticoagulation, higher risk of ARIA with the use of monoclonal antibodies targeting β-amyloid). As a consequence, brain imaging with MRI or CT is appropriate for all cognitive evaluations, even in the absence of focal neurological deficits. Using imaging as a quantitative biomarker to measure lesions adds value. For example, the Evans' index (the ratio of the maximum width of the frontal horns of the lateral ventricles and the maximal internal diameter of the skull at the same level) can show that ventricular enlargement is out of proportion to brain atrophy sug-

Table 2.3 Typical biomarker results in common cognitive disorders

Alzheimer's disease
Brain MRI
Atrophy of the entorhinal cortex, hippocampus, amygdala, parahippocampus, diffuse cerebral cortical atrophy
Clinical subtypes: Hemispheric asymmetric, occipital atrophy
Molecular imaging
Positive amyloid PET, positive tau PET (e.g., Flortaucipir), FDG-PET—predominant posterior cingulate gyrus and bilateral temporoparietal hypometabolism
Clinical subtypes: Progressive aphasia, posterior cortical atrophy
CSF
Low Aβ42, or low Aβ42/Aβ40 ratio
Elevated total and phosphorylated tau
Frontotemporal degeneration
Brain MRI
Atrophy of the frontal and anterior temporal cortices
Clinical subtypes: Asymmetric
Molecular imaging
Negative amyloid PET, FDG-PET with predominant frontal, anterior cingulate and anterior temporal hypometabolism
Clinical subtypes: Progressive aphasia, behavioral variant frontotemporal degeneration, symmetric and asymmetric hypometabolism
Dementia with Lewy bodies
Brain MRI
Gray matter atrophy in the posterior parietal cortices, absent swallow tail in the substantia nigra
Molecular imaging
Dopaminergic imaging with reduced presynaptic dopaminergic transporter, FDG-PET with high ratio of glucose metabolism in the posterior cingulate region compared with the precuneus and cuneus (cingulate island sign), cardiac sympathetic denervation by MIBG SPECT
Skin biopsy
Immunofluorescence for α-synuclein and PGP9.5 in skin nerve fibers

gesting normal pressure hydrocephalus in a patient with gait disturbance, cognitive impairment, and impaired bladder control.

White matter changes also contribute to cognitive impairment in AD and, if severe and in the right setting, can suggest vascular dementia. Sometimes, the pattern of white matter abnormality is diagnostic, such as in multiple sclerosis,

Table 2.4 Typical biomarker results in common movement disorders

Parkinson's disease

Molecular imaging

Dopaminergic imaging with reduced presynaptic dopaminergic transporter, cardiac sympathetic denervation by MIBG SPECT

Skin biopsy

Immunofluorescence for α-synuclein and PGP9.5 in skin nerve fibers

Others

Hyperechogenicity of the substantia nigra on transcranial ultrasound

Quantitative olfactory testing: Hyposmia/anosmia

Multiple system atrophy

Brain MRI

Atrophy of the putamen with a hyperintense T2 border of the lateral putamen and T2 hypointensity of the body of the putamen. Atrophy of the middle cerebellar peduncle, pons, or cerebellum (MSA-P and MSA-C). Hot cross bun sign (MSA-C)

Molecular imaging

Reduced presynaptic dopaminergic transporter with dopaminergic imaging (MSA-P > MSA-C), FDG-PET with hypometabolism in the putamen, brainstem, or cerebellum, preserved cardiac sympathetic innervation by MIBG SPECT

Skin biopsy

Immunofluorescence for α-synuclein and PGP9.5 in skin nerve fibers

Others

Autonomic function testing with autonomic failure

Sphincter electromyogram with evidence of denervation and reinnervation, urodynamic testing with neurogenic bladder and postvoid residual >100 mL

Quantitative olfactory testing: Preserved sense of smell

Supine plasma norepinephrine level > 200 pg/mL

Progressive supranuclear palsy

Brain MRI

Midbrain atrophy (hummingbird sign)

Molecular imaging

Reduced presynaptic dopaminergic transporter with dopaminergic imaging, positive tau PET, FGD PET: Asymmetrical or bilateral hypometabolism has been reported in the prefrontal cortices, the anterior cingulate gyrus, and the midbrain, preserved cardiac sympathetic innervation by MIBG SPECT

Corticobasal degeneration

Brain MRI

Asymmetric cortical atrophy, focal atrophy predominantly involves the posterior frontal and parietal regions, along with dilatation of the lateral ventricles. T2-signal hyperintensity of the atrophic cortex and underlying white matter

Table 2.4 (continued)

Molecular imaging

Reduced presynaptic dopaminergic transporter with dopaminergic imaging, FDG-PET with asymmetrical hypometabolism was observed in the central region, the putamen and thalamus

autoimmune encephalitis, and metabolic leukoencephalopathies. Cerebral autosomal dominant arteriopathy with subcortical infarcts and leukoencephalopathy (CADASIL) is associated with widespread confluent white matter hyperintensities, particularly in the anterior temporal lobe. The Fazekas scale is a four-level score to quantify white matter hyperintensities, but its added value in the clinical setting is not well established.

Brain volume measurements are also valuable. Accumulating evidence from quantitative MRI studies shows that hippocampal atrophy is present before dementia onset and progresses with conversion to clinically apparent AD. However, because there is overlap between aging- and AD-associated focal hippocampal atrophy, this finding can only be considered supportive and not diagnostic. In the behavioral variant of FTD, there is predominantly atrophy of the frontal and temporal lobes with relative preservation of posterior areas, whereas the atrophy is predominantly left-sided in inferior-frontal and insular cortices in the nonfluent variant of primary progressive aphasia, and asymmetrical (commonly left-sided) anteroinferior temporal lobe and temporal gyrus atrophy is seen in the semantic variant of primary progressive aphasia.

There are no easily identifiable MRI features to support the diagnosis of DLB. The mesial temporal lobe and hippocampi remain relatively normal in size DLB, helping to distinguish it from AD [20], whereas gray matter atrophy in the posterior parietal cortices is more common in DLB than AD [21]. Other brain MRI abnormalities in DLB include atrophy of the frontal lobes and parietotemporal regions, enlargement of the lateral ventricles, and absent swallow-tail sign in the substantia nigra pars compacta (also seen in PD) [20, 22]. Brain MRI is not necessary for the diagnosis of PD. Progressive accumulation of iron in the substantia nigra and caudal putamen has been reported with specialized MRI techniques, but further studies are needed for validation.

A variety of focal lesions can be seen in less common movement disorders. In multiple system atrophy (MSA), brain MRI may vary based on the clinical subtype. In MSA-P, the brain MRI frequently reveals atrophy of the putamen with a hyperintense T2 border of the lateral putamen and T2 hypointensity of the body of the putamen. Atrophy of the middle cerebellar peduncle, pons, or cerebellum can be seen in MSA-P and MSA-C. The hot cross bun sign is the classic sign in patients with MSA-C and refers to cruciform T2 hyperintensities of the pons [23]. Predominant midbrain atrophy (the hummingbird sign) increases the diagnostic confidence in patients diagnosed with progressive supranuclear palsy (PSP) based on clinical features. Early in corticobasal degeneration, brain imaging may be normal [24]. As the disease progresses, asymmetric cortical atrophy is observed in up to half of patients [25]. Focal atrophy predominantly involves the posterior frontal and parietal regions, with dilatation of the lateral ventricles. On T2-weighted images, there is hyperintensity of the atrophic cortex and underlying white matter [26].

Heavy metal deposition in the brain can be seen in rare forms of parkinsonism (e.g., manganese-induced parkinsonism, neurodegeneration with brain iron accumulation, Wilson's disease).

Transcranial ultrasound of the substantia nigra is another imaging technique that can reveal focal lesions. Hyperechogenicity of the substantia nigra is characteristic of PD, whereas normal echogenicity suggests atypical parkinsonism and poorer response to levodopa treatment. Hyperechogenicity does not correlate well with disease severity or change with disease progression [27]. Limitations of this technique include the requirements for an experienced examiner and a sufficient bone window [28].

Is There Cerebral Cortical or Subcortical Hypometabolism?

Neurodegenerative diseases have typical regional patterns of hypometabolism, and FDG-PET imaging can be helpful to distinguish different forms of dementia or atypical parkinsonian syndromes. AD shows hypometabolism in the bilateral temporal lobes (middle and inferior temporal gyri), limbic system (parahippocampal gyrus and posterior cingulate gyrus), parietal lobe, and, rarely, occipital structures [29]. Early in FTD by contrast, glucose hypometabolism is limited to the frontal and anterior temporal lobes. As the disease progresses, pathologic changes spread into the prefrontal, parietal, and temporal regions. The pattern of hypometabolism on FDG-PET can help distinguish between the different variants of primary progressive aphasia. In progressive non-fluent aphasia, hypometabolism is most pronounced in the left anterior insula and frontal opercular region, whereas in semantic dementia decreased glucose metabolism is seen in the bilateral anterior temporal lobes (worse on the left side) and logopenic progressive aphasia demonstrates left posterior perisylvian or parietal hypometabolism.

The cingulate island sign, where individuals with DLB have a high ratio of glucose metabolism in the posterior cingulate region compared with the precuneus and cuneus, may be demonstrated on FDG-PET imaging [21]. Occipital hypoperfusion is also more common in DLB when compared to AD, affecting both primary visual cortex and visual association areas, including the precuneus [30]. Hypometabolism in the putamen, brainstem, or cerebellum is seen in MSA, whereas asymmetrical or bilateral hypometabolism in the prefrontal cortices, the anterior cingulate gyrus, and the midbrain is common in PSP. In corticobasal syndrome, asymmetrical hypometabolism is observed in the central region, the putamen, and the thalamus [31]. By contrast, no FDG-PET abnormalities would be expected in functional cognitive disorder or psychiatric illness.

Is There Amyloid or Tau Pathology?

The presence of amyloid pathology is necessary but insufficient alone for a clinical diagnosis of AD MCI or dementia. Instead, most evidence indicates accumulation of amyloid occurs early and often does not cause symptoms, sometimes preceding dementia by 10–20 years [32, 33]. The research framework for AD uses biomarkers to characterize the pathological characteristics of A/T/N where "A" refers to the positive or negative results of a β-amyloid biomarker, "T," of a tau biomarker, and "N," to a biomarker of neurodegeneration or neuronal injury. While amyloid does not correlate with the severity of symptoms, the distribution and severity of tau pathology and neuronal/synaptic loss do. When there is uncertainty about the diagnosis of AD or whether MCI is due to AD pathology, AD biomarkers are valuable. When it is important to have very high diagnostic confidence to imitate appropriate therapy, accuracy of PET amyloid imaging and dopaminergic imaging biomarkers compared to neuropathology is nearly 100%. Conversely, amyloid imaging is unlikely to distinguish between DLB and AD as amyloid pathology is common in both. Tau PET ligands bind to different sites with 18F-flortaucipir specific for tau in AD and 18F-PI-2620 binding tau in PSP (the latter drug is not yet FDA approved) [34, 35]. Alternatively, amyloid and tau biomarkers can be measured in the CSF. Several forms of tau can be assessed in biofluids: total tau (t-tau), phosphorylated tau (p-tau), and tau phosphorylated at different threonines: p-tau181, p-tau217, and p-tau231. Phosphorylated tau is more specific for AD pathology, and p-tau217 appears to have the best diagnostic accuracy [36]. Plasma versions of these assays currently are under development. Changes in amyloid and tau PET imaging also have been used to assess response to investigational drug treatments, and amyloid and tau drug response biomarkers will likely be adopted in clinical practice when disease-modifying drugs become available.

Is There a Loss of Presynaptic Striatal Dopaminergic Innervation?

Imaging of presynaptic dopaminergic transporter with dopaminergic imaging can assist in making a correct diagnosis in patients with suspected parkinsonian syndromes [37]. However, dopaminergic imaging is not helpful to differentiate between neurodegenerative parkinsonian syndromes. There is evidence of denervation in PD and all cases of MSA-P, whereas relative preservation of dopaminergic terminals is observed in MSA with cerebellar features [38]. Presynaptic dopamine transporter imaging is also abnormal in PSP and corticobasal syndrome [39]. Dopaminergic imaging may be helpful in the evaluation of patients who present with action tremor and subtle features of parkinsonism. Imaging of presynaptic dopamine transporter is normal or reveals only a small degree of dopaminergic degeneration in essential tremor [40], contrasting the typical pattern of pronounced posterior putamen reductions of radiotracer binding observed in PD [41]. Dopaminergic imaging may also be helpful to distinguish drug-induced parkinsonism from PD. In the assessment of patients with dementia, dopaminergic imaging should not be ordered if there is clear objective evidence of parkinsonism. A positive dopamine scan can help diagnose DLB, particularly if parkinsonism is equivocal on examination. The effectiveness of presynaptic dopaminergic transporter imaging in the distinction between DLB and AD was confirmed in an autopsy study with 88% sensitivity and 100% specificity [42]. Patients need to discontinue medications that interfere with presynaptic dopamine transporter binding before dopaminergic imaging.

Is There Loss of Cardiac Postganglionic Sympathetic Innervation?

Evidence of cardiac sympathetic denervation by imaging has been studied as a diagnostic tool in patients with dementia to distinguish between DLB and AD. Studies have reported a high correlation between abnormal cardiac sympathetic activity evaluated with MIBG myocardial scintigraphy and a clinical diagnosis of DLB [43, 44]. Reduced MIBG uptake is an "indicative" biomarker in the research criteria for the diagnosis of prodromal DLB [45].

Neuroimaging evidence of cardiac sympathetic denervation in PD was first reported by Goldstein and collaborators using 18-fluorodopamine cardiac PET imaging [46]. Numerous studies have confirmed these findings using MIBG cardiac single-photon emission computed tomography (SPECT) imaging [47–49]. In clinical practice, MIBG cardiac SPECT is most useful to differentiate patients with PD and orthostatic hypotension from patients with MSA. Most MSA patients have biomarkers of intact cardiac sympathetic innervation; however, rare cases of MSA with neuroimaging evidence of cardiac noradrenergic deficiency have been reported [46, 50, 51]. Cardiac sympathetic innervation is usually preserved in PSP and CBD, although patients with PSP may exhibit a mild decrease in MIBG [52]. In the USA, MIBG scanning is not done for this purpose, despite being available at most academic centers and used for other indications such as the diagnostic evaluation of pheochromocytoma. A major reason is due to the lack of coverage by third-party payers.

Is There Central or Peripheral Autonomic Failure?

Autonomic function testing in MSA reveals evidence of central autonomic dysfunction. Cardiovascular adrenergic failure is usually severe and frequently the most pronounced finding [53, 54]. The thermoregulatory sweat test is abnormal in most patients with MSA and often demonstrates the involvement of predominantly preganglionic fibers; however, this test is only available in a few specialized centers and its diagnostic performance relative to pathologic diagnosis is unknown. Urodynamic investigations in MSA reveal large postvoid residuals (>100 mL), absence of detrusor-sphincter coordination, and atonic bladder with low urethral pressure [55]. Thus, specialized autonomic testing can be helpful to better characterize the severity and distribution of autonomic impairment, however, these tests are not widely available.

What Are the Neurophysiological Characteristics of the Tremor?

Tremor is vastly heterogeneous often making it difficult to distinguish the cause based on clinical characteristics alone. A functional tremor may co-exist in essential tremor or PD. Many patients with PD also exhibit postural tremor. In a population-based setting, resting tremor was a common clinical feature in patients with essential tremor, with prevalence reaching nearly 50% [56]. Patients with essential tremor also can exhibit slowness of movements reminiscent of the bradykinesia seen in PD. Furthermore, epidemiological studies suggest that essential tremor populations have an increased risk of developing PD [57]. Electrophysiological biomarkers with analysis of tremor frequencies and amplitude provide clinicians objective evidence for identifying the cause of the tremor [58]. Surface electromyography and accelerometry define the neurophysiological characteristics of functional tremor and have good sensitivity and specificity in diagnosis [59].

Is There Evidence of Alpha-Synuclein Pathology?

Visualization of synuclein aggregates by immunofluorescence on skin biopsy is available to clinicians in the USA and can be helpful when patients do not improve with an appropriate trial of levodopa or when MSA is suspected [60]. Synuclein in the skin indicates the possibility of MSA, whereas its absence raises suspicion for a tauopathy or a non-degenerative parkinsonian syndrome such as drug-induced parkinsonism. Available testing does not distinguish between the different synucleinopathies.

Polysomnography showing REM-sleep behavior disorder (RBD) is indirect evidence of a synucleinopathy such as PD or DLB. In clinical practice, physicians often rely on questionnaires without objective testing for RBD and literature suggests a high correlation of polysomnogram-proven RBD with the RBD questionnaire results [61].

Factors Affecting Biomarker Interpretation

The interpretation of a biomarkers result must consider the clinical context and question being asked. Prior probability of a positive test result strongly influences the statistical characteristics of a test. Avoiding indiscriminate testing helps distinguish important results from incidental findings and biomarker findings of uncertain clinical significance. An elevated CSF 14-3-3 supports a diagnosis of CJD, but it is not always abnormal in this disease and can be elevated in other disorders [62]. Likewise, the significance of "borderline" results can be overlooked if it is inconsistent with other evidence but can also be extremely helpful if positivity is consistent with a confluence of other evidence.

Clinicians share the responsibility with laboratories and imaging centers for accurate interpretation of biomarker results. Clinicians are responsible for deciding which biomarker is tested based upon their understanding of biomarker performance, availability, acceptability to patients, convenience, and cost. Clinicians do not control biomarker measurement; that is the responsibility of specialists at laboratories and imaging centers. However, clinicians affect biomarker measurement by determining how the patient is prepared for testing, how the sample is collected, and the information provided to the laboratory and imaging center. Misinterpretation of brain scans performed in patients with FTD in one study certainly was due in part to only information about clinical history being provided in only 11 of 40 MRI requests [3]. Clinicians should temper their interpretation of results with an understanding of factors affecting biomarker measurement, including patient factors, technical considerations, and statistical characteristics of the biomarker in relevant clinical populations. Patient factors and technical considerations include intra-assay variability of measurement, method of sample collection and handling, and potential methodological pitfalls (Table 2.5).

Table 2.5 Patient and technical factors to consider

Brain MRI
Patient factors
• Cooperation of patient is necessary to avoid motion artifact
• Precautions are necessary with cardiac implantable electronic devices, cochlear implants, drug infusion pumps, cerebral artery aneurysm clips, magnetic dental implants, hearing aids
• Contraindicated in patients with metallic intraocular foreign bodies. Orbit X-ray must be taken and reviewed by the radiologist for approval before the MRI if there is a history of facial injury or trauma
• MRI contrast agents rarely cause allergic reactions
• Patients with a history of renal disease or on dialysis need to be evaluated carefully before injection of gadolinium for MRI procedure
Technical factors
• Imaging acquisition: High resolution, isovoxel
• Slice thickness should be standardized
• Periodic use of phantoms
• Semi-quantitative or quantitative analyses should be performed if possible to help answer the clinical question
PET/SPECT imaging
Patient factors
• Cooperation of patient is necessary to avoid motion artifact
• Drugs that could interfere with tracer binding to presynaptic dopamine transporters should be discontinued before dopaminergic imaging
• Drugs that could interfere with glucose uptake in the brain should be discontinued before FDG-PET (i.e., insulin)
• For cardiac sympathetic neuroimaging, patients should be screened for conditions known to cause cardiac denervation such as diabetes mellitus, heart failure. Screening for coronary artery disease is important because perfusion imaging is not routinely done with cardiac MIBG SPECT. Medications that can interfere with the uptake of MIBG should be discontinued
• No drug withdrawal is recommended at this time for amyloid PET imaging
Technical factors
• Careful selection of region of interest for comparison with cerebral cortical metabolism in FDG-PET or with striatal dopamine transporter binding in dopaminergic imaging
CSF
Patient factors
• Cooperation of patient is necessary. Sedation may be required

(continued)

Table 2.5 (continued)

• Patient's anatomy may require fluoroscopy-guided lumbar puncture

Technical factors

• Pre-analytical sample handling and storage play an important role in the reliable measurement of CSF biomarkers in AD
• CSF amyloid beta (Aβ)1–42 and tau should be measured in fresh, non-processed CSF collected in low-binding opaque polystyrene rather than clear polypropylene tubes
• Transport and storage of the sample at 2–8 °C for up to 15 days or 20–25 °C for up to 48 h

Skin biopsy

Technical factors

• Local anesthesia should be used and is best achieved by subcutaneous infiltration with lidocaine
• 3.0 mm punch skin biopsy performed at three sites: Posterior cervical, distal thigh, and distal leg
• Biopsy samples are stored in a container with a mixture of water and formaldehyde (formalin) or some other fluid to preserve the specimens
• Specimens should be analyzed by a laboratory with expertise in dual immunostaining for protein gene product 9.5 and phosphorylated α-synuclein

Patient and Technical Factors Affecting Interpretation of Imaging Biomarkers

Clinicians ordering imaging biomarkers must consider many patient factors. Medications such as steroids, level of hydration, and environmental and cognitive stimuli affect biomarker measurement of brain volume, metabolism, and blood flow (particularly functional MRI). Stable blood glucose levels are essential to meet the assumptions underlying FDG-PET imaging. Because many drugs, particularly psychoactive medications, alter dopaminergic imaging, clinicians should carefully review the patient's medication list and discontinue the interfering drugs for a sufficient half-life before tracer administration. Patients with pacemakers, intracranial clips, and other metallic implants are inappropriate for MRI imaging. Patient cooperation also must be considered. Minimizing head movement is critical for imaging biomarkers, using sedation or head immobilization, if necessary.

Radiologists and nuclear medicine specialists must pay attention to many technical details to ensure that imaging biomarkers are reliable. Imaging acquisition (ideally high resolution, iso-voxel) and instrument characteristics are critical. For example, slice thickness of images substantially affects the measured size of a tumor [63]. Periodic use of phantoms and imaging protocols assure quality control and consistent quantification of acquired images.

A large number of image analysis methods are available. The simplest imaging biomarkers to implement clinically are semi-quantitative scoring systems developed to achieve more standardized visual assessment. The Fazekas 0–3 rating of white matter hyperintensities is a widely used example, and semi-quantitative ratings also have been developed for global and medial temporal atrophy brain atrophy, and other metrics [64]. With adherence to standardized image acquisition protocols, software analysis can yield much more sensitive quantitative measures. Commercial image analysis software is available for MRI volumetric analysis of total brain and individual anatomic regions, with hippocampal volume being particularly relevant for dementing diseases [65]. FDG-PET and amyloid PET automated analysis software are also commercially available. These software packages have the marked advantage of comparing results against reference populations, such as cognitively normal individuals in the same age range and using different internal reference regions. For example, the pons is often used for comparison with cerebral cortical metabolism in FDG-PET because it is not affected in most dementing diseases and the cerebellum is often used for comparison with cerebral cortical binding of amyloid imaging because neuritic amyloid plaques are not found there. In special circumstances when these rules are not applicable, the software can allow the selection of an alternative reference region.

A significant issue with imaging biomarkers is the large number of potential biomarkers. Functional MRI has had difficulty finding clinical applications because of the large number of variables considered simultaneously, making replication difficult. The solution is to pre-specify the imaging variable that will be considered and use other imaging outcomes as supportive.

Composite biomarkers such as hippocampal volume/total brain volume can function like composite fluid biomarkers to account for known technical and patient factors.

As new biomarkers are being developed and brought to the clinic, physicians should remain aware of methodological limitations and vigilant and critical about the results.

Patient and Technical Factors Affecting Interpretation of Fluid Biomarkers

Clinicians ordering fluid biomarkers also must consider patient factors that can affect intra-assay variability. There is less concern about the effects of medication and there are few contraindications than imaging biomarkers, but fluid biomarkers can be affected by contaminants, pre-analytic specimen collection and handling. For CSF studies a traumatic tap should be avoided but the susceptibility of biomarker result to this contaminant is often not known. The possible effects of pre-analytic and assay methods are perhaps best exemplified by the challenges of measuring Aβ 1–42, which is reliably reduced in the presence of AD plaque pathology [66]. With a lack of an approved reference method and the variability of cut-off values in different studies, detailed protocols have been developed to limit the contributions of specimen collection and handling [67]. The practical importance of variables such as time of day for collection, CSF volume collected, and number of freeze/thaw cycles is unclear, but the type of collection tube has been found to significantly alter affect the measurement of CSF Aβ 1–42 levels. Aβ protein binds to the surface of polystyrene collection tubes found on most hospital and clinic CSF procedure trays. If unrecognized, an artifactually low Aβ 1–42 result could be interpreted as indicating AD pathology. To address this problem low binding, opaque polypropylene rather than clear polystyrene collection tubes always should be used, and measuring the ratio of Aβ 1–42/Aβ 1–40 minimizes this effect and is a more robust biomarker.

Assay methods used in biomarker measurement also affect interpretation and inter-assay variability in the measurement of a biomarker is significant. Clinicians may need to inquire about the method used by the laboratory and its statistical characteristics for the question being asked. Depending upon the circumstances an alternative assay method should be requested. Continuing to use the measurement of Aβ 1–42 for illustration, the performance of five different CSF immunoassays differed significantly, and all performed worse than an antibody-independent mass spectrometry procedure [68]. Using a ratio of Aβ 1–42/Aβ 1–40 or a ratio with tau levels did not alter these findings. Measurement of biomarkers in plasma would be logistically easier and more acceptable to patients but requires much more sensitive assays that have only recently become available. Head-to-head comparison of eight different plasma Aβ 1–42 measures showed considerable variation, again finding more technically demanding and expensive mass spectroscopy methods performing best [69]. Automated analysis methods may prove to give more consistent results, but the variability of biofluid assays has shown that so far amyloid PET is the gold standard for assessing AD Aβ plaque pathology because it correlates highly with postmortem brain histopathology [70].

Accurate identification of phosphorylated α-synuclein within cutaneous nerves should be assessed by the biopsy at three different sites (posterior cervical, distal thigh, and distal leg) to increase diagnostic accuracy. Biopsy samples should then be stored in a container with a mixture of water and formaldehyde (formalin) or some other fluid to preserve the specimens and analyzed by a laboratory with expertise in dual immunostaining for protein gene product 9.5 and phosphorylated α-synuclein.

Statistical Characteristics

Interpretation of a biomarker result must consider its statistical characteristics (Table 2.6). Results of diagnostic biomarkers are typically dichotomous, i.e., either positive or negative,

Table 2.6 Statistical characteristics of diagnostic biomarkers

- Receiver operator characteristic (ROC) statistic to determine the cut-off for a positive test
- Prior probability of a positive test in the population receiving the test

Affected by the prevalence of disease in the population being tested

- Accuracy = proportion of the time a test result is correct (true positive + true negative/total cases)
- False positive rate = proportion with a positive test without the disease
- False negative rate = proportion with the disease that have a positive test
- Positive predictive value = proportion with a positive test who have disease
- Negative predictive value = proportion with a negative test without disease
- Positive likelihood ratio = how much prior probability of a disease is increased with a positive test
- Negative likelihood ratio = how much prior probability of no disease is increased with a negative test

Independent of the prevalence of disease in the population being tested

- Sensitivity = proportion of those with the condition who have a positive test result
- Specificity = proportion of those without the condition who have a negative test result
- Diagnostic odds ratio = (True positives/false positives)/(false negatives/true negatives)
- Upper and lower assay method technical limits of detection (e.g., pg/mL)

based upon a cut-off value determined by a receiver operating characteristic curve (ROC) area under the curve statistic that best discriminates cases from non-cases. Sometimes the alternative of a "borderline" result is provided, with the implicit understanding that less extreme values are less likely to be clinically significant. The prior probability or base rate of biomarker positivity in the population receiving the test profoundly affects the accuracy (false positive and false negative rates) and the positive and negative predictive value of a test result. This is the most compelling reason to avoid indiscriminate use of biomarkers: only using biomarkers after a comprehensive clinical assessment to answer relevant questions markedly increases accuracy of the result. Positive and negative likelihood ratios are

useful in comparing the value of different tests in a specific population [71].

Although they are not as relevant to diagnostic decision-making, sensitivity and specificity are commonly used to describe the statistical characteristics of a test because they are unaffected by the prevalence of disease in the population being studied. Note, however, that sensitivity and specificity depend on what populations are being compared. Often sensitivity and specificity are reported for comparison of a population with one disease compared to normal controls. This is not as relevant as sensitivity and specificity compared to clinical populations such as distinguishing AD among those with dementia. For example, a dopamine scan measuring the integrity of dopamine transporters is highly accurate, specific, and sensitive in distinguishing essential tremor and PD, but does not help differentiate PD from PSP. Also notice that a "gold standard" has to be used to identify those with and without disease in computing these statistical characteristics. A limitation of most diagnostic biomarkers is that clinical rather than neuropathological diagnosis is used as the "gold standard." If knowledge of the biomarker result has not been rigorously withheld by those making a clinical diagnosis, all measures can be inflated because of "circular reasoning," i.e., the biomarker is accurate because the diagnosis was based on the biomarker. Autopsy-validated biomarkers are PET amyloid imaging with AD pathology [70], FDG-PET in distinguishing AD from FTD [72] and AD from DLB [73]. Autopsy-validated biomarkers are imperfect as a diagnostic "gold standard" and will yield lower sensitivity and specificity then neuropathological diagnoses. Nevertheless, validated PET biomarkers are frequently used to assess the performance of new biomarkers making it possible to include hundreds of samples in a short time [74].

Statistical tests relevant for biomarkers that intended for purposes other than diagnosis may be different. The validity of disease monitoring and drug response biomarkers may be evaluated by comparing results with categorical severity of impairment, rate of change in a cognitive measure, or the proportion of those improving with treatment. Prognostic and risk biomarkers may compare proportions of the population reaching a specified outcome. Safety biomarkers are always imperfect, and it may be sufficient to show that a negative biomarker reduces the chance of an adverse event.

Errors and Misuse of Biomarkers in Clinical Care

Biomarkers are subject to errors and misuse (Table 2.7). The most common and damaging are overdependence and underuse. Overdependence occurs because of shortcuts taken in a diagnostic evaluation. It can be simpler to order tests and see what shows up than the exacting task of a comprehensive evaluation where multiple lines of evidence must be integrated into a confident and exact diagnosis. Failing to consider prior probabilities it is tempting to accept a positive result of a single test and overlook or not collect inconsistent evidence. Underuse also causes similar problems. Once again inconsistent evidence is overlooked and not tested with biomarkers. Overreliance on clinical judgment unaided by any testing is often in error and ultimately serves the best interests of neither the clinician or patient. Diagnostic uncertainty is common, and diagnostic excellence needs to be managed, including the ethical duty to communicate uncertainty honestly to patients and families [75]. Referral to specialty care is an alternative to shortcuts for those unfamiliar with the diagnosis and management of neurodegenerative diseases but often causes misuses of biomarkers.

A positive biomarker of one type of pathology (e.g., β-amyloid, α-synuclein, etc.) does not necessarily reflect the underlying cause of a patient's disease. The contribution of α-synuclein, β-amyloid, and tau aggregation in PD and AD is still a matter of debate. Importantly, one cannot ignore the fact that α-synuclein, β-amyloid, and tau aggregation are frequent "co-pathologies" in neurodegenerative diseases [76, 77], and these proteins can also be found in the brain of individuals without dementia or parkinsonism [78]. Autopsy studies have found that most elderly subjects have more than one brain pathology present, even asymptomatic individuals [79].

Table 2.7 Potential errors and misuses of biomarkers

Utilization errors and misuse
• Overuse—Needlessly repeating studies or obtaining imaging and biomarker studies unlikely to contribute to a diagnosis, thus causing excessive costs without additional clinical benefit
• Underuse—Failure to utilize the imaging modality that could provide critical information for diagnosis
• Omission—Failure to incorporate significant imaging and biomarker findings in diagnosis and management
• Overdependence—Using biomarkers to decide whether there is a neurodegenerative disease when clinical assessment alone is reliable, or basing decisions only on biomarker results without utilizing other relevant clinical evidence
• Indiscriminate or inappropriate use—"Ornamental" testing without intending to use results in clinical decision-making, using biomarkers as an alternative to reasoned clinical assessment

Interpretation errors
• Overinterpretation—Assigning a diagnosis based on clinically insignificant imaging findings or borderline biomarker results inconsistent with other evidence
• Misinterpretation—Failing to recognize the presence of clinically significant lesions, causing errors in radiographic diagnosis
• Inconsistent interpretation—Variability between radiologists or in patient to patient descriptions and clinical significance ascribed to identical imaging findings

Technical errors
• Lack of reliability—Inappropriate patient preparation, inconsistent acquisition or processing of imaging data, causing misinterpretation
• Artifact—Failure to prevent or identify image acquisition or analysis errors, sample contamination or mishandling that prevent the accurate interpretation of scans

Moreover, indirect evidence from human studies suggests protein aggregation in sporadic cases may be protective and not capable of discriminating clinical disease subtypes [80].

Future Biomarkers

Remarkable advances in the understanding of the pathology of neurodegenerative diseases offer the promise that future biomarkers will fulfill still unmet clinical needs. We do not yet have imaging or biofluid biomarkers for α-synuclein, TDP-43, activated microglia, or the multiple isoforms and configurations of tau [81]. Detection of α-synuclein in plasma-derived extracellular vesicles has shown promise as a potential diagnostic biomarker for PD [82]. Protein misfolding cyclic amplification or real-time quaking-induced conversion measured in CSF are promising tools to identify different patterns of α-synuclein aggregation in different synucleinopathies [83, 84]. The use of this technology is also a promising tool for the identification of synucleinopathies at the prodromal stage [85]. PET ligands for tau appear to have different affinities that could be exploited to differentiate between tauopathies [86].

Increasingly, we will call upon biomarkers to predict disease onset in pre-symptomatic and prodromal phases. Proteins and metabolites such as neurofilament light chain, amyloid precursor protein soluble metabolites, and α-synuclein may allow earlier identification of a neurodegenerative disorder. Plasma biomarkers using new analytic techniques able to detect much lower protein concentrations make early detection more feasible. Imaging biomarkers may predict disease complications, such as distinguishing AD that is likely or unlikely to develop behavioral complications [87].

Biomarker panels may solve some of the limitations of targeted biomarkers. Proteomics, metabolomics, and transcriptomics are powerful tools capable of simultaneous analysis of multiple constituents to identify small changes in protein, metabolites, or RNA profiles. Metabolomics profiling in particular holds great promise in providing unique insights into molecular pathogenesis and identifying candidate biomarkers for clinical detection and therapies. As illustrated by the A/T/N biomarker classification of cognitive disorders [88], combinations of biomarkers can lead to the clinical recognition of diseases previously recognized only with postmortem examination and co-pathologies, such as limbic-predominant age-related TDP-43 encephalopathy (LATE) and primary age-related tauopathy (tangle-only dementia, PART) [89, 90].

Recognizing these less understood disorders and their presence as co-pathologies may explain some of the heterogeneity of progression of the dementing disease and become important in prognosis and treatment planning [91, 92].

Imaging and fluid biomarkers for neurodegenerative diseases are here to stay and will be an increasingly important requirement for providing optimal clinical care. The principles of appropriate use cut through the challenges of misuse and cost that otherwise undermine the clinical application of significant scientific advances.

References

1. Biomarker Working Group F-NB. Biomarkers, endpoints, and other tools. In: Spring S, editor. BEST (biomarkers, endpoints, and other tools). Silver Spring: FDA-NIH; 2016.
2. Herzog R, Elgort DR, Flanders AE, Moley PJ. Variability in diagnostic error rates of 10 MRI centers performing lumbar spine MRI examinations on the same patient within a 3-week period. Spine J. 2017;17(4):554–61.
3. Suárez J, Tartaglia MC, Vitali P, Erbetta A, Neuhaus J, Laluz V, et al. Characterizing radiology reports in patients with frontotemporal dementia. Neurology. 2009;73(13):1073–4.
4. Kinahan PE, Perlman ES, Sunderland JJ, Subramaniam R, Wollenweber SD, Turkington TG, et al. The QIBA profile for FDG PET/CT as an imaging biomarker measuring response to cancer therapy. Radiology. 2020;294(3):647–57.
5. Skillbäck T, Rosén C, Asztely F, Mattsson N, Blennow K, Zetterberg H. Diagnostic performance of cerebrospinal fluid total tau and phosphorylated tau in Creutzfeldt-Jakob disease: results from the Swedish Mortality Registry. JAMA Neurol. 2014;71(4):476–83.
6. Bergeron D, Beauregard JM, Guimond J, Fortin MP, Houde M, Poulin S, et al. Clinical impact of a second FDG-PET in atypical/unclear dementia syndromes. J Alzheimers Dis. 2016;49(3):695–705.
7. Tolosa E, Borght TV, Moreno E, DaTSCAN Clinically Uncertain Parkinsonian Syndromes Study Group. Accuracy of DaTSCAN (123I-ioflupane) SPECT in diagnosis of patients with clinically uncertain parkinsonism: 2-year follow-up of an open-label study. Mov Disord. 2007;22(16):2346–51.
8. Taswell C, Villemagne VL, Yates P, Shimada H, Leyton CE, Ballard KJ, et al. 18F-FDG PET improves diagnosis in patients with focal-onset dementias. J Nucl Med. 2015;56(10):1547–53.
9. Mesulam MM, Coventry C, Kuang A, Bigio EH, Mao Q, Flanagan ME, et al. Memory resilience in

Alzheimer disease with primary progressive aphasia. Neurology. 2021;96(6):e916–e25.

10. Taylor-Rubin C, Azizi L, Croot K, Nickels L. Primary progressive aphasia education and support groups: a clinical evaluation. Am J Alzheimers Dis Other Dement. 2020;35:1533317519895638.

11. Kuhl DE, Koeppe RA, Minoshima S, Snyder SE, Ficaro EP, Foster NL, et al. In vivo mapping of cerebral acetylcholinesterase activity in aging and Alzheimer's disease. Neurology. 1999;52(4):691–9.

12. Marek K, Jennings D, Seibyl J. Imaging the dopamine system to assess disease-modifying drugs: studies comparing dopamine agonists and levodopa. Neurology. 2003;61(6 Suppl 3):S43–8.

13. Mintun MA, Lo AC, Duggan Evans C, Wessels AM, Ardayfio PA, Andersen SW, et al. Donanemab in early Alzheimer's disease. N Engl J Med. 2021;384(18):1691–704.

14. Marshall GA, Monserratt L, Harwood D, Mandelkern M, Cummings JL, Sultzer DL. Positron emission tomography metabolic correlates of apathy in Alzheimer disease. Arch Neurol. 2007;64(7):1015–20.

15. Blazhenets G, Ma Y, Sörensen A, Schiller F, Rücker G, Eidelberg D, et al. Predictive value of (18) F-Florbetapir and (18)F-FDG PET for conversion from mild cognitive impairment to Alzheimer dementia. J Nucl Med. 2020;61(4):597–603.

16. Salloway S, Chalkias S, Barkhof F, Burkett P, Barakos J, Purcell D, et al. Amyloid-related imaging abnormalities in 2 phase 3 studies evaluating Aducanumab in patients with early Alzheimer disease. JAMA Neurol. 2022;79(1):13–21.

17. Elias-Sonnenschein LS, Viechtbauer W, Ramakers IH, Verhey FR, Visser PJ. Predictive value of APOE-ε4 allele for progression from MCI to AD-type dementia: a meta-analysis. J Neurol Neurosurg Psychiatry. 2011;82(10):1149–56.

18. Albert MS, DeKosky ST, Dickson D, Dubois B, Feldman HH, Fox NC, et al. The diagnosis of mild cognitive impairment due to Alzheimer's disease: recommendations from the National Institute on Aging-Alzheimer's Association workgroups on diagnostic guidelines for Alzheimer's disease. Alzheimers Dement. 2011;7(3):270–9.

19. Smith EE, Egorova S, Blacker D, Killiany RJ, Muzikansky A, Dickerson BC, et al. Magnetic resonance imaging white matter hyperintensities and brain volume in the prediction of mild cognitive impairment and dementia. Arch Neurol. 2008;65(1):94–100.

20. Whitwell JL, Weigand SD, Shiung MM, Boeve BF, Ferman TJ, Smith GE, et al. Focal atrophy in dementia with Lewy bodies on MRI: a distinct pattern from Alzheimer's disease. Brain. 2007;130(Pt 3):708–19.

21. Scamarcia PG, Agosta F, Caso F, Filippi M. Update on neuroimaging in non-Alzheimer's disease dementia: a focus on the Lewy body disease spectrum. Curr Opin Neurol. 2021;34(4):532–8.

22. Shams S, Fällmar D, Schwarz S, Wahlund LO, van Westen D, Hansson O, et al. MRI of the swallow tail sign: a useful marker in the diagnosis of Lewy body dementia? AJNR Am J Neuroradiol. 2017;38(9):1737–41.

23. Palma JA, Norcliffe-Kaufmann L, Kaufmann H. Diagnosis of multiple system atrophy. Auton Neurosci. 2018;211:15–25.

24. Mahapatra RK, Edwards MJ, Schott JM, Bhatia KP. Corticobasal degeneration. Lancet Neurol. 2004;3(12):736–43.

25. Hauser RA, Murtaugh FR, Akhter K, Gold M, Olanow CW. Magnetic resonance imaging of corticobasal degeneration. J Neuroimaging. 1996;6(4):222–6.

26. Soliveri P, Monza D, Paridi D, Radice D, Grisoli M, Testa D, et al. Cognitive and magnetic resonance imaging aspects of corticobasal degeneration and progressive supranuclear palsy. Neurology. 1999;53(3):502–7.

27. Berg D, Behnke S, Seppi K, Godau J, Lerche S, Mahlknecht P, et al. Enlarged hyperechogenic substantia nigra as a risk marker for Parkinson's disease. Mov Disord. 2013;28(2):216–9.

28. Saeed U, Lang AE, Masellis M. Neuroimaging advances in Parkinson's disease and atypical parkinsonian syndromes. Front Neurol. 2020;11:572976.

29. Mosconi L. Brain glucose metabolism in the early and specific diagnosis of Alzheimer's disease. FDG-PET studies in MCI and AD. Eur J Nucl Med Mol Imaging. 2005;32(4):486–510.

30. Lobotesis K, Fenwick JD, Phipps A, Ryman A, Swann A, Ballard C, et al. Occipital hypoperfusion on SPECT in dementia with Lewy bodies but not AD. Neurology. 2001;56(5):643–9.

31. Beyer L, Meyer-Wilmes J, Schönecker S, Schnabel J, Brendel E, Prix C, et al. Clinical routine FDG-PET imaging of suspected progressive supranuclear palsy and corticobasal degeneration: a gatekeeper for subsequent tau-PET imaging? Front Neurol. 2018;9:483.

32. Hof PR, Glannakopoulos P, Bouras C. The neuropathological changes associated with normal brain aging. Histol Histopathol. 1996;11(4):1075–88.

33. Bateman RJ, Xiong C, Benzinger TL, Fagan AM, Goate A, Fox NC, et al. Clinical and biomarker changes in dominantly inherited Alzheimer's disease. N Engl J Med. 2012;367(9):795–804.

34. Ossenkoppele R, Rabinovici GD, Smith R, Cho H, Schöll M, Strandberg O, et al. Discriminative accuracy of [18F]flortaucipir positron emission tomography for Alzheimer disease vs other neurodegenerative disorders. JAMA. 2018;320(11):1151–62.

35. Brendel M, Barthel H, van Eimeren T, Marek K, Beyer L, Song M, et al. Assessment of 18F-PI-2620 as a biomarker in progressive Supranuclear palsy. JAMA Neurol. 2020;77(11):1408–19.

36. Leuzy A, Janelidze S, Mattsson-Carlgren N, Palmqvist S, Jacobs D, Cicognola C, et al. Comparing the clinical utility and diagnostic performance of CSF P-Tau181, P-Tau217, and P-Tau231 assays. Neurology. 2021;97(17):e1681–e94.

37. Bega D, Kuo PH, Chalkidou A, Grzeda MT, Macmillan T, Brand C, et al. Clinical utility of DaTscan in patients with suspected Parkinsonian syn-

drome: a systematic review and meta-analysis. NPJ Parkinsons Dis. 2021;7(1):43.

38. Pirker W, Asenbaum S, Bencsits G, Prayer D, Gerschlager W, Deecke L, et al. [123I]beta-CIT SPECT in multiple system atrophy, progressive supranuclear palsy, and corticobasal degeneration. Mov Disord. 2000;15(6):1158–67.

39. Kaasinen V, Kankare T, Joutsa J, Vahlberg T. Presynaptic striatal dopaminergic function in atypical Parkinsonism: a metaanalysis of imaging studies. J Nucl Med. 2019;60(12):1757–63.

40. Gerasimou G, Costa DC, Papanastasiou E, Bostanjiopoulou S, Arnaoutoglou M, Moralidis E, et al. SPECT study with I-123-Ioflupane (DaTSCAN) in patients with essential tremor. Is there any correlation with Parkinson's disease? Ann Nucl Med. 2012;26(4):337–44.

41. Waln O, Wu Y, Perlman R, Wendt J, Van AK, Jankovic J. Dopamine transporter imaging in essential tremor with and without parkinsonian features. J Neural Transm. 2015;122(11):1515–21.

42. Walker Z, Jaros E, Walker RW, Lee L, Costa DC, Livingston G, et al. Dementia with Lewy bodies: a comparison of clinical diagnosis, FP-CIT single photon emission computed tomography imaging and autopsy. J Neurol Neurosurg Psychiatry. 2007;78(11):1176–81.

43. Kim JS, Park HE, Oh YS, Song IU, Yang DW, Park JW, et al. (123)I-MIBG myocardial scintigraphy and neurocirculatory abnormalities in patients with dementia with Lewy bodies and Alzheimer's disease. J Neurol Sci. 2015;357(1–2):173–7.

44. Estorch M, Camacho V, Paredes P, Rivera E, Rodríguez-Revuelto A, Flotats A, et al. Cardiac (123)I-metaiodobenzylguanidine imaging allows early identification of dementia with Lewy bodies during life. Eur J Nucl Med Mol Imaging. 2008;35(9):1636–41.

45. McKeith IG, Ferman TJ, Thomas AJ, Blanc F, Boeve BF, Fujishiro H, et al. Research criteria for the diagnosis of prodromal dementia with Lewy bodies. Neurology. 2020;94(17):743–55.

46. Goldstein DS, Holmes C, Cannon RO III, Eisenhofer G, Kopin IJ. Sympathetic cardioneuropathy in dysautonomias. N Engl J Med. 1997;336(10):696–702.

47. Treglia G, Stefanelli A, Cason E, Cocciolillo F, Di Giuda D, Giordano A. Diagnostic performance of iodine-123-metaiodobenzylguanidine scintigraphy in differential diagnosis between Parkinson's disease and multiple-system atrophy: a systematic review and a meta-analysis. Clin Neurol Neurosurg. 2011;113(10):823–9.

48. Treglia G, Cason E, Stefanelli A, Cocciolillo F, Di Giuda D, Fagioli G, et al. MIBG scintigraphy in differential diagnosis of Parkinsonism: a meta-analysis. Clin Auton Res. 2012;22(1):43–55.

49. Suzuki M, Kurita A, Hashimoto M, Fukumitsu N, Abo M, Ito Y, et al. Impaired myocardial 123I-metaiodobenzylguanidine uptake in Lewy body disease: comparison between dementia with

50. Cook GA, Sullivan P, Holmes C, Goldstein DS. Cardiac sympathetic denervation without Lewy bodies in a case of multiple system atrophy. Parkinsonism Relat Disord. 2014;20(8):926–8.

51. Lamotte G, Holmes C, Sullivan P, Lenka A, Goldstein DS. Cardioselective peripheral noradrenergic deficiency in Lewy body synucleinopathies. Ann Clin Transl Neurol. 2020;7:2450.

52. Kamada T, Miura S, Kida H, Irie KI, Yamanishi Y, Hoshino T, et al. MIBG myocardial scintigraphy in progressive supranuclear palsy. J Neurol Sci. 2019;396:3–7.

53. Goldstein DS, Holmes C, Li ST, Bruce S, Metman LV, Cannon RO III. Cardiac sympathetic denervation in Parkinson disease. Ann Intern Med. 2000;133(5):338–47.

54. Norcliffe-Kaufmann L, Kaufmann H, Palma JA, Shibao CA, Biaggioni I, Peltier AC, et al. Orthostatic heart rate changes in patients with autonomic failure caused by neurodegenerative synucleinopathies. Ann Neurol. 2018;83(3):522–31.

55. Shin JH, Park KW, Heo KO, Chung SJ, Choo MS. Urodynamic study for distinguishing multiple system atrophy from Parkinson disease. Neurology. 2019;93(10):e946–e53.

56. Louis ED, Hernandez N, Michalec M. Prevalence and correlates of rest tremor in essential tremor: cross-sectional survey of 831 patients across four distinct cohorts. Eur J Neurol. 2015;22(6):927–32.

57. Tarakad A, Jankovic J. Essential tremor and Parkinson's disease: exploring the relationship. Tremor Other Hyperkinet Mov (N Y). 2018;8:589.

58. Wang X, Cao Z, Liu G, Liu Z, Jiang Y, Ma H, et al. Clinical characteristics and electrophysiological biomarkers of Parkinson's disease developed from essential tremor. Front Neurol. 2020;11:582471.

59. Thomsen BLC, Teodoro T, Edwards MJ. Biomarkers in functional movement disorders: a systematic review. J Neurol Neurosurg Psychiatry. 2020;91(12):1261–9.

60. Gibbons CH, Wang N, Kim JY, Campagnolo M, Freeman R. Skin biopsy in evaluation of autonomic disorders. Continuum (Minneapolis, Minn). 2020;26(1):200–12.

61. Chahine LM, Daley J, Horn S, Colcher A, Hurtig H, Cantor C, et al. Questionnaire-based diagnosis of REM sleep behavior disorder in Parkinson's disease. Mov Disord. 2013;28(8):1146–9.

62. Geschwind MD, Martindale J, Miller D, DeArmond SJ, Uyehara-Lock J, Gaskin D, et al. Challenging the clinical utility of the 14-3-3 protein for the diagnosis of sporadic Creutzfeldt-Jakob disease. Arch Neurol. 2003;60(6):813–6.

63. Sullivan D, Jackson E. Quantitative imaging: images to numbers. In: Samei E, Krupinski E, editors. The handbook of medical image perception and techniques. Cambridge: Cambridge University Press; 2018. p. 407–14.

64. Wahlund LO, Westman E, van Westen D, Wallin A, Shams S, Cavallin L, et al. Imaging biomarkers of dementia: recommended visual rating scales with teaching cases. Insights Imaging. 2017;8(1):79–90.

65. Jack CR Jr, Barkhof F, Bernstein MA, Cantillon M, Cole PE, Decarli C, et al. Steps to standardization and validation of hippocampal volumetry as a biomarker in clinical trials and diagnostic criterion for Alzheimer's disease. Alzheimers Dement. 2011;7(4):474–85.e4.

66. Engelborghs S, De Vreese K, Van de Casteele T, Vanderstichele H, Van Everbroeck B, Cras P, et al. Diagnostic performance of a CSF-biomarker panel in autopsy-confirmed dementia. Neurobiol Aging. 2008;29(8):1143–59.

67. Vanderstichele HM, Janelidze S, Demeyer L, Coart E, Stoops E, Herbst V, et al. Optimized standard operating procedures for the analysis of cerebrospinal fluid Aβ42 and the ratios of Aβ isoforms using low protein binding tubes. J Alzheimers Dis. 2016;53(3):1121–32.

68. Janelidze S, Pannee J, Mikulskis A, Chiao P, Zetterberg H, Blennow K, et al. Concordance between different amyloid immunoassays and visual amyloid positron emission tomographic assessment. JAMA Neurol. 2017;74(12):1492–501.

69. Janelidze S, Teunissen CE, Zetterberg H, Allué JA, Sarasa L, Eichenlaub U, et al. Head-to-head comparison of 8 plasma amyloid-β 42/40 assays in Alzheimer disease. JAMA Neurol. 2021;78(11):1375–82.

70. Clark CM, Schneider JA, Bedell BJ, Beach TG, Bilker WB, Mintun MA, et al. Use of florbetapir-PET for imaging beta-amyloid pathology. JAMA. 2011;305(3):275–83.

71. Qizilabash N, Qizilabash N. Evidence-based diagnosis. Evidence-based dementia practice. Oxford: Blackwell Science; 2002. p. 18–25.

72. Foster NL, Heidebrink JL, Clark CM, Jagust WJ, Arnold SE, Barbas NR, et al. FDG-PET improves accuracy in distinguishing frontotemporal dementia and Alzheimer's disease. Brain. 2007;130(Pt 10):2616–35.

73. Minoshima S, Foster NL, Sima AA, Frey KA, Albin RL, Kuhl DE. Alzheimer's disease versus dementia with Lewy bodies: cerebral metabolic distinction with autopsy confirmation. Ann Neurol. 2001;50(3):358–65.

74. Li Y, Schindler SE, Bollinger JG, Ovod V, Mawuenyega KG, Weiner MW, et al. Validation of plasma amyloid-β 42/40 for detecting Alzheimer disease amyloid plaques. Neurology. 2022;98(7):e688–e99.

75. Dahm MR, Crock C. Understanding and communicating uncertainty in achieving diagnostic excellence. JAMA. 2022;327:1127.

76. Irwin DJ, Grossman M, Weintraub D, Hurtig HI, Duda JE, Xie SX, et al. Neuropathological and genetic correlates of survival and dementia onset in synucleinopathies: a retrospective analysis. Lancet Neurol. 2017;16(1):55–65.

77. Karanth S, Nelson PT, Katsumata Y, Kryscio RJ, Schmitt FA, Fardo DW, et al. Prevalence and clinical phenotype of quadruple misfolded proteins in older adults. JAMA Neurol. 2020;77(10):1299–307.

78. Wallace LMK, Theou O, Godin J, Andrew MK, Bennett DA, Rockwood K. Investigation of frailty as a moderator of the relationship between neuropathology and dementia in Alzheimer's disease: a cross-sectional analysis of data from the rush memory and aging project. Lancet Neurol. 2019;18(2):177–84.

79. Beach TG, Adler CH, Sue LI, Serrano G, Shill HA, Walker DG, et al. Arizona study of aging and neurodegenerative disorders and brain and body donation program. Neuropathology. 2015;35(4):354–89.

80. Espay AJ, Vizcarra JA, Marsili L, Lang AE, Simon DK, Merola A, et al. Revisiting protein aggregation as pathogenic in sporadic Parkinson and Alzheimer diseases. Neurology. 2019;92(7):329–37.

81. Shi Y, Zhang W, Yang Y, Murzin AG, Falcon B, Kotecha A, et al. Structure-based classification of tauopathies. Nature. 2021;598(7880):359–63.

82. Stuendl A, Kraus T, Chatterjee M, Zapke B, Sadowski B, Moebius W, et al. α-Synuclein in plasma-derived extracellular vesicles is a potential biomarker of Parkinson's disease. Mov Disord. 2021;36(11):2508–18.

83. Shahnawaz M, Mukherjee A, Pritzkow S, Mendez N, Rabadia P, Liu X, et al. Discriminating α-synuclein strains in Parkinson's disease and multiple system atrophy. Nature. 2020;578(7794):273–7.

84. Bargar C, Wang W, Gunzler SA, LeFevre A, Wang Z, Lerner AJ, et al. Streamlined alpha-synuclein RT-QuIC assay for various biospecimens in Parkinson's disease and dementia with Lewy bodies. Acta Neuropathol Commun. 2021;9(1):62.

85. Iranzo A, Fairfoul G, Ayudhaya ACN, Serradell M, Gelpi E, Vilaseca I, et al. Detection of α-synuclein in CSF by RT-QuIC in patients with isolated rapid-eye-movement sleep behaviour disorder: a longitudinal observational study. Lancet Neurol. 2021;20(3):203–12.

86. Leuzy A, Chiotis K, Lemoine L, Gillberg PG, Almkvist O, Rodriguez-Vieitez E, et al. Tau PET imaging in neurodegenerative tauopathies-still a challenge. Mol Psychiatry. 2019;24(8):1112–34.

87. Therriault J, Pascoal TA, Savard M, Benedet AL, Chamoun M, Tissot C, et al. Topographic distribution of amyloid-β, tau, and atrophy in patients with behavioral/dysexecutive Alzheimer disease. Neurology. 2021;96(1):e81–92.

88. Jack CR Jr, Bennett DA, Blennow K, Carrillo MC, Dunn B, Haeberlein SB, et al. NIA-AA research framework: toward a biological definition of Alzheimer's disease. Alzheimers Dement. 2018;14(4):535–62.

89. Nelson PT, Dickson DW, Trojanowski JQ, Jack CR, Boyle PA, Arfanakis K, et al. Limbic-predominant age-related TDP-43 encephalopathy (LATE): consensus working group report. Brain. 2019;142(6):1503–27.

90. Crary JF, Trojanowski JQ, Schneider JA, Abisambra JF, Abner EL, Alafuzoff I, et al. Primary age-related tauopathy (PART): a common pathology

associated with human aging. Acta Neuropathol. 2014;128(6):755–66.

91. Nag S, Yu L, Wilson RS, Chen EY, Bennett DA, Schneider JA. TDP-43 pathology and memory impairment in elders without pathologic diagnoses of AD or FTLD. Neurology. 2017;88(7):653–60.

92. Boyle PA, Yang J, Yu L, Leurgans SE, Capuano AW, Schneider JA, et al. Varied effects of age-related neuropathologies on the trajectory of late life cognitive decline. Brain. 2017;140(3):804–12.

Victor W. Pike

Preamble

Well-designed radiotracers for molecular imaging provide a means to obtain important insights into the unfolding of neurodegenerative disorders and to assist in the development of new therapeutic strategies. Certain radiotracers may also become tools for disease diagnosis. Positron emission tomography (PET) now dominates over single-photon emission computerized tomography (SPECT) for brain imaging in human subjects. This is not least because modern radiochemistry with positron-emitting carbon-11 ($t_{1/2}$ = 20.4 min) and fluorine-18 ($t_{1/2}$ = 109.8 min) offers greater flexibility and possibility to design brain-penetrant radiotracers than does γ-emitting iodine-123 ($t_{1/2}$ = 13.2 h). This chapter provides an overview of prominent and clinically available radiotracers for the study of neurodegenerative disorders from a chemical and radiochemical perspective, particularly from the perspectives of their design, synthesis, and production. Emphasis is on an increasingly broad spectrum of clinically useful PET radiotracers, although a few important SPECT radiotracers are also considered. Useful radiotracers may be broadly classified into two types, those that depend on enzymic modification for retention in brain and those which are designed to bind avidly and revers-

ibly to specific proteins. The ensuing discussion is organized according to these two types of radiotracers.

Radiotracers Acting Through Brain Metabolic Pathways

Historically, radiotracers for imaging metabolic pathways were among the first to emerge as being useful for studying neurodegenerative disorders in the PET imaging field. Most notably, these include [^{18}F]FDG for the study of brain regional glucose metabolism and [^{18}F]FDOPA for the study of striatal dopaminergic neurons. These two radiotracers continue to be broadly applied in clinical settings. They are discussed here as the two main examples of radiotracers acting through metabolic pathways.

[^{18}F]FDG for Measuring Regional Brain Glucose Metabolism

The brain uses glucose almost exclusively as its fuel for energy production [1]. Glucose arrives in brain from plasma with the assistance of specific transporters at the blood–brain barrier. Within the brain, glucose is first phosphorylated at its 6-position by hexokinase before undergoing all the remaining enzyme-mediated steps of glycolysis and concomitant energy production.

V. W. Pike (✉)
Molecular Imaging Branch, National Institute of
Mental Health, Bethesda, MD, USA
e-mail: pikev@mail.nih.gov

© The Author(s), under exclusive license to Springer Nature Switzerland AG 2023
D. J. Cross et al. (eds.), *Molecular Imaging of Neurodegenerative Disorders*,
https://doi.org/10.1007/978-3-031-35098-6_3

Neurodegeneration is strongly associated with decreased brain glycolysis. Hence, it was early realized that an ability to measure glycolysis in vivo could have importance for the study of neurodegeneration and its possible diagnosis. The development of [^{18}F]2-fluoro-2-deoxy-D--glucose ([^{18}F]FDG) as a radiotracer for measuring regional glucose metabolism stems from pioneering work on [^{14}C]2-deoxy-D-glucose ([^{14}C]DG). Although [^{14}C]DG mimics glucose with regard to both brain entry and phosphorylation by hexokinase, the charged product [^{14}C]DG-6-phosphate is inert to further glycolysis because of the missing 2-hydroxy group. [^{14}C]DG-6-phosphate therefore accumulates within cells and enables glucose metabolism to be measured by autoradiography [2].

In some senses, PET may be considered to be autoradiography in vivo. Therefore, the possibility to develop an analogous technique for monitoring brain glucose metabolism in health and disease in living humans was pursued as a major goal upon the arrival of PET technology in the late 1970s. Although procedures for the synthesis of [^{11}C]DG quickly became known, it was early realized that the short half-life of carbon-11 ($t_{1/2}$ = 20.4 min) would prevent broad radiotracer application in PET and that a longer-lived fluorine-18 ($t_{1/2}$ = 109.8 min) label would be preferred.

A fluorine atom is almost isosteric with a hydrogen atom and can also serve as a bioisostere for a hydroxy group. Therefore, it was predicted and quickly found that replacement of the 2-hydroxy group in glucose with fluorine-18 would retain the important properties of DG, namely an ability to readily enter brain, avid substrate behavior for hexokinase, and accumulation within cells as the membrane-impermeable 6-phosphate (Fig. 3.1). This became the founding example of Gallagher's principle of metabolic trapping within the PET imaging field [3]. This principle has later been exploited in the design of some other PET radiotracers, such as labeled substrates for acetylcholinesterase (see later).

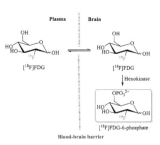

Fig. 3.1 Gallagher's principle of metabolic trapping, as exemplified with [^{18}F]FDG

[^{18}F]FDG was first synthesized in 1978 by treating 3,4,6-*tri-O*-acetyl-D-glucal with [^{18}F] fluorine (^{18}F-F) from the ^{20}Ne(d,α)^{18}F reaction on neon containing added fluorine, separating the ^{18}F-labeled 1,2-difluoro-glucose from its co-produced 1,2-difluoro-mannose epimer and finally removing the acetyl and 1-fluoro groups under acidic conditions. This "electrophilic" method is overall very low-yielding [4]. Mainly this is because the nuclear reaction is intrinsically low-yielding and because half of the starting radioactivity is unavoidably wasted. Notwithstanding, it soon became apparent that the rate of [^{18}F]FDG trapping in vivo was indeed proportional to glucose metabolism and that decreased regional trapping in brain could be interpreted as being due to synaptic and neuronal damage. Regional metabolic rate for glucose could be estimated by compartmental modeling or graphical analysis in tandem with a "lumped constant" to convert obtained values from [^{18}F]FDG into those for glucose itself.

Studies revealed that [^{18}F]FDG was excreted in urine with the desirable effect of generally depleting background radiotracer uptake in the body. This behavior, coupled with high uptake in rapidly growing tumors because of enhanced glycolysis, underpins the current use of [^{18}F]FDG as a major radiotracer in cancer diagnosis and management. Thus, [^{18}F]FDG rapidly gained value for imaging in both neurology and oncology. This culminated in the approval of [^{18}F]FDG by the Food and Drug Administration (FDA) and by the Centers for Medicare and Medicaid Services for insurance reimbursement in the USA in the 1990s. The global market for [18F]-labeled tracers for medical imaging has swelled to well over $1.5bn and continues to be dominated by [18F] FDG. Tremendous advances in [18F]FDG synthesis, fluorine-18 production, and PET imaging technology facilitated this commercial development and enabled the very significant contribution that it has made to improved healthcare.

A major advance in [18F]FDG synthesis came with a straightforward and efficient "nucleophilic" synthesis based on treatment of 3,4,5,6-tetra-acetyl-D-mannose triflate from [18F] fluoride produced by the proton irradiation of [18O]water according to the high-yielding $^{18}O(p.n)^{18}F$ reaction [5] (Fig. 3.2). Nowadays, several Curies of [18F]fluoride can be obtained from this nuclear reaction and [18F]FDG is produced for commercial distribution in multi-Ci batches by basically the same nucleophilic method with only relatively minor refinements. By comparison with this high production level, a PET scan in a single human patient requires only a relatively small dose of [18F]FDG (5–10 mCi) [6]. Millions of [18F]FDG administrations now occur annually. Several automated modules have become commercially available for safe high-level [18F]FDG production under "Current Good Manufacturing Practice" (cGMP) conditions.

Advances in radiochemical methodology seen in the production of [18F]FDG from no-carrier-added [18F]fluoride have been readily exploited for the high-activity production of many other clinically useful PET radiotracers. In particular, commercially available modules for [18F]FDG synthesis have been readily adapted to the high yield syntheses of many other radiotracers that are based on nucleophilic substitution reactions with [18F]fluoride (see examples in Table 3.1).

[18F]FDOPA for Imaging Striatal Dopaminergic Neurons

Dopamine is a major neurotransmitter that plays important roles in the brain "reward system," in bodily movement control, and in cognition. Dopamine is synthesized within nerve cells from L-tyrosine. This amino acid enters brain from plasma with the aid of the stereospecific L-aromatic amino acid transporter (AAAT). The first step of dopamine synthesis is rate-limiting and is catalyzed by tyrosine 3-monoxygenase (tyrosine hydroxylase; TH). The second step is catalyzed by aromatic L-amino acid decarboxylase (L-DOPA decarboxylase; AAAD or AADC). In parts of the nervous system that can release dopamine as a neurotransmitter, no further metabolism occurs. These dopaminergic neurons are principally located in the striatum. Any dopamine that accumulates in the synapse during neurotransmission can be recycled for storage in presynaptic vesicles by virtue of the dopamine reuptake transporter (DAT) and the vesicular monoamine transporter type 2 (VMAT-2).

Orally administered L-DOPA is itself able to enter brain from periphery with the aid of AAAT. L-DOPA is widely used as a drug to increase dopamine neurotransmission and thereby to relieve the debilitating motor symptoms accompanying Parkinson's disease and related syndromes. [18F]6-Fluoro-L-DOPA ([18F]FDOPA) is a simple labeled analog of L-DOPA that is likewise able to enter brain from plasma with the aid of AAAT. This tracer is converted into [18F]6-fluorodopamine ([18F]FDA) by AAAD and is retained as such in striatum (Fig. 3.3). [18F]FDA can be methylated by catechol-O-methyltransferase (COMT) to [18F]3-O-methyl-6-fluoro-L-DOPA ([18F]3-OMFD), which becomes uniformly distributed at a low level throughout brain. [18F]FDA is also metabolized to a lesser extent by monoamine oxidase (MAO) to [18F]6-fluoro-3,4-dihydroxyphenylacetic acid ([18F]FDOPAC) and subsequently by COMT to [18F]6-fluorochromovanillic acid ([18F]FHVA). AAAD and COMT are also present in peripheral tissues such as liver, kidneys, and lungs. Thus, [18F]3-OMFD is also produced in periphery and is able to enter brain from plasma. Despite this pharmacokinetic and metabolic complexity, [18F] FDOPA-brain PET well reflects radiotracer transport into the neurons, DOPA decarboxylation, and dopamine storage capacity.

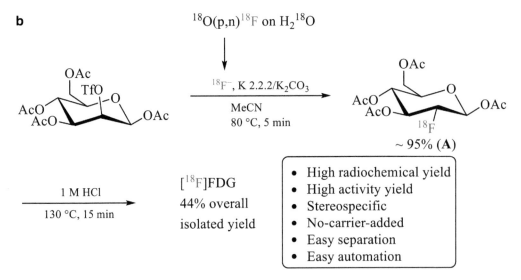

Fig. 3.2 Representative early ("electrophilic") and late ("nucleophilic") radiosyntheses of [^{18}F]FDG. (**a**) Original 'electrophilic' synthesis of [^{18}F]FDG. (**b**) Prototypical nucleophilic synthesis of [^{18}F]FDG

Table 3.1 Prominent radiotracers produced for clinical studies of neurodegeneration based on reversible binding to protein targets

Radiotracer	Structure	Favored labeling method	Protein target	Notes
Radiotracers for studying DAT and VMAT2 in Parkinson's disease				
[^{11}C]PE2I		Methylation of a carboxylic acid with [^{11}C]methyl triflate	DAT	
[^{18}F]FE-PE2I		Substitution of a tosylate group with [^{18}F] fluoride	DAT	
DaTscan (Ioflupane ^{123}I injection; [^{123}I]FP-CIT)		Radioiodination of a trialkylstannyl precursor	DAT	Approved by FDA
[^{11}C]DTBZ		Methylation of a phenol precursor with [^{11}C]methyl triflate	VMAT2	
[^{18}F]AV133		Substitution of a tosylate group with [^{18}F] fluoride	VMAT2	
Radiotracers for imaging the cholinergic system in dementia				
[^{11}C]Donepezil		Methylation of a phenol precursor with [^{11}C]methyl iodide	AChE	Racemic radiotracer

(continued)

Table 3.1 (continued)

Radiotracer	Structure	Favored labeling method	Protein target	Notes
[¹²³I]IBVM		Radioiodination of a tributylstannyl precursor	VAChT	
[¹⁸F]FEOBV		Substitution of a tosylate group with [¹⁸F] fluoride	VAChT	
[¹²³I]5-IA ([¹²³I]5-IA-85380)		Radioiodination of a Boc-protected trimethylstannyl precursor	$\alpha_4\beta_2$ nAChR	
[¹⁸F]2-FA (2-[¹⁸F] fluoro-A-85380)		Substitution of an Me_3N^+ group in an N-Boc protected precursor with [¹⁸F] fluoride	$\alpha_4\beta_2$ nAChR	$K_d = 1.33$ nM
[¹⁸F](−)Flubatine		Substitution of an Me_3N^+ group with [¹⁸F] fluoride in N-Boc-protected precursor	$\alpha_4\beta_2$ nAChR	The higher affinity (+)-enantiomer has also recently been introduced.
[¹⁸F]AZAN		Substitution of a bromo group with [¹⁸F] fluoride	$\alpha_4\beta_2$ nAChR	$K_d = 0.26$ nM
[¹⁸F]XTRA		Substitution of a bromo group with [¹⁸F] fluoride	$\alpha_4\beta_2$ nAChR	$K_d = 0.06$ nM suitable for extra-thalamic imaging

[18F]ASEM		Substitution of a nitro group with [18F] fluoride	α7nAChR	Very high molar activity is required
Radiotracers for TSPO in neuroinflammation				
(R)-[11C]PK11195		Methylation of a nor-precursor with [11C] methyl iodide	TSPO in all genotypes	First generation
[11C]PBR28		Methylation of a phenolic hydroxyl group with [11C]methyl iodide	TSPO in HABs and MABs only	Second generation
[18F]FBR ([18F]PBR06)		Substitution of a bromo group with [18F] fluoride	TSPO in HABs and MABs only	Second generation
[18F]FEPPA		Radiofluorination of a tosylate precursor	TSPO in HABs and MABs only	Second generation

(continued)

Table 3.1 (continued)

Radiotracer	Structure	Favored labeling method	Protein target	Notes
[¹¹C]DPA-713		Methylation of a phenolic hydroxyl group with [¹¹C]methyl iodide	TSPO in HABs and MABs only	Second generation
[¹⁸F]DPA-714		Radiofluorination of a tosylate precursor	TSPO HABs and MABs only	Second generation
[¹¹C]ER176		Methylation of a nor-precursor with [¹¹C] methyl iodide	TSPO in all genotypes	Third generation
Radiotracers for imaging cyclooxygenases in neuroinflammation				
[¹¹C]PS13		Methylation of a phenol precursor with [¹¹C]methyl iodide	COX-1	First in class Substantial signal
[¹¹C]MC1		Methylation of a phenol precursor with [¹¹C]methyl iodide	COX-2	First in class Low signal

Radiotracers for imaging β-amyloid in dementia

Compound	Structure	Target	Synthesis	Notes
[11C]PiB ([11C]Pittsburg compound B)		β-Amyloid	Methylation of a nor-precursor with [11C] methyl triflate	"Gold standard" radiotracer
[18F]Flutemetamol ([18F]GE067; [18F]3′-F-PiB; Vizamyl™)		β-Amyloid	Substitution of nitro group in protected precursor with [18F]fluoride	GE Healthcare FDA approved
[18F]Florbetapen (F-BAY94-9172; Neuraceq™)		β-Amyloid	Substitution of a mesylate group with [18F]fluoride	Piramal Imaging FDA approved
[18F]Florbetapir ([18F]AV-45; Amyvid™)		β-Amyloid	Substitution of a tosylate group in an N-Boc protected precursor with [18F]fluoride	Eli Lilly FDA approved
[18F]NAV4694 ([18F]AZD4694; Flutafuranol)		β-Amyloid	Substitution of a nitro group in a protected precursor with [18F]fluoride	
[18F]FIBT		β-Amyloid	Reaction of [18F]2-fluoroethyl tosylate with a phenol precursor	Provides selective high contrast image in AD

Radiotracers for imaging tau in dementia

Compound	Structure	Target	Synthesis	Notes
[11C]PBB3		Tau	Methylation of a nor-precursor with [11C] methyl triflate	
[18F]THK5351		Tau	Substitution of tosylate in an O-pyranyl protected precursor with [18F]fluoride	

(continued)

Table 3.1 (continued)

Radiotracer	Structure	Favored labeling method	Protein target	Notes
[18F]Flortaucipir ([18F]AV1451; [18F]T807; Tauvid™)		Substitution of an Me_3N^+ group in an N-Boc protected precursor with [18F]fluoride	Tau	Eli Lilly Approved by FDA
[18F]MK-6240		Substitution of a nitro group in an di-N-Boc protected precursor with [18F]fluoride	Tau	
Radiotracer for imaging OGA enzyme				
[18F]LSN3316612		Substitution of a nitro group with [18F]fluoride	OGA	LSN3316612 can be labeled with carbon-11
Radiotracers for imaging SV2A synaptic density				
[11C]UCB-J		Pd-mediated 11C-methylation of a bromo precursor with [11C]methyl iodide	SV2A	Alternative 18F-labeling is low yielding
[18F]UCB-H		Treatment of a diaryliodonium salt with [18F]fluoride	SV2A	Robust high-activity yield synthesis

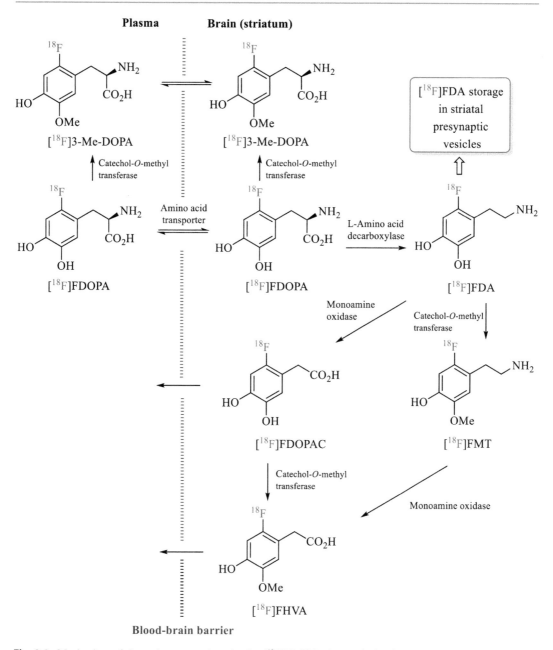

Fig. 3.3 Mechanism of dopamine neuron imaging by [^{18}F]FDOPA. Anatomical sub-compartments in the brain are ignored with the exception of [^{18}F]FDA, which is protected from metabolism by vesicular storage

Consequently, this radiotracer can be used to evaluate the dopaminergic function of presynaptic neurons in Parkinson's disease.

To improve image quality in clinical PET studies, the availability of [^{18}F]FDOPA for the brain from plasma may be enhanced by inhibiting AAAD with carbidopa and COMT with entacapone or nitecapone. Striatal-to-occipital radioactivity ratio and influx constant K_{iocc} are commonly used as analytical outputs in PET studies with [^{18}F]FDOPA. Both parameters are useful for discriminating Parkinson's disease patients from healthy individuals. [^{18}F]FDOPA was approved by the FDA in 2019 for assisting the early diagnosis of Parkinson's disease and has been commercially available in EU countries since as early as 2006.

The earliest syntheses of [^{18}F]FDOPA were inefficient carrier-added "electrophilic" methods. They used [^{18}F]fluorine or [^{18}F]acetyl hypofluorite ([^{18}F]MeCOOF), a readily prepared derivative with similar reactivity, as the labeling agent for reaction on L-DOPA or a protected derivative. In some cases, this resulted in difficult to separate 2-, 5-, and 6-[^{18}F]regioisomers. The 6-[^{18}F]fluoro isomer is however the preferred radiotracer. In this isomer, the fluorine atom is most distal from the two hydroxy groups and has least influence on the acidity and nucleophilicity of the 3-hydroxy group for methylation by COMT, resulting in the lowest background level of radiometabolites in brain.

Numerous methods for [^{18}F]FDOPA synthesis have been reported over recent decades [7].

Whereas much improved and regiospecific electrophilic methods emerged quite quickly and are still used in some laboratories [8] (Fig. 3.4), major advances have also taken place to enable [^{18}F]FDOPA to be prepared in very high yield from nucleophilic methods using [^{18}F]fluoride. Some earlier nucleophilic methods were challenging multi-step syntheses based on aromatic substitution of a good leaving group (e.g., F, NO$_2$, or Me$_3$N$^+$), usually in a hydroxy-protected benzaldehyde derivative. In these methods, the formyl group serves as a necessary but temporary electron-withdrawing group for activation of the leaving group for substitution by [^{18}F] fluoride. The amino acid side chain has then to be built up from the formyl group through multiple chemical steps. One such method has been implemented to produce [^{18}F]FDOPA at the Curie level [9] (Fig. 3.4a). More recently, simpler methods that require only two steps, radiofluorination and deprotection, have come to the fore based on the use of hypervalent iodine, stannyl, or boronic acid ester precursors [7]. These methods are readily automated on commercial apparatus for producing high activities of [^{18}F]FDOPA at high molar activity. However, the optimal method for broad utilization is still undecided. Figure 3.4 compares some examples of cGMC-compliant electrophilic and nucleophilic methods known to be in current use [10, 11]. By taking advantage of the high yield ^{18}O(p,n)^{18}F reaction, multi-dose preparation of [^{18}F]FDOPA is possible by either radiochemical approach (Fig. 3.4a, b).

a

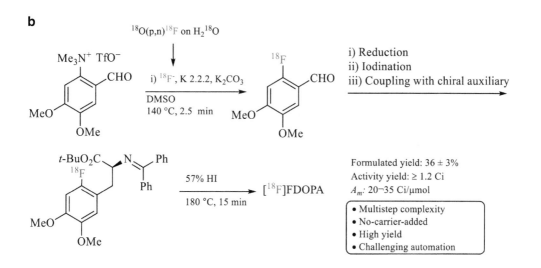

^{20}Ne(d,α)^{18}F on Ne-F$_2$ (Method **A**), or
^{18}O(p,n)^{18}F on ^{18}O-^{18}O (Method **B**) (2-shot method)

i) ^{18}F-F

CHCl$_3$ (− 20 °C)
ii) evaporate
iii) 47% HBr
130 °C, 5 min

[^{18}F]FDOPA

- Difficult ^{18}F-F production
- Carrier-added
- Easily automated

Formulated yield: 15 ± 5% (**A**); 23 ± 4% (**B**)
Activity yield: 14 ± 5 mCi (**A**); Activity yield: 122 ± 26 mCi (**B**);
A_m: 0.23 ± 0.09 mCi/μmol (**A**); A_m: 3.27 ± 0.27 mCi/μmol (**B**)

b

^{18}O(p,n)^{18}F on H$_2$^{18}O

i) ^{18}F$^-$, K 2.2.2, K$_2$CO$_3$

DMSO
140 °C, 2.5 min

i) Reduction
ii) Iodination
iii) Coupling with chiral auxiliary

57% HI

180 °C, 15 min

[^{18}F]FDOPA

Formulated yield: 36 ± 3%
Activity yield: ≥ 1.2 Ci
A_m: 20‒35 Ci/μmol

- Multistep complexity
- No-carrier-added
- High yield
- Challenging automation

c

^{18}O(p,n)^{18}F on H$_2$^{18}O

i) ^{18}F$^-$, Bu$_4$NOTf/Cs$_2$CO$_3$

CuPy$_4$OTf$_2$,
Pyridine, DMF
110 °C, 20 min
ii) 12 M HCl, ascorbic acid
100 °C, 10 min

MOMO = Methoxymethyl ether

[^{18}F]FDOPA

Formulated yield: 6 ± 1%
Activity yield: 104 ± 16 mCi
A_m: 3.8 ± 2.1 Ci/μmol

- Two efficient steps in one pot
- No-carrier-added
- Easily automated

Fig. 3.4 Examples of "electrophilic" and "nucleophilic" syntheses of [^{18}F]FDOPA in current clinical use. (Data from references [8–11]). (**a**) An 'electrophilic' synthesis of [^{18}F]FDOPA from [^{18}F]fluorine for cGMP production. (**b**) A multi-step 'nucleophilic' synthesis of [^{18}F]FDOPA from [^{18}F]fluoride for cGMP production. (**c**) A two-step 'nucleophilic' synthesis of [^{18}F]FDOPA from [^{18}F]fluoride for cGMP production

Radiotracers Aimed at Reversibly Binding Specific Proteins in Brain

Many radiotracers for the study of neurodegeneration rely on a common mechanism of action, namely selective and reversible binding of the radiotracer to a target protein within brain as a means to report on its available regional distribution, density, and interaction with pharmacological agents. The target proteins may be, for example, neurotransmitter receptors, transporters, enzymes, or abnormal protein deposits. These imaging targets generally exist at very low densities. The design features and properties required for such successful radiotracers have been discussed at length [12].

The first requirement of any radiotracer intended to image a protein in brain is an ability to enter the brain freely from plasma by passive diffusion (Fig. 3.5). A radioactivity uptake in brain exceeding one standardized uptake value (SUV), where 1 SUV would represent a theoretical average radioactivity distribution throughout the subject, is desirable within a few minutes of intravenous injection. This ability to cross the blood–brain barrier is fostered by relatively low molecular weight (<500 Da), moderate lipophilicity (a $\log D$ value between 1 and 3 at physiological pH), low topological polar surface area,

(<80 Å^2), an accurately measurable high plasma free fraction, and an absence of efflux transporter liability. Once inside brain, the radiotracer should bind avidly but reversibly to the target protein and not to any others. This is usually assured by a dissociation constant (K_d) in the low nanomolar range such that K_d (nM)/B_{max} (nM) is >5, where B_{max} is the density of the target protein. Generally, non-specific (weak and non-saturable) binding to brain tissue should be relatively low. This is usually the case if $\log D$ is kept within a moderate range. Radioactivity in brain should represent the radiotracer itself and not any radiometabolite that enters from the periphery or that may be formed in the brain itself [12, 13]. Finally, the radiotracer should be readily labeled at high molar activity (A_m) with carbon-11 or fluorine-18 by methods that are readily transferable to cGMP conditions on commercially available automated radiosynthesis platforms.

Favored methods of radiosynthesis include single-step methylation of heteroatoms (e.g., O or N) or carbon with [^{11}C]methyl iodide or [^{11}C]methyl triflate, and nucleophilic substitution reactions with [^{18}F]fluoride on aryl or alkyl precursors carrying good leaving groups (Table 3.1). ^{11}C-Methylation at an aryl oxygen or primary amino group often succeeds in avoiding troublesome radiometabolites because demethylation

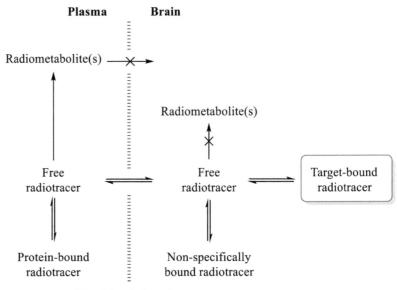

Fig. 3.5 Idealized behavior of a PET radiotracer intended to bind reversibly to a target protein in brain. The imaging goal is to attain a high proportion of radioactivity in the target-bound compartment

ultimately gives [^{11}C]carbon dioxide which does not stay in brain. [^{18}F]Fluoride can be troublesome as a radiometabolite by binding to skull and compromising quantification of PET data acquired in nearby cortical regions. Radiofluorination at an aryl or hetaryl carbon almost always avoids this issue. Some [^{18}F]fluoroalkyl groups resist radiodefluorination, in particular the [^{18}F]2-fluoroethoxy group and longer "PEGylated" alkyl groups, such as the [^{18}F]$F(C_2H_4O)_3-$ group, seen in some prominent radiotracers (Table 3.1). Successful radiotracers should provide robust output measures such as the binding potential (BP_{ND}) or total volumes of distribution (V_T) for the target protein.

The radiotracer design principles outlined above have been successfully implemented in the development of abroad arsenal of radiotracers for imaging protein targets of relevance to the study of neurodegeneration (Table 3.1). Currently, major areas of interest [14, 15] are the imaging of: (1) TSPO as a biomarker of neuroinflammation [16, 17], (2) β-amyloid and tau in dementia [18], and (3) SV2A protein as a marker of synaptic density [19]. Recently cyclooxygenases have also become of interest for the study of neuroinflammation [20]. Other types of radiotracers that have long drawn attention for the study of neurodegeneration include radiotracers for imaging the presynaptic dopamine system (DAT, VMAT2) [21], the cholinergic system (the vesicular acetylcholine transporter (VAChT) and nicotinic receptors) [22] (Table 3.1). A brief discussion of reversibly binding radiotracers in clinical use in each area now follows, highlighting particular issues and achievements.

Radiotracers for Imaging DAT and VMAT2

DAT is an important regulator of synaptic dopamine level. The presynaptic localization of DAT makes it a useful marker of neuron integrity and density. Therefore, DAT imaging can be useful in the diagnosis of neurodegenerative disorders, such as Parkinson's disease. Both SPECT and PET tracers have been developed for DAT imag-

ing [21]. The most effective and most widely radiotracers used for clinical imaging of DAT are based on the core tropane structure of cocaine. A SPECT radiotracer DaTscan (Ioflupane 123-I) has been in clinical use for over two decades and is an important tool for assisting the diagnosis of neurodegenerative Parkinsonian syndrome. Important radiotracers for the clinical imaging of DAT with PET are close analogs of DaTscan and include [^{11}C]PE2I and [^{18}F]FE-PE2I (Table 3.1).

VMAT2 is a vesicle membrane-bound presynaptic protein responsible for the transfer of dopamine and other monoamine neurotransmitters from cytosol into storage vessels. The two radiotracers which have found most use for clinical imaging of VMAT2 are [^{11}C]dihydrotetrabenazine ([^{11}C]DTBZ) and an [^{18}F]3-fluoropropyl analog ([^{18}F]]AV-133) (Table 3.1) [21]. VMAT2 location is not limited to dopaminergic neurons but PET images predominantly reflect dopaminergic neurons in striatum.

Radiotracers for Imaging the Cholinergic System

Interest in the molecular imaging of the cholinergic system stems from the cholinergic hypothesis of dementia, namely that the loss of brain cholinergic neurons results in impaired memory function [22]. Early radiotracers for imaging the cholinergic system were designed to estimate acetylcholinesterase (AChE) activity and were [N-methyl-^{11}C]N-methyl-piperidinol esters of short chain carboxylic acids. The action of AChE on these substates in cholinergic neurons releases [N-methyl-^{11}C]N-methyl-piperidinol which then accumulates because of its hydrophilicity (c.f., Gallagher's principle of metabolic trapping, as described earlier). The acetate ([^{11}C]AMP) and propionate ([^{11}C]PMP) esers have been the most studied radiotracers in human.

More recent radiotracers are designed to bind to AChE in the synaptic space to provide a measure of the integrity of presynaptic nerve terminals. The best known of these radiotracers is [^{11}C]donepezil (Table 3.1). Donepezil itself is a reversibly binding inhibitor of AChE and an important drug for the treatment of AD. In general, PET radiotracers should not be administered as racemates because enantiomers may show possible differences in pharmacokinetics, metabolism, and binding to proteins, thereby adding to the challenge of the biomathematical analysis of PET data. This principle is nullified in the case of [11C]donepezil because its enantiomers interconvert in vivo and have unequally high affinity. Therefore, this radiotracer is used as the racemate. Successful quantification of [11C]donepezil binding in human brain has been reported.

Radiotracers have been developed to image the vesicular acetylcholine transporter (VAChT) with SPECT and PET, notably [123I]IBVM and [18F]FEOBV, respectfully (Table 3.1). Cholinergic neurotransmission is mediated by ionotropic nicotinic cholinergic and muscarinic cholinergic receptors. Various radiotracers have been developed for clinical imaging of certain nicotinic receptor subtypes. These include [123I]5-IA, [18F]2-FA, the enantiomers of [18F]flubatine, [18F]AZAN, and [18F]XTRA for the α4β2 nicotinic subtype, and [18F]ASEM for the α7 subtype (Table 3.1). The very low density of α4β2 nicotinic receptors requires that the radiotracers have high affinity and that they be produced and used at very high molar activities. The exceptionally high affinity of [18F]XTRA (K_d, 0.06 nM) provides measurable PET signal in extra-thalamic regions unlike lower affinity radiotracers that are mainly useful for thalamic imaging.

Radiotracers for Imaging TSPO

Neuroinflammation is a possible contributing factor in several brain disorders, including neurodegeneration. Translocator protein 18 kDa (TSPO) has steadily become a recognized biomarker of neuroinflammation. In brain, this protein is located at outer mitochondrial membranes, mainly on microglia but also on astrocytes. TSPO density increases in response to a wide range of acute and chronic neuroinflammatory insults. Therefore, PET imaging of TSPO has broad scope for the investigations of a wide range of neurodegenerative disorders.

Racemic [11C]PK11195 (Table 3.1) emerged in the 1980s as the prototypical radiotracer for the PET imaging of TSPO. This radiotracer has later been used as its somewhat higher affinity R-enantiomer but still provides low signal-to-noise and poor ability to detect subtle changes in TSPO density. These deficiencies have prompted strenuous efforts over many years to find improved radiotracers, culminating in several clinically more useful radiotracers, such as [11C]PBR28, [11C]DPA-713, [18F]FEPPA, [18F]PBR06 ([18F]FBR), and [18F]DPA-714 (Table 3.1) [16, 17]. However, these "second-generation" radiotracers turn out to be variously sensitive to a polymorphism (rs6971) in the TSPO gene having about 30% prevalence in Caucasians, 25% in Africans, and 4% in Japanese, and 2% of Han Chinese. Individuals with two copies of the minor allele (low affinity binders; LABs) bind these radiotracers with lower affinity than those with two copies of the major allele (high affinity binders; HABs). Heterozygotes (mixed affinity binders; MABs) equally express the high and low binding sites. Individuals with the same overall TSPO density but different genotypes will produce different size PET signals. Therefore, burdensome genotyping is required for correction of acquired binding potential data. For some radiotracers, such as [11C]PBR28, imaging of TSPO in LABs is not even possible. Despite its poor imaging performance, (R)-[11C]PK11195 accounted for almost half (47%) of all TSPO radiotracer administrations to patients (3914) up to the year 2020. [11C]PBR28 accounted for 24% of administrations in the same period.

Effort has been placed on developing "third generation" radiotracers that may reduce or avoid issues in earlier generation radiotracers. One such radiotracer is [11C]ER176 (Table 3.1). [11C]ER176 is a less lipophilic structural congener of (R)-[11C]PK11195 because of the extra ring nitrogen in its structure. ER176 shows high TSPO affinity and low human genotype sensitivity in vitro. [11C]ER176 provides robust PET signal-to-noise ratios in all human genotypes, but subjects do still require genotyping. The cGMP-compliant production of [11C]ER176, like that of (R)-[11C]PK11195 itself, is based on methylation of the secondary amide precursor with [^{11}C]methyl iodide. This production has recently been described along with many details that are also relevant to the cGMP-compliant production of a wide range of radiotracers produced by ^{11}C-methylation reactions [23].

No ^{18}F-labeled analog of ER176 has yet entered clinical evaluation, although encouraging preclinical evaluations have been reported. The ^{18}F-labeled TSPO radiotracer with most clinical use is [^{18}F]FEPPA (in 11% of patients up to 2020), followed by [^{18}F]DPA714 (5%), and [^{18}F] PBR06. Each of these radiotracers is readily prepared by automated and efficient single-step nucleophilic substitution reactions with [^{18}F] fluoride.

Radiotracers for Imaging Cyclooxygenases

Cyclooxygenases (COXs) catalyze an early step in the biotransformation of arachidonic acid into various prostaglandins and thromboxanes that are recognized to be major inflammatory mediators. The constitutively expressed COX-1 isoform maintains the physiological integrity of major organs, such as stomach and kidney. Several studies now suggest that COX-1 may also play a pro-inflammatory role in various pathologic conditions, including neurodegeneration. The inducible COX-2 isoform is associated with responses to external injury or stimuli, including inflammation and pain. These enzymes might therefore serve as surrogate markers for the progression of diseases with a neuroinflammatory component.

There is growing interest in developing PET radiotracers for brain COX-1 and COX-2 [20]. Recently, [^{11}C]PS13 (Table 3.1) has been shown to image constitutively abundant COX-1 in healthy human brain. Much less abundant COX-2 has been detected in healthy human with low signal from the radiotracer [^{11}C]MC1 (Table 3.1). Both [^{11}C]PS13 and [^{11}C]MC1 are produced by ^{11}C-methylation of phenol precursors by readily automated cGMP-compliant procedures. ^{18}F-Labeled radiotracers are not presently available for imaging COXs.

Radiotracers for Imaging β-Amyloid

The most widely applied PET radiotracer for imaging the appearance of β-amyloid plaques in Alzheimer's disease (AD) is [^{11}C]PiB or [^{11}C] Pittsburg Compound B. This radiotracer was developed from the pathologic stain, thioflavin-T, which was known to bind avidly to β-pleated sheet aggregates of amyloid-beta (Aβ) peptide in vitro. Key steps in this development were to remove the N-methyl group from the dye to render it structurally neutral and therefore to be more capable of crossing the blood–brain barrier and to improve affinity for β-amyloid aggregates by further modest structural changes. This gave a large range of benzothiazoleanilines (BTAs). Among these compounds, [^{11}C]PiB ([^{11}C]6-OH-BTA-1) (Table 3.1) appeared outstanding in showing about 200-fold higher binding affinity to Aβ plaques (K_d 1.4 nM in brain homogenates) than thioflavin-T, very low binding affinity to aggregated tau, and good entry into brain followed by fast clearance as a result of desirably moderate lipophilicity. Radiolabeling was simply achieved by N-methylation of nor-precursor with [^{11}C]methyl iodide [24]. The regional distribution of [^{11}C]PiB in AD brain was found to be very similar to that of Aβ deposits observed postmortem. PET imaging with [^{11}C]PiB readily identified patients with high amyloid β-plaque deposition [25].

[^{11}C]PiB is now regarded as the "gold standard" radiotracer for β-amyloid imaging and has been used for thousands of administrations. However, the short half-life limits its widespread use. Therefore, development of a β-amyloid tracer with a fluorine-18 label has been strenuously pursued by various pharma companies. Three radiotracers with imaging performance similar to that of [^{11}C]PiB have now been approved by the FDA for clinical use, namely [^{18}F]flutemetamol (Vizamyl™), [^{18}F]florbetapir (Amyvid™), and [^{18}F]florbetaben (Neuraceq™) (Table 3.1). Binding of β-amyloid PET radiotracers to white matter can potentially hinder identification in early-onset AD. To address this issue, Astra Zeneca developed [^{18}F]AZD4694, now called [^{18}F]NAV4694 or Flutafuranol (Table 3.1).

In AD patients this radiotracer selectively labels Aβ-amyloid deposits in gray matter with only a low level of non-displaceable binding in plaque-devoid white matter. Another promising radiotracer is [^{18}F]FIBT (Table 3.1) which shows high selectivity for Aβ-amyloid fibrils in vitro and high imaging contrast in AD in vivo.

Radiotracers for Imaging Tau

Tau is a phosphoprotein which normally functions to stabilize brain microtubules. Six isoforms of tau exist with either three (3R) or four repeats (4R) of the microtubule-binding domain. Abnormal deposits of hyperphosphorylated tau generate neurofibrillary tangles (NFTs) and neuropil threads that cluster around β-amyloid plaques in patients with AD. Tau deposits also appear in several other neurodegenerative diseases named tauopathies, such as sporadic corticobasal degeneration, progressive supranuclear palsy, and Pick's disease. Neurodegeneration and cognitive impairment have been found to be significantly correlated when assessed by measuring NFT density postmortem. NFTs are not found appreciably in persons with nil to minimal cognitive decline, in contrast to β-amyloid plaque deposition which can still be present.

Aggregated tau proteins are mainly located intracellularly. Candidate tau radiotracers target their β-sheet domains. Because other misfolded proteins have similar structures, high selectivity for aggregated tau is a prerequisite. Different ligands may bind to different loci on NFT structures. Moreover, tau aggregates exist at lower concentrations than Aβ plaques. Therefore, tau deposits are a very demanding target for PET radiotracer development with necessary selectivity being particularly challenging to achieve. For many tau radiotracers, lack of an adequate tau selectivity has only become clear following early clinical use.

The development of candidate tau radiotracers has been very actively pursued, based on various chemotypes [14, 15]. A **p**henyl**b**utadienyl**b**enzothiazole, named [^{11}C]PBB3 (Table 3.1), was one of the first to appear. However, this radiotracer was found to have major deficiencies, including off-target binding to MAO-B in basal ganglia and to unidentified sites in venous sinus and choroid plexus. Radiometabolites were also taken up by brain, compromising robust quantification. Moreover, the butadienyl substructure is easily photo-isomerized. Careful shielding of the radiotracer from light during production and use is therefore necessary.

Subsequent efforts have been mainly directed at producing ^{18}F-labeled tau radiotracers [^{18}F]THK5351 (Table 3.1), a high affinity (K_d, 2.9 nM) radiotracer from an arylquinoline series, was taken into advanced clinical trials, but was found to bind to MAO-B in basal ganglia and to MAO-B and neuromelanin in mid-brain, thalamus, and hippocampus. This radiotracer is no longer considered useful. In 2020, a pyridoindole, [^{18}F]flortaucipir ([^{18}F]T807; [^{18}F]AV1451; Tauvid™) (Table 3.1) became the first and so far only radiotracer to be approved for tau imaging by the FDA. This radiotracer shows favorable kinetics and high affinity (K_d, 14.6 nM) for the 3R/4R tau isoform combination that is typically found in AD. However, this radiotracer also shows considerable off-target binding, in this case to MAO-B in basal ganglia, neuromelanin in mid-brain, and unidentified sites in choroid plexus.

Many newer radiotracer candidates continue to emerge, such as the azaindole isoquinoline, [^{18}F]MK-6240 (Table 3.1). Although the available data on this and other recent tau PET radiotracers are encouraging, their utilities still need to be demonstrated in large clinical trials.

Imaging of O-GlcNAcase

The attachment of O-linked β-N-acetylglucosamine (O-GlcNAc)) at serine and threonine residues modifies the key hyperphosphorylated protein involved in tauopathies. Two enzymes, O-GlcNAc transferase and O-GlcNAc hydrolase (O-GlcNAcase; OGA), control this process by catalyzing the attachment and detachment of O-GlcNAc, respectively. O-GlcNAcylation hinders abnormal phosphorylation and aggregation of tau, thus stabilizing the microtubule-associated tau protein. Tau-specific O-GlcNAc appears decreased in AD brain. Moreover, in preclinical studies, upregulation of O-GlcNAcylation by OGA inhibitors reduces pathologic tau phosphorylation and aggregation and prevents neurodegeneration. These findings suggest that OGA inhibition can be a strategy for treating tauopathies. Recently, a radiotracer for O-GlcNAcase, namely [^{18}F]LSN 3316612 (Table 3.1), has been reported and evaluated in human [26]. This radiotracer has potential for assisting drug discovery and for studies in neurodegeneration.

Radiotracers for Imaging Synaptic Density

Many neurodegenerative disorders are accompanied by reduced synaptic densities, as shown postmortem. The brain synaptic vesicle glycoprotein 2A is expressed throughout the brain and has been identified as the binding site for the anti-epileptic drug, levetiracetam. PET radiotracers that target SVA2 have been developed recently and have enabled the quantification of regional synaptic density in vivo [19]. [^{11}C]UCB-J (Table 3.1) has gained the most prominence for PET imaging of SV2A and has clear potential for assessing synaptic density decline in neurodegenerative disorders.

[^{11}C]UCB-J was originally synthesized through palladium-mediated cross-coupling of an aryl trifluoroborate precursor with [^{11}C]methyl iodide in THF-water [27]. However, attempts to establish this method in other laboratories for clinical use incurred considerable difficulties that have spurred the development of improved methods [28, 29]. It seems that the trifluoroborate precursor is not reactive and needs conversion to some of the more reactive arylboronic acid in situ. Deliberate inclusion of a few percent of the boronic acid in the tetrafluoroborate results in more reaction reproducibility. Finally, a stable and pure bromo precursor has become commercially available and has been shown to react effectively in palladium-mediated coupling with [^{11}C]methyl iodide to produce [^{11}C]UCB-J in adequate yields for clinical studies (personal communication; Dr. Meixiang Yu; Southern Methodist University TX). The method can be rendered cGMP-compliant and has been adopted in at least two laboratories.

The labeling of UCB-J with fluorine-18 has been tested by different methods. However, only very low yields have been obtained. Nonetheless, the structurally related but less well-performing [^{18}F]UCB-H (Table 3.1) has been produced regularly and reliably in greater than 1 Curie activity yield for clinical studies. The radiosynthesis is based on single-step radiofluorination of a bench-stable aryl(pyridinyl)iodonium salt precursor [30].

Final Remarks

A wide range of radiotracers for an increasing number of molecular targets is now available for studying, investigating and, in some cases, diagnosing neurodegeneration. Radiotracers labeled with no-carrier-added carbon-11 find utility in PET imaging near cyclotrons that are able to produce this radionuclide according to the ^{14}N(p,α)^{11}C reaction. They are mostly labeled by relatively simple ^{11}C-methylation procedures. These radiotracers have played important roles in "proof-of-concept" imaging studies. Where molecular imaging targets are of interest for study or evaluation in large numbers of subjects, fluorine-18 labeled radiotracers become desirable. In many cases, they can become accessible in high activities for broad distribution from cyclotron-produced [^{18}F]fluoride. Major progress can be expected in the near future with regard to satisfying many unmet needs for robust imaging of new imaging targets associated with neurodegeneration.

Acknowledgments VWP was supported by the Intramural Research Program of the National Institutes of Health (National Institute of Mental Health, Project ZIA-MH002793). VWP thanks Dr. Shuiyu Lu (NIMH) for reading and checking the manuscript.

References

1. Sokoloff L. Circulation and energy metabolism of the brain. In: Siegel GJ, Albers RW, Katzman R, Agranoff BW, editors. Brain Neurochemistry. 2nd ed. Boston: Little Brown; 1976. p. 388–413.

2. Sokoloff L, Reivich M, Kenendy C, Des Rosiers MH, Patlak CS, Pettigrew KD, Sakurada O, Shinohara M. The [^{14}C]deoxyglucose method for the measurement of local cerebral glucose utilization: theory, procedure, and normal values in the conscious and anesthetized albino rat. J Neurochem. 1977;28:897–916.

3. Gallagher BM, Fowler JS, Gutterson NI, MacGregor RR, Wan C-N, Wolf AP. Metabolic trapping as a principle of radiopharmaceutical design: some factors responsible for the biodistribution of [F]2-deoxy 2-fluoro-D-glucose. J Nucl Med. 1978;10:1154–61.

4. Fowler JS, Ido T. Initial and subsequent approach for the synthesis of ^{18}FDG. Semin Nucl Med. 2002;32:6–12. https://doi.org/10.1053/snuc.2002.29270.

5. Hamacher K, Coenen HH, Stöcklin G. Efficient stereospecific synthesis of NCA 2-[^{18}F]fluoro-2-deoxy-2-glucose. J Nucl Med. 1986;27:235–8.

6. Sowa AR, Jackson IM, Desmond TJ, Alicea J, Mufarreh AJ, Pham JM, Stauff J, Winton WP, Fawaz MV, Henderson BD, Hockley BG, Rogers VE, Koeppe RA, Scott PJH. Futureproofing [^{18}F]fludeoxyglucose manufacture at an academic medical center. EJNMMI Radiopharm Chem. 2018;3:12. https://doi.org/10.1186/s41181-018-0048-x.

7. Neves ACB, Hrynchak I, Fonseca I, Alves VHP, Pereira MM, Falcão A, Abrunhosa AJ. Advances in the automated synthesis of 6-[^{18}F]fluoro-L-DOPA. EJNMMI Radiopharm Chem. 2021;6:11. https://doi.org/10.1186/s41181-021-00126-z.

8. Luurtsema G, Boersma HH, Schepers M, de Vries AMT, Maas B, Zijlma R, de Vries EFJ, Elsinga PH. Improved GMP-compliant multi-dose production and quality control of 6-[^{18}F]fluoro-L-DOPA. EJNMMI Radiopharm Chem. 2016;1:7. https://doi.org/10.1186/s41181-016-0009-1.

9. Libert LC, Franci X, Plenevaux AR, Oui T, Maruoka K, Luxen AJ. Production at the Curie level of no-carrier-added 6-^{18}F-fluoro-L-dopa. J Nucl Med. 2013;54:1154–61.

10. Andersen VL, Soerensen MA, Dam JH, Langkjaer N, Petersen H, Bender DA, Fugloe D, Huynh THV. GMP production of 6-[^{18}F]fluoro-DOPA for PET/CT imaging by different synthetic routes: a three center experience. EJNMMI Radiopharm Chem. 2021;6:21. https://doi.org/10.1186/s41181-021-00135-y.

11. Mossine AV, Tanzey SS, Brooks AF, Makaravage KJ, Ichiishi N, Miller JM, Henderson BD, Erhard T, Bruetting C, Skaddan MB, Sanford MS, Scott PJH. Synthesis of high-molar-activity [^{18}F]6-fluoro-L-DOPA suitable for human use via Cu-mediated fluorination of a BPin precursor. Nat Protoc. 2020;15:1742–59. https://doi.org/10.1038/s41596-020-0305-9.

12. Pike VW. Considerations in the development of reversibly binding PET radioligands for brain imaging. Curr Med Chem. 2016;23:1818–69. https://doi.org/10.2174/0929867323666160418114826.

13. Pike VW. PET radiotracers: crossing the blood–brain barrier and surviving metabolism. Trends Pharmacol Sci. 2009;30:431–40.

14. Tiepolt S, Patt M, Aghakhanyan G, Meyer PM, Hesse S, Barthel H, Sabri O. Current radiotracers to image neurodegenerative diseases. EJNMMI Radiopharm Chem. 2019;4:17. https://doi.org/10.1186/s41181-019-0070-7.

15. Young PNE, Estarallas M, Coomans E, Srikrishna M, Beaumont H, Maass A, Venkataraman AV, Lissaman R, Jiménez D, Betts MJ, McGlinchey E, Berron D, O'Connor A, Fox NC, Pereira JB, Jagust W, Carter SF, Paterson RW, Schöll M. Imaging biomarkers in neurodegeneration: current and future practices. Alzheimers Res Therapy. 2020;12:49. https://doi.org/10.1186/s13195-020-00612-7.

16. Chauveau F, Becker G, Boutin H. Have (R)-[^{11}C] PK11195 challengers fulfilled the promise? A scoping review of clinical TSPO PET studies. Eur J Nucl Med Mol Imaging. 2021;49:201–20. https://doi.org/10.1007/s00259-021-05425-w.

17. Viviano M, Barresi E, Siméon FG, Costa B, Taliani S, Da Settimo F, Pike VW, Castellano S. Essential principles and recent progress in the development of TSPO PET ligands for neuroinflammation imaging. Curr Med Chem. 2022;29:4862. https://doi.org/10.2174/0929867329666220329204054.

18. Uzuegbunam BC, Librizzi D, Yousefi BH. PET radiopharmaceuticals for Alzheimer's disease and Parkinson's disease, the current and future landscape. Molecules. 2020;25:977. https://doi.org/10.3390/molecules25040977.

19. Becker G, Dammico S, Bahri MA, Salmon E. The rise of synaptic density PET imaging. Molecules. 2020;25:2303. https://doi.org/10.3390/molecules25102303.

20. Kenou BV, Manly LS, Rubovits SB, Umeozulu SA, Van Buskirk MG, Zhang AS, Pike VW, Zanotti-Fregonara P, Henter ID, Innis RB. Cyclooxygenases as potential PET imaging biomarkers to explore neuroinflammation in dementia. J Nucl Med. 2022;63:53S.

21. Kilbourn MR. ^{11}C- and ^{18}F-radiotracers for in vivo imaging of the dopamine system: past, present and future. Biomedicine. 2021;9:108. https://doi.org/10.3390/biomedicines9020108.

22. Bohnen NI, Kanel P, Müller MLTM. Molecular imaging of the cholinergic system in Parkinson's disease. Int Rev Neurol. 2018;141:211–50. https://doi.org/10.1016/bs.irn.2018.07.027.

23. Hong J, Telu S, Zhang Y, Miller WH, Shetty HU, Morse CL, Pike VW. Translation of ^{11}C-labeled tracer synthesis to a CGMP environment as exemplified by [^{11}C]ER176 for PET imaging of human TSPO. Nat

Protoc. 2021;16:4419–45. https://doi.org/10.1038/s41596-021-00584-4.

24. Mathis CA, Wang Y, Holt DP, Huang G-F, Debnath ML, Klunk WE. Synthesis and evaluation of ¹¹C-labeled 6-substituted 2-aryl benzothiazoles as amyloid imaging agents. J Med Chem. 2003;46:2740–54.

25. Klunk WE, Engle H, Nordberg A, Wang Y, Blomqvist G, Holt DP, Bergström M, Savitcheva I, Huang GF, Estrada S, Ausén B, Debnath ML, Barletta J, Price JC, Sandell J, Lopresti BJ, Wall A, Koivisto P, Antoni G, Mathis CA, Långström B. Imaging brain amyloid in Alzheimer's disease with Pittsburgh compound-B. Ann Neurol. 2004;55:306–19.

26. Lu S, Haskali MB, Ruley KM, Dreyfus NJF, DuBois SL, Paul S, Liow J-S, Morse CL, Kowalski A, Gladding RL, Gilmore J, Mogg AJ, Michelle Morin SM, Lindsay-Scott PJ, Ruble JC, Kant NA, Shcherbinin S, Barth VN, Johnson MP, Cuadrado M, Jambrina E, Mannes AJ, Nuthall HN, Zoghbi SS, Jesudason CD, Innis RB, Pike VW. PET ligands [¹⁸F]LSN3316612 and [¹¹C]LSN3316612 quantify O-linked-β-N-acetyl-glucosamine hydrolase in the brain. Sci Transl Med. 2020;12:eaau2939. https://doi.org/10.1126/scitranslmed.aau2939.

27. Nabulsi NB, Mercier J, Holden D, Carré S, Najafzadeh S, Vandergeten M-C, Lin S, Deo A, Price N, Wood M, Lara-Jaime T, Montel F, Laruelle M, Carson RE, Hannestad J, Huang Y. Synthesis and preclinical evaluation of ¹¹C-UCB-J as a PET tracer for imaging the synaptic vesicle glycoprotein 2A in the brain. J Nucl Med. 2016;5:777–84.

28. Rokka J, Schlein E, Eriksson J. Improved synthesis of SV2A targeting radiotracer [¹¹C]UCB-J. EJNMMI Radiopharm Chem. 2019;4:30. https://doi.org/10.1186/s41181-019-0080-5.

29. Sephton SM, Miklovicz T, Russell JJ, Doke A, Li L, Boros I, Aigbirhio FI. Automated radiosynthesis of [¹¹C]UCB-J for imaging synaptic density by positron emission tomography. J Label Compd Radiopharm. 2020;63:151–6. https://doi.org/10.1002/jlcr.3828.

30. Warnier C, Lemaire C, Becker G, Zaragoza G, Giacomelli F, Aerts J, Otabashi M, Bahri MA, Mercier J, Plenevaux A, Luxen A. Enabling efficient positron emission tomography (PET) imaging of synaptic vesicle glycoprotein 2A (SV2A) with a robust and one-step radiosynthesis of a highly potent ¹⁸F-labeled ligand ([¹⁸F]UCB-H). J Med Chem. 2016;59:8955–66.

Satoshi Minoshima, Tanyaluck Thientunyakit, Donna J. Cross, and Karina Mosci

Introduction

Since the development of [F-18]fluorodeoxyglucose (FDG) in the 1970s, FDG PET has been used extensively for research and clinical applications in dementia [1]. In the USA, FDG PET has been reimbursed for the differential diagnosis of Alzheimer's disease (AD) versus frontotemporal dementia (FTD). Although approval for reimbursement varies from country to country, FDG PET has become a critical tool for the clinical evaluation of dementing disorders. Owing to regional perfusion—metabolic coupling in neurodegenerative disorders, perfusion SPECT can provide imaging features of dementing disorders similar to those seen on FDG PET and has been used routinely in clinical practice. However, the image quality of SPECT is typically limited in comparison to that of FDG PET due to differences in instrumentation.

Brain FDG PET in Dementia: What Have We Learned?

Over the past four decades of FDG PET applications to dementia, FDG PET has unveiled key features of glucose metabolic changes in neurodegenerative dementias. The number of publications concerning FDG PET in dementia is currently the third largest in the literature (Fig. 4.1). General findings of FDG PET in neurodegenerative dementia are briefly summarized in Table 4.1.

S. Minoshima (✉) · D. J. Cross
Department of Radiology and Imaging Sciences, University of Utah, Salt Lake City, UT, USA
e-mail: sminoshima@hsc.utah.edu; d.cross@utah.edu

T. Thientunyakit
Division of Nuclear Medicine, Department of Radiology, Faculty of Medicine Siriraj Hospital, Mahidol University, Bangkok, Thailand
e-mail: tanyaluck.thi@mahidol.ac.th

K. Mosci
Department of Nuclear Medicine, Hospital das Forças Armadas (HFA), Brasilia, Distrito Federal, Brazil
e-mail: karina.mosci@gruposanta.com.br

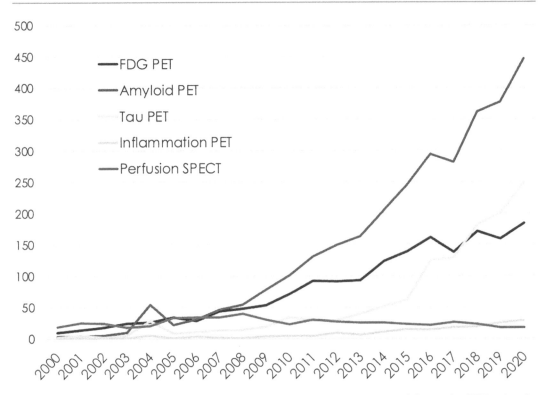

Fig. 4.1 The number of publications concerning FDG PET, amyloid PET, tau PET, neuroinflammation PET, and perfusion SPECT in dementia, from 2000 to 2020. (Search data from PUBMED https://pubmed.ncbi.nlm.nih.gov)

Table 4.1 Brain FDG PET in neurodegenerative dementias: what have we learned?

- FDG PET findings represent not only local neuronal injuries, but also remote effects
- Regional FDG PET abnormalities generally correlate with specific clinical symptoms
- The metabolic changes seen in AD are distinct from those seen in normal aging
- The spatial extent of FDG PET abnormalities provides differential diagnostic clues
- Statistical mapping significantly improves the diagnostic accuracy of brain FDG PET
- Medial temporal lobe is only mildly affected in AD despite atrophy
- The posterior cingulate cortex and precuneus are often affected in early AD
- What used to be called 'subcortical dementia' has cortical abnormalities
- Younger patients tend to exhibit more prominent FDG PET abnormalities
- The clinical subtypes of AD and FTLD exhibit unique FDG PET abnormalities
- Amyloid deposition and FDG PET abnormalities have a minimal correlation in AD
- Cortical tau deposition and FDG PET changes seem to have a good correlation in AD
- The severity of FDG PET abnormalities provides a prognostic value
- New neurodegenerative dementias with associated FDG PET findings
- The significance of co-pathologies in elderly dementia patients

Indications of FDG PET in Dementia Evaluation and Challenges

Owing to widespread use for cancer staging in Nuclear Medicine practice, FDG PET has become a commonly available and relatively inexpensive imaging test particularly when compared to the recently developed proteomic imaging techniques such as amyloid and tau PET imaging. The imaging protocol for brain FDG PET is well established and standardized [2]. The general indications for FDG PET in the evaluation of dementia are summarized in Table 4.2.

One of the important applications of FDG PET in dementia has been to assist in the differential diagnosis of neurodegenerative disorders. Although the ability to differentiate dementing disorders is still an important clinical use of FDG PET, the field is evolving with new observations from more widespread applications of FDG PET to clinical patients, data available from clinicopathologic correlations, and evolving and new definitions of neurodegenerative diseases. Requirements for FDG PET interpretation in dementia patients are evolving as well. For example, cases referred from specialized cognitive disorder clinics are often complex, with discordance between imaging findings and even autopsy results. New pathologic markers have been identified, and previously published studies in the literature may or may not have employed an appropriate and modern panel of pathologic stains, which can limit the validity of imaging findings that have been reported with "autopsy" or "pathology" confirmation. "Textbook" cases capture only a portion of such diverse patients as we encounter in the clinic (Fig. 4.2), and there are many unknowns despite the increasing number of biomarkers, which are available for investigations and clinical evaluations. Continuing efforts are needed to better characterize neurodegenerative dementing disorders via clinico-imaging-pathologic correlation studies.

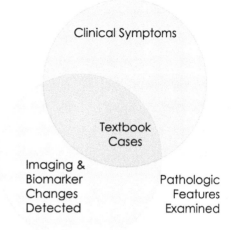

Fig. 4.2 The relationship between the clinical symptoms, imaging and biomarker changes detected, and pathologic features examined. It is important to note that 'textbook' cases represent only a fraction of dementia cases we encounter in the clinic and in investigational studies. Imaging findings can be discordant with clinical features, and pathologic examinations may or may not detect all of the pathologic changes, particularly if new markers are not used. One or limited types of imaging or pathologic examinations do not exclude co-pathologies

Table 4.2 Value of FDG PET in dementia evaluation

Differential diagnosis of suspected neurodegenerative dementias
Detection of early neurodegenerative dementias
Detection of possible co-pathologies
Prognostic evaluation

Statistical Mapping of Brain FDG PET

Since our development of statistical mapping technology based on normal database for brain FDG PET [3], several statistical mapping technologies for FDG PET have become available on workstations in a clinical setting (Fig. 4.3). When used appropriately, image interpretation using statistical mapping of FDG PET can achieve a positive likelihood ratio of AD similar to that of amyloid PET [4]. It is important to note that the interpretation of brain FDG PET for dementia evaluation needs to rely on the spatial extent of

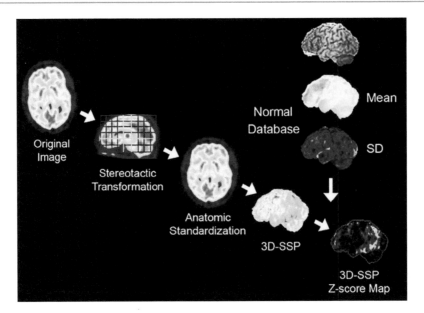

Fig. 4.3 Statistical Z-score mapping, 3D-SSP, to improve interpretation of FDG PET. The technique automatically transforms an individual FDG PET scan to a standard stereotactic space, compares the transformed individual scan with a normal database in the stereotactic space using Z-score mapping, and produces a 3-dimensional map for interpretation [3]. This technique significantly enhances the consistent detection of metabolic changes on FDG PET (or other brain PET studies such as amyloid PET) and improves the diagnostic accuracy [4]

the changes in the FDG uptake, not just the regional values of the z-scores or the standard uptake value (SUV or SUVr). The use of scientifically validated software and quality control for each case is equally critical for the reliable interpretation of brain FDG PET.

Pretest Probability and Referral Bias

The positive predictive value (PPV) indicates the probability that patients with an abnormal test result have the disease. The negative predictive value (NPV) indicates the probability that patients with a negative test result do not actually have the disease. These two descriptive statistics are useful when interpreting the significance of the test results. The PPV and NPV of imaging tests also depend on the prevalence of the disease in the test population [5]. When the pretest probably for the disease increases, the PPV increases while the NPV decreases. Therefore, an understanding of the prevalence of the disease in a test population referred from specific clinics or by providers becomes an important consideration when translating imaging findings to clinical value. For example, patients referred from cognitive disorder clinics or by dementia specialists tend to have positive and often complex, pathology, which can increase the PPV and decrease the NPV. In contrast, for patients referred from general clinics or from a non-dementia specialist without a careful clinical evaluation, the pretest probability for the disease tends to be lower, and thus the PPV decreases, and the NPV increases. A pretest probability of disease that is around 56%–58%, achieves the maximum diagnostic gain for brain FDG PET (Fig. 4.4) [6].

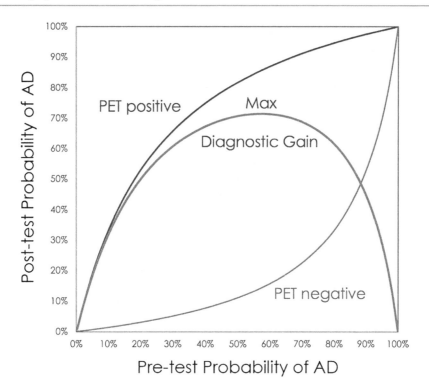

Fig. 4.4 Pretest probability/post-test probability and diagnostic gain by FDG PET in the detection of AD. FDG PET sensitivity and specificity to detect AD is assumed to be 90% and 80%, respectively, in this analysis. The maximum diagnostic gain by PET for the detection of AD is for a pretest probability of 56–58%. This suggests that FDG PET may not add a diagnostic value in the clinical assessment if clinical suspicion for AD is very high (typical clinical presentation) or suspicion is too low (such as subjective memory complaint, which cannot be confirmed by objective assessments)

Differential Diagnosis of AD, FTD, and DLB: Standard of Imaging Practice

FDG PET can provide differential diagnostic clues for three major neurodegenerative dementias, namely, AD, FTD, and dementia with Lewy bodies (DLB) (Table 4.3). The differential diagnosis of these disorders is often a critical clinical question since (1) most commonly prescribed cholinesterase inhibitors are effective for AD and DLB, but not necessarily for FTD; (2) neuroleptic/antipsychotic medications, which are often used to treat the behavioral and psychological symptoms in moderately advanced dementia patients, can cause a severe reaction in DLB; and (3) can result in changes in clinical management and prognosis [6]. FDG PET has been considered generally appropriate for the differentiation of these three diseases as well as for atypical dementias such as suspected Creutzfeldt-Jakob Disease [7].

AD A typical feature of AD on FDG PET is decreased FDG uptake in the parietal and temporal association cortices, posterior cingulate cortex and precuneus, as well as the frontal association cortex, which is in contrast to the relative preservation of FDG uptake in the primary sensorimotor cortex, primary visual cortex, basal ganglia, thalamus, brainstem, and cerebellum (Fig. 4.5). Asymmetric involvement is not uncommon. Decreased FDG uptake in the posterior cingulate cortex and precuneus can be more readily appreciated by statistical mapping analysis. Early-onset patients (onset age younger than 65 years old) tend to show more prominent reductions compared to late-onset patients.

Table 4.3 AD, DLB, FTLD/FTD, and newly recognized neurodegenerative disorders

- Alzheimer's disease (AD)
  - Posterior cortical atrophy (PCA)
  - Behavioral variant AD, frontal variant AD (fvAD)
  - Logopenic-variant PPA (lvPPA)
- Dementia with Lewy bodies (DLB)
- Frontotemporal lobar degeneration (FTLD)/frontotemporal dementia (FTD)
  - Behavioral variant FTD (bvFTD)/Pick's disease (PiD)
  - Primary progressive aphasia (PPA)
    Semantic dementia (SD)/semantic-variant primary progressive aphasia (svPPA)
    Nonfluent-variant primary progressive aphasia (nfvPPA)
    Logopenic-variant primary progressive aphasia (lvPPA)
  - Movement disorders/atypical Parkinsonian syndrome
    Progressive supranuclear palsy (PSP)
    Corticobasal degeneration (CBD)
    Atypical multiple system atrophy (MSA)
- Newly recognized neurodegenerative diseases
  - Limbic-predominant age-related TDP-43 encephalopathy (LATE)
  - FTLD with fused in sarcoma (FUS)

Right   Left

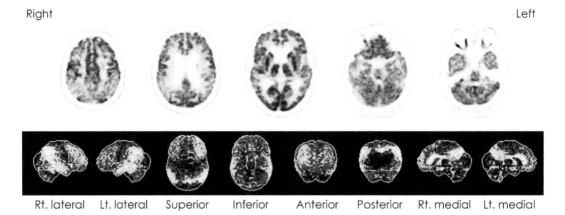

Rt. lateral   Lt. lateral   Superior   Inferior   Anterior   Posterior   Rt. medial   Lt. medial

Fig. 4.5 Alzheimer's disease (AD). FDG PET transaxial images (top row) and 3D-SSP Z-score maps (bottom row)

DLB FDG PET findings for DLB is somewhat similar to those seen with AD, but DLB patients often show decreased FDG uptake in the primary visual cortex of the occipital lobe (Fig. 4.6). This finding is considered as a "supportive" biomarker for DLB [8]. It is important to note that decreased uptake in the visual association cortex can also be seen in AD, and it should not be taken as a DLB sign. Relatively preserved FDG uptake in the posterior cingulate cortex in DLB has been reported ("Cingulate Island" sign), though autopsy validation of this finding is limited. Dopamine transporter SPECT ([I-123]ioflupane SPECT) shows decreased striatal uptake equiva-

lent to the findings typically seen in idiopathic Parkinson's disease (Fig. 4.6).

FTD Frontotemporal lobar degeneration (FTLD) encompasses various neurodegenerative diseases that primarily affect the frontal and temporal lobes of the brain. FTD represents the clinical manifestation of FTLD. The classic FTD, Pick's disease (PiD), is considered a behavioral variant of FTD (bvFTD) (Fig. 4.7). Clinical and pathologic categorization of FTLD and FTD are still evolving. PiD/bvFTD demonstrates decreased FDG uptake in the frontal as well as anterior temporal lobes. The frontal involvement

Right   Left

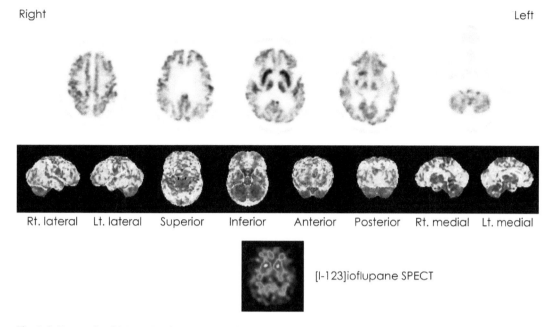

Rt. lateral   Lt. lateral   Superior   Inferior   Anterior   Posterior   Rt. medial   Lt. medial

[I-123]ioflupane SPECT

Fig. 4.6 Dementia with Lewy bodies (DLB). FDG PET transaxial images (top row) and 3D-SSP Z-score maps (middle row), and [I-123]ioflupane (DaTscan) SPECT (bottom row)

Right   Left

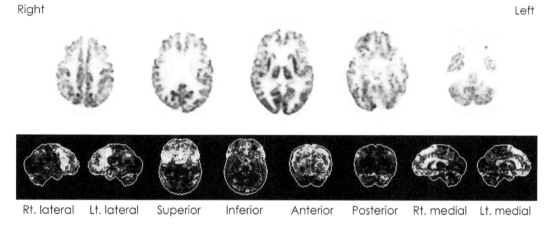

Rt. lateral   Lt. lateral   Superior   Inferior   Anterior   Posterior   Rt. medial   Lt. medial

Fig. 4.7 Behavioral variant of frontotemporal dementia (bvFTD)/Pick's disease (PiD). FDG PET transaxial images (top row) and 3D-SSP Z-score maps (bottom row)

is often sharply demarcated. The FDG uptake in the caudate nucleus is also often decreased. In contrast to AD, where the mid-to-posterior temporal lobe is typically involved, the anterior temporal lobe is involved in PiD/bvFTD. Similarly to AD, the FDG uptake in the primary sensorimotor and primary visual cortices is relatively preserved, and asymmetric hemispheric involvement is common.

Recognition of Subtypes of FTLD/FTD and AD

There have been efforts to subcategorize FTLD/FTD as well as AD, based on clinical symptoms and pathologic findings (Table 4.3). In particular, the subcategories of FTLD/FTD have evolved continuously over the past few decades. Each subcategory of FTLD/FTD is associated with somewhat unique FDG PET findings, such as described for PiD/bvFTD above. It is becoming a prerequisite for Nuclear Medicine physicians and radiologists to recognize such patterns for FDG PET interpretation in dementia work up.

Posterior Cortical Atrophy (PCA)

Patients with PCA present progressive impairments in visuospatial and visuoperceptual functions while vision itself is intact [9]. In the early stages of the disease, memory and language are relatively preserved. Onset of the disease before the age of 65 is common and the clinical diagnosis is not straightforward [10]. MRI often shows accentuated atrophy in the occipital lobe while other cortices such as parietal lobe are often involved. FDG PET shows decreased uptake in the medial and lateral occipital association cortices, in addition to decreased uptake in other neocortical areas such as the parietal and posterior temporal cortices, which are also often involved in AD (Fig. 4.8, *PCA*) [11]. Amyloid PET images are often positive. The most common underlying

pathology is AD, and PCA is often considered a variant of AD. The pattern of decreased FDG uptake as well as amyloid tracer uptake in the occipital lobe overlaps between PCA and DLB [12, 13], although the clinical features between PCA and DLB are often distinct.

The Behavioral Variant of AD (bvAD)/ Frontal Variant of AD (fvAD)

The behavioral variant of AD (bvAD) (or frontal variant of AD, fvAD [14]) is characterized by early and predominant behavioral deficits caused by AD pathology [15]. Amyloid and tau pathologies do not differ significantly between the bvAD and typical AD. Significantly decreased FDG uptake in the frontal and anterior temporal lobes, in addition to varying degrees of decreased FDG uptake in the parietal and posterior temporal cortices, typical of AD, are often seen in the bvAD as well (Fig. 4.8, bvAD). Differentiation between the bvAD, bvFTD, and mixed dementia/co-pathologies of AD + FTLD is often not straightforward on FDG PET.

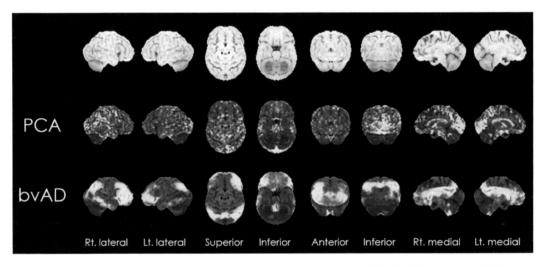

Fig. 4.8 AD variants. Posterior cortical atrophy (PCA) and behavioral variant of AD (bvAD). Reference MRI images (top row), FDG PET transaxial images (middle row), and 3D-SSP Z-score maps (bottom row)

Primary Progressive Aphasia (PPA)

PPA is subcategorized into the following three subtypes, which have distinct clinical features, FDG PET findings (Fig. 4.9), and underlying pathologies.

Semantic Dementia (SD)/Semantic-Variant PPA (svPPA)

SD or svPPA manifests with impaired semantic memory in verbal and nonverbal domains. FDG PET findings of SD/svPPA are fairly characteristic, involving the anterior temporal lobe bilaterally, but often the left temporal lobe more severely than the right. The involvement of the temporal lobe is anterior compared to the mid-to-posterior region as often seen in AD.

Nonfluent (Agrammatic)-Variant PPA (nfvPPA)

nfvPPA manifests as increasing difficulty in speaking, speech apraxia, and impaired comprehension of complex sentences, as well as difficulty in swallowing and other motor symptoms. Decreased FDG uptake is seen predominantly in the left lateral posterior frontal cortex, superior medial frontal cortex, and insula, which is distinct from the pattern seen in SD or svPPA above.

Logopenic-Variant PPA (lvPPA)

lvPPA manifests as impairments in naming and sentence repetition, and patients progressively exhibit an inability to retain complex verbal information. lvPPA more often manifests with cognitive and behavioral symptoms as compared to other PPAs.

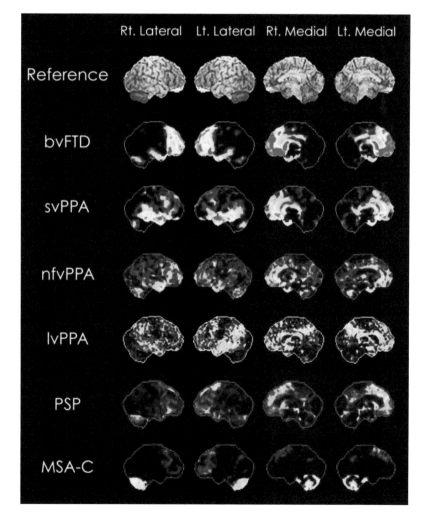

Fig. 4.9 FDG PET 3D-SSP Z-score maps of subtypes of frontotemporal lobar degeneration (FTLD)/ frontotemporal dementia (FTD)

FDG PET shows decreased uptake in the lateral temporal cortex and inferior parietal lobule, with patterns somewhat similar to those seen in Alzheimer's disease, and often the left hemisphere is more severely affected than the right.

Movement Disorder/Atypical Parkinsonian Syndrome

Some movement disorders and atypical Parkinson syndromes affect the frontal and temporal lobes and are considered within the spectrum of FTLD/FTD.

Progressive Supranuclear Palsy (PSP) PSP manifests with abnormalities in movement, gate, vision, speech, and swallowing, as well as in mood and behavior. The clinical differential diagnosis of AD, PSP, PD, vs. other FTLD/FTD is often not straightforward. FDG PET shows focally decreased FDG uptake in the midbrain as well as more diffuse decreases in the medial frontal and anterior cingulate cortices. Decreased uptake in the midbrain in PSP is often seen before MRI or structural imaging shows atrophy of midbrain tegmentum, i.e., the "Hummingbird sign."

Corticobasal Degeneration (CBD) CBD is another rare neurodegeneration characterized by motor abnormalities (such as "alien limb syndrome"). Decreased FDG uptake is seen in the frontoparietal regions without sparing of the sensorimotor cortex, basal ganglia, and thalamus (as often spared in AD). FDG PET findings are often asymmetric relative to the clinical symptoms.

PSP and CBD as well as MSA are atypical Parkinsonian syndromes in which dopamine transporter SPECT imaging shows decreased striatal uptake. However, while dopamine transporter SPECT alone cannot differentiate PSP, CBD, and MSA, the spatial patterns of altered FDG uptake can provide a clue for the differential diagnosis among these disorders.

FTLD Subtypes: Underlying Proteinopathies

One important reason for the clinical subclassification in FTLD is to determine the different underlying pathologies and proteinopathies responsible for the clinical symptoms. Predominant types of abnormal protein aggregates have been identified for FTLD subtypes (Table 4.4). When new treatments specific for proteinopathies are developed, it will be important to differentiate such FTLD subcategories. One challenge for FTLD subcategorization is that there is limited one-to-one correspondence between the underlying pathology, clinical symptoms, imaging findings, and clinically defined subtypes of FTLD. This is in part due to the operational definitions of the FTLD subtypes, but also attests to the heterogeneous and complex clinicopathologic features of FTLD.

Table 4.4 Major abnormal protein aggregates found in FTLD

Aggregates	Clinical features
Amyloid	lvPPA
Tau	bvFTD/PiD, PSP, CBD, nfvPPA, svPPA/AD
TDP-43	svPPA/SD, lvPPA
FUS	bvFTD, CBD

TDP-43 transactive response DNA binding protein of 43 kDa, *FUS* fused in sarcoma

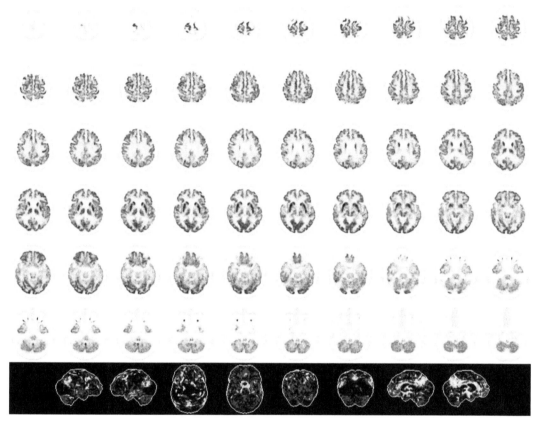

Fig. 4.10 Patient with mild cognitive impairment (MCI). It is difficult to detect, visually, decreased FDG uptake on the transaxial images (black and while images on the top rows). 3D-SSP Z-score maps (bottom row), however, show decreased FDG uptake in the precuneus/posterior cingulate cortex as well as lateral parietal association cortex bilaterally that can be confirmed retrospectively on the transaxial images. Statistical mapping improves accuracy and consistency of FDG PET interpretation especially when clinical symptoms are mild or a very early stage of diseases is suspected

Mild Cognitive Impairment (MCI) and Early Diagnosis

FDG PET has been used for patients who are suffering from mild cognitive impairment (MCI) [16] or mild dementia. FDG PET can (1) detect patterns of regional metabolic changes that indicate the presence of neurodegenerative disorders and (2) provide prognostic implications (such as conversion from MCI to AD or normal to MCI) [17–21]. These cited studies also indicated the value of combining FDG PET and ApoE genotypes as well as cerebrospinal fluid biomarkers such as amyloid and tau for the prediction of cognitive decline.

When applying FDG PET to patients with MCI or mild dementia, regional metabolic changes can be subtle. Statistical mapping greatly helps detect such subtle changes more consistently (Fig. 4.10) [22].

Newly Recognized Neurodegenerative Dementing Disorders

New forms of neurodegeneration have been recently recognized owing to advancements in proteomic research, longitudinal cohort studies, and clinicopathologic correlations. When interpreting brain FDG PET, the recognition of such diseases has become critical, since some of them are particularly prevalent among elderly patients, and there is limited evidence regarding effectiveness of conventional and new treatments with these disorders.

Limbic-Predominant Age-Related TDP-43 Encephalopathy (LATE) The high prevalence of neurodegenerative dementia characterized by transactive response DNA binding protein of 43 kDa (TDP-43) proteinopathy has been recently recognized as a new disease entity [23]. Phosphorylated TDP-43 was initially identified in FTLD and amyotrophic lateral sclerosis (ALS), and subsequently identified in patients with AD and hippocampal sclerosis particularly among elderly patients (age above 80 years). Its public health impact is estimated to be as significant as AD. MRI findings of LATE can include profound atrophy in the hippocampus, often more significant than that seen in AD. Clinically, LATE is difficult to differentiate from AD. FDG PET findings often show (1) significantly decreased FDG uptake in the medial temporal lobe including hippocampus (hippocampal FDG uptake in AD is mildly decreased) and (2) additional decreased FDG uptake in the orbital frontal and prefrontal cortices (Figs. 4.11 and 4.12, *LATE*). However, the specificity of these findings to LATE has not been established. Currently, there is no imaging biomarker specific for TDP-43.

FTLD with Fused in Sarcoma (FUS), A New Subtype of FTLD FUS is a ubiquitously expressed protein, and mutations of FUS gene on chromosome 16 have been linked to ALS and FTD. FUS has structural and functional similarities with TDP-43. FUS might define the majority of tau/TDP-43-negative FTLD cases [24, 25]. Reports of FDG PET findings are still limited, but based on our experience with autopsy confirmation, FTLD with FUS demonstrates decreased FDG uptake in the lateral and medial frontal cortex, orbital frontal cortex, and anterior temporal lobe (Fig. 4.12, *FUS*). These findings are consistent with those seen with the FTLD spectrum.

Right   Left

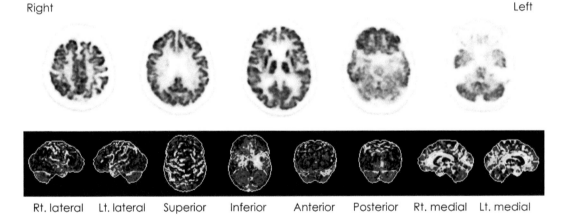

Rt. lateral   Lt. lateral   Superior   Inferior   Anterior   Posterior   Rt. medial   Lt. medial

Fig. 4.11 Limbic-predominant age-related TDP-43 encephalopathy (LATE). FDG PET transaxial images (top row) and 3D-SSP Z-score maps (bottom row)

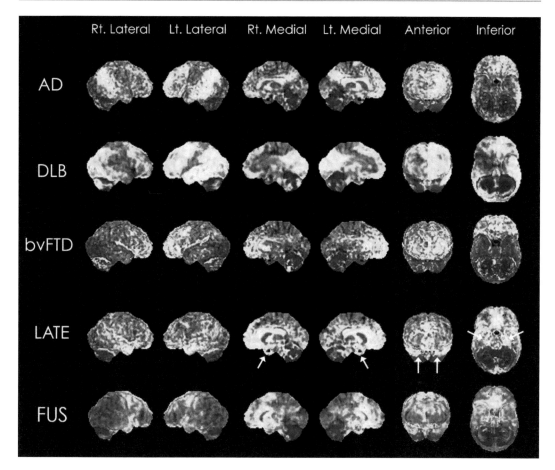

Fig. 4.12 FDG PET 3D-SSP Z-score maps of various neurodegenerative dementias, AD, DLB, bvFTD, LATE, and FUS. LATE shows distinct hypometabolism in the medial temporal lobe (white arrows). Decreased FDG uptake is more prominent in the posterior part of the brain among AD and DLB, while decreased FDG uptake is more prominent in the anterior part of the brain among bvFTD, LATE, and FUS (FTLD spectrum)

Recognition of Mixed Dementia and Co-pathologies

It is well known that AD and Vascular Dementia (VaD), two common dementing disorders, often co-exist and are termed "mixed dementia." The presence of one disease does not exclude the presence of other causes of dementia. Co-pathologies are common across neurodegenerative diseases, particularly in elderly patients, owing to advancements in proteinomics, molecular imaging, and clinicopathologic correlation (Fig. 4.13). A recent autopsy investigation demonstrated that a large fraction of elderly patients with cognitive impairment showed up to four co-existing pathologies [26]. There is an increasing number of autopsy studies reporting various co-pathologies and mixed dementia (Table 4.5). When FDG PET demonstrates atypical findings or when the multimodal imaging results are incongruent, mixed dementia or multiple co-pathologies should be suspected. FDG PET may be able to confirm the clinically relevant cause of dementia, even with the presence of co-pathologies [27].

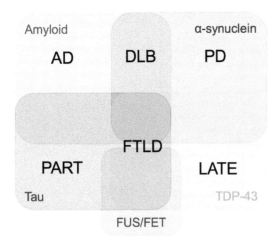

Fig. 4.13 Neurodegenerative dementias and overlapping proteinopathies—amyloid, tau, a-synuclein, TDP-43, and FUS. Emerging proteinopathies such as fused in sarcoma (FUS), EWS, TAF15 in the FET family of proteins have been identified in FTLD. Recent clinicopathologic investigations have revealed a frequent occurrence of co-pathologies involving multiple proteinopathies in elderly patients. A traditional 'dichotomous' differential diagnosis does not capture the complex nature of neurodegeneration, clinical symptoms, imaging findings, and underlying pathologies

Table 4.5 Examples of co-pathologies in dementing disorders

AD and TDP-43, cerebral amyloid angiopathy
AD and tauopathy, TDP-43
AD and DLB with TDP-43, tau, α-synuclein pathologies
AD and corticobasal syndrome, FTLD-TDP, Lewy body disease
AD and CBD
DLB and AD pathology
FTLD-tau and AD and vascular co-pathologies
PiD and AD
PiD and AD, cerebral amyloid angiopathy, Lewy body disease
PiD and PSP
PSP and AD
PSP and AD and PD
PSP and AD, AGD, CBD, Lewy body disease

Table modified from [1]

Clinical Interpretation of FDG PET for Dementia Evaluation

FDG PET can detect early metabolic changes associated with neurodegenerative diseases prior to the structural changes seen on CT or MRI. More recently, the differential diagnosis of neurodegenerative dementias can be complemented by the detection of specific proteinopathies using imaging biomarkers such as amyloid PET, tau PET, or dopamine transporter SPECT. FDG PET is relatively inexpensive, widely available, and can differentiate multiple neurodegenerative disorders in a single test when images are interpreted accurately by trained clinicians using validated statistical mapping technology.

The categorical or dichotomous distinction between AD, DLB, and FTD by FDG PET is no longer sufficient or possible, given the recognition of overlapping co-pathologies particularly in elderly patients. Also, the presence of amyloid deposition confirmed by amyloid PET or fluid biomarkers does not exclude presence of significant co-pathologies. We still do not have reliable or available imaging or fluid biomarkers for alpha-Synuclein, TDP-43, or emerging proteinopathies such as FUS, and FDG PET may be able to identify new diseases such as LATE, based on the features and patterns of altered FDG uptake.

For the clinical interpretation of FDG PET, it becomes less relevant to fit FDG PET findings into a single category of neurodegeneration when the findings are not "typical" for known neurodegenerative patterns. Instead, it is important to recognize potential co-pathologies and describe findings that are responsible for clinical symptoms and relevant for possible treatment/management approaches. Complex or atypical clinical presentations are often referred for advanced imaging by dementia specialists.

There have been extensive efforts to develop effective anti-amyloid treatments for AD. When such treatments become widespread, the detection of significant co-pathologies in patients with amyloid positive PET may become critical, since anti-amyloid monotherapy in such situations is likely to have limited efficacy. The use of imaging as well as non-imaging biomarkers will provide insight into the underlying causes of the clinical presentation, and identify concurrent neurodegenerative disorders, thus helping to guide the use of disease specific therapeutics.

References

1. Minoshima S, Cross D, Thientunyakit T, Foster NL, Drzezga A. (18)F-FDG PET imaging in neurodegenerative dementing disorders: insights into subtype classification, emerging disease categories, and mixed dementia with copathologies. J Nucl Med. 2022;63:2s–12s.
2. Guedj E, Varrone A, Boellaard R, et al. EANM procedure guidelines for brain PET imaging using [(18) F]FDG, version 3. Eur J Nucl Med Mol Imaging. 2022;49:632–51.
3. Minoshima S, Frey KA, Koeppe RA, Foster NL, Kuhl DE. A diagnostic approach in Alzheimer's disease using three-dimensional stereotactic surface projections of Fluorine-18-FDG PET. J Nucl Med. 1995;36:1238–48.
4. Frisoni GB, Bocchetta M, Chetelat G, et al. Imaging markers for Alzheimer disease: which vs how. Neurology. 2013;81:487–500.
5. Bours MJ. Bayes' rule in diagnosis. J Clin Epidemiol. 2021;131:158–60.
6. Minoshima S, Mosci K, Cross D, Thientunyakit T. Brain [F-18]FDG PET for clinical dementia workup: differential diagnosis of Alzheimer's disease and other types of dementing disorders. Semin Nucl Med. 2021;51:230–40.
7. American College of Radiology ACR Appropriateness Criteria. Dementia. https://acsearch.acr.org/docs/3111292/narrative/.
8. McKeith IG, Boeve BF, Dickson DW, et al. Diagnosis and management of dementia with Lewy bodies: fourth consensus report of the DLB consortium. Neurology. 2017;89:88–100.
9. Crutch SJ, Lehmann M, Schott JM, Rabinovici GD, Rossor MN, Fox NC. Posterior cortical atrophy. Lancet Neurol. 2012;11:170–8.
10. Yong KXX, Graff-Radford J, Ahmed S, et al. Diagnosis and management of posterior cortical atrophy. Curr Treat Options Neurol. 2023;25:23–43.
11. Shir D, Graff-Radford J, Machulda MM, et al. Posterior cortical atrophy: primary occipital variant. Eur J Neurol. 2022;29:2138–43.
12. Whitwell JL, Graff-Radford J, Singh TD, et al. (18) F-FDG PET in posterior cortical atrophy and dementia with Lewy bodies. J Nucl Med. 2017;58:632–8.
13. Nedelska Z, Josephs KA, Graff-Radford J, et al. (18) F-Av-1451 uptake differs between dementia with Lewy bodies and posterior cortical atrophy. Mov Disord. 2019;34:344–52.
14. Lehingue E, Gueniat J, Jourdaa S, et al. Improving the diagnosis of the frontal variant of Alzheimer's disease with the Daphne Scale. J Alzheimers Dis. 2021;79:1735–45.
15. Ossenkoppele R, Singleton EH, Groot C, et al. Research criteria for the behavioral variant of Alzheimer disease: a systematic review and meta-analysis. JAMA Neurol. 2021;79(1):48–60.
16. Petersen RC, Caracciolo B, Brayne C, Gauthier S, Jelic V, Fratiglioni L. Mild cognitive impairment: a concept in evolution. J Intern Med. 2014;275:214–28.
17. De Leon MJ, Convit A, Wolf OT, et al. Prediction of cognitive decline in normal elderly subjects with 2-[(18)F]fluoro-2-deoxy-D-glucose/positron-emission tomography (FDG/PET). Proc Natl Acad Sci U S A. 2001;98:10966–71.
18. Mosconi L, Perani D, Sorbi S, et al. MCI conversion to dementia and the APOE genotype: a prediction study with FDG-PET. Neurology. 2004;63:2332–40.
19. Chetelat G, Eustache F, Viader F, et al. FDG-PET measurement is more accurate than neuropsychological assessments to predict global cognitive deterioration in patients with mild cognitive impairment. Neurocase. 2005;11:14–25.
20. Drzezga A, Grimmer T, Riemenschneider M, et al. Prediction of individual clinical outcome in mci by means of genetic assessment and (18)F-FDG PET. J Nucl Med. 2005;46:1625–32.
21. Fellgiebel A, Scheurich A, Bartenstein P, Muller MJ. FDG-PET and CSF phospho-tau for prediction of cognitive decline in mild cognitive impairment. Psychiatry Res. 2007;155:167–71.
22. Burdette JH, Minoshima S, Vander Borght T, Tran DD, Kuhl DE. Alzheimer disease: improved visual interpretation of PET images by using three-dimensional stereotaxic surface projections. Radiology. 1996;198:837–43.
23. Nelson PT, Dickson DW, Trojanowski JQ, et al. Limbic-predominant age-related Tdp-43 encephalopathy (late): consensus working group report. Brain. 2019;142:1503–27.
24. Neumann M, Rademakers R, Roeber S, Baker M, Kretzschmar HA, Mackenzie IR. A new subtype of frontotemporal lobar degeneration with Fus pathology. Brain. 2009;132:2922–31.
25. Urwin H, Josephs KA, Rohrer J, et al. Fus pathology defines the majority of tau- and Tdp-43-negative frontotemporal lobar degeneration. Acta Neuropathol. 2010;120:33–41.
26. Boyle PA, Yu L, Wilson RS, Leurgans SE, Schneider JA, Bennett DA. Person-specific contribution of neuropathologies to cognitive loss in old age. Ann Neurol. 2018;83:74–83.
27. Mesulam MM, Dickerson BC, Sherman JC, et al. Case 1-2017. A 70-year-old woman with gradually progressive loss of language. N Engl J Med. 2017;376:158–67.

Alexander Drzezga and Kathrin Giehl

Introduction

Today, direct and noninvasive detection of amyloid plaque pathology in the brain is possible by means of PET imaging using commercially available and approved PET tracers [1, 2]. The employment of these imaging biomarkers may allow to overcome several limitations currently hampering clinical/neuropsychological assessment of neurodegenerative disorders such as Alzheimer's disease. Of these limitations, reliable etiological classification of the underlying pathology is particularly relevant [3–6]. It is commonly accepted today that the clinical/symptomatic appearance of neurodegenerative disorders not necessarily reflects a specific neuropathology, but rather the topography of neuronal dysfunction and damage. Thus, reliable differential diagnosis between different etiological forms of neurodegeneration is hardly possible on the basis of clinical assessment, only. Also, clinical assessment does not warrant reliable early diagnosis of disease, since accumulation of disease pathology in the brain begins many years before the first clinically detectable symptoms appear [7, 8]. Therefore, recently developed diagnostic criteria, e.g., from the National Institute on Aging and the Alzheimer's Association, divide Alzheimer's disease—the most common form of neurodegenerative dementia—into different stages, i.e., a preclinical, prodromal, and dementing phase [9–11]. Finally, symptom-oriented diagnosis limits follow-up and therapy control, due to the usually slow and fluctuating symptomatic progression and its variable correlation to the quantity of pathological features in the brain.

These shortcomings have led to increased efforts with the aim of introducing suitable diagnostic biomarkers to optimize diagnostic workup. With regard to Alzheimer's disease, this has resulted in the introduction of the so-called A/T/N classification. This framework distinguishes three main categories of pathologies and corresponding biomarkers: Markers of amyloid pathology (A), markers of tau pathology (T), and markers of neuronal injury (N). Among these factors, interstitial deposition of ß-amyloid peptides in the form of

A. Drzezga (✉)
Department of Nuclear Medicine, Faculty of Medicine and University Hospital Cologne, University of Cologne, Cologne, Germany

German Center for Neurodegenerative Diseases (DZNE), Bonn-Cologne, Germany

Institute of Neuroscience and Medicine (INM-2), Molecular Organization of the Brain, Jülich, Germany
e-mail: alexander.drzezga@uk-koeln.de

K. Giehl
Department of Nuclear Medicine, Faculty of Medicine and University Hospital Cologne, University of Cologne, Cologne, Germany

Institute of Neuroscience and Medicine (INM-2), Molecular Organization of the Brain, Jülich, Germany
e-mail: kathrin.giehl@uk-koeln.de

the so-called amyloid plaques in the brain represent one of the core neuropathological features of Alzheimer's disease, required for a definite diagnosis [12]. Previously, this was only possible by means of histopathological post-mortem detection in brain tissue but, obviously, amyloid imaging now offers an optimal method to directly asses the "A" status in the living brain (Fig. 5.1).

Several tracers for amyloid imaging have been approved and are commercially available today. Their function and utility have been documented in extensive studies, including large-scale prospective trials such as "IDEAS" (imaging dementia, evidence for amyloid scanning) [13]. The practical

need for reliable in vivo biomarkers of amyloid pathology has further increased with the development of therapeutic trials directly aiming at amyloid deposition as a central therapeutic target. Many of these studies were initially unsuccessful [5], which may have in part been due to the inclusion of patients without definite evidence of the target pathology [5, 14]. However, some successful results have been reported for some representatives of the newer generation of monoclonal antibodies [15] and in 2021 with aducanumab (Aduhelm™), the first amyloid-targeting antibody therapy receiving FDA-approval in the USA. Thus, it can be expected that molecular imaging will play an increasingly important role with regard to patient selection suitable for modern therapeutic approaches and therapy response assessment.

In this chapter, we aim to summarize the current status of amyloid imaging with regard to indications, application, and interpretation.

Theoretical Background on the Clinical Value of Amyloid Imaging

Reliable Diagnosis and Differential Diagnosis of Alzheimer's Disease

As mentioned above, clinical-symptomatic appearance of neurodegenerative disorders does not correspond reliably with underlying neuropathology. Reliable diagnosis of Alzheimer's disease has particular practical relevance with regard to (A) detection of atypical forms of Alzheimer's disease as well as (B) identification of cases clinically appearing like Alzheimer's disease on the basis of a different pathology (Fig. 5.2):

A: With regard to the first group, several atypical subtypes of Alzheimer's disease have been described, clinically not fulfilling the typical features of the disease while exhibiting characteristic AD-neuropathology [16]. Clinical appearance and patterns of neuronal dysfunction (e.g., measured with [18F]FDG-PET) of these subtypes differ considerably. However, reliable assignment of these subtypes to the category of Alzheimer's disease has relevant consequences regarding

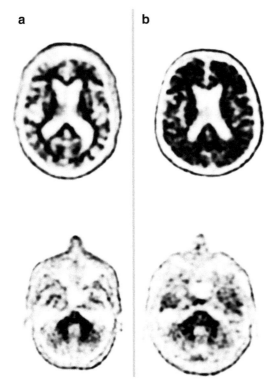

a   b

Fig. 5.1 Amyloid-PET ([18F]-Florbetaben) findings in (**a**) amyloid-negative subject and (**b**) an amyloid-positive patient with Alzheimer's disease. Top row: cortical tracer distribution pattern. No specific cortical tracer uptake is present in (**a**), only white matter uptake can be detected. In (**b**), specific cortical tracer accumulation is observed, resulting in blurred/missing contrast between white and gray matter. Bottom row: imaging results on the level of the cerebellum. Both in (**a**) and (**b**) non-specific white matter uptake is observed in the cerebellar crus, whereas no specific tracer uptake is found in the cerebellar hemispheres neither in (**a**) nor (**b**)

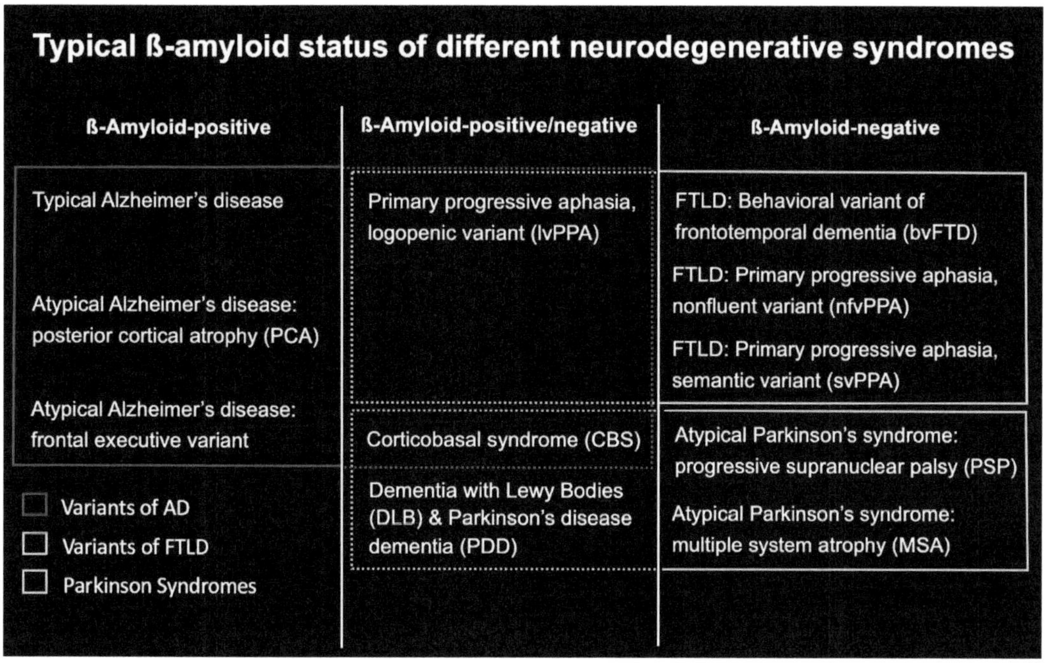

Typical ß-amyloid status of different neurodegenerative syndromes

ß-Amyloid-positive	ß-Amyloid-positive/negative	ß-Amyloid-negative
Typical Alzheimer's disease	Primary progressive aphasia, logopenic variant (lvPPA)	FTLD: Behavioral variant of frontotemporal dementia (bvFTD)
Atypical Alzheimer's disease: posterior cortical atrophy (PCA)		FTLD: Primary progressive aphasia, nonfluent variant (nfvPPA)
		FTLD: Primary progressive aphasia, semantic variant (svPPA)
Atypical Alzheimer's disease: frontal executive variant	Corticobasal syndrome (CBS)	Atypical Parkinson's syndrome: progressive supranuclear palsy (PSP)
☐ Variants of AD	Dementia with Lewy Bodies (DLB) & Parkinson's disease dementia (PDD)	Atypical Parkinson's syndrome: multiple system atrophy (MSA)
☐ Variants of FTLD		
☐ Parkinson Syndromes		

Fig. 5.2 Typically amyloid-positive and amyloid-negative symptomatic disease entities. Left column: Syndromes that usually present amyloid-positive. Right column: Syndromes that usually present amyloid-negative. Middle column: Syndromes in which both amyloid-positive and negative cases can be observed in relevant frequency. Importantly, clinical appearance does not allow reliable conclusions on amyloid status

treatment, further diagnostic workup and therapy approaches. Three dominant subtypes have been described:

1. Posterior Cortical Atrophy

   These patients often present with relatively isolated problems in their visual functions, while memory and other cognitive functions may initially remain preserved [17, 18]. Particularly in later stages of disease, a pronounced cortical atrophy has been described in posterior parietal and occipital regions, which eventually coined the designation of this disease as "posterior cortical atrophy." It has been demonstrated that a large proportion of patients exhibiting this syndrome are suffering from Alzheimer's disease, when assessed by histopathology [19]. However, clinical evaluation alone is not sufficient to reach an etiological diagnosis, as other disorders such as corticobasal degeneration, Lewy body disease and even prion diseases may mimic the symptomatic phenomenon of posterior cortical atrophy [20]. Consequently, verification of amyloid deposition by means of amyloid PET imaging may be of great clinical value [19, 21].

2. Logopenic/Aphasic Atypical Variant of AD

   The logopenic variant of primary progressive aphasia is characterized by language deficits, especially concerning word-finding difficulties. The syndrome has usually been assigned to the primary progressive aphasias and, thus, to the complex of frontotemporal lobar degeneration (FTLD). However, by means of neuropathological assessment as well as by in vivo amyloid imaging, it has been demonstrated that in even up to 50% of patients with logopenic aphasia amyloid plaque pathology can be identified as an underlying neuropathological feature [3, 16, 22–24]. However, also amyloid negative cases occur, which may show other pathologies such as TDP43 or tau aggregates [25]. With regard to the high-frequency of amyloid-positive cases, these are today considered a logopenic/aphasic variant of Alzheimer's disease.

3. Frontal/Executive Atypical Variant of AD

The fronal/executive variant of Alzheimer's disease is clinically characterized by symptoms usually associated with FTLD subtypes such as the behavioral variant of frontotemporal dementia (bvFTD). These symptoms include disturbed executive functions such as abstract reasoning, structured planning as well as behavioral abnormalities [26]. Amyloid imaging can be helpful to distinguish these cases by proving evidence for the presence of amyloid in the cases of atypical AD and/or by demonstrating amyloid negativity in cases of bvFTD (which are usually not associated with relevant amyloid plaque pathology) [3, 26–28].

Apart from these three well-described entities of atypical AD, it has been demonstrated that amyloid pathology can also occur in the symptomatic appearance of other typical neurodegenerative diseases, such, e.g., the corticobasal syndrome but also in other subtypes of FTLD [3, 29, 30]. Again, amyloid imaging may play an essential role in detecting these cases [31].

B: Apart from cases of atypical AD, a second group of cases can be challenging regarding differential diagnosis. This refers to conditions symptomatically resembling Alzheimer's disease, while being caused by other underlying neuropathologies. Again amyloid imaging can be of relevant value also for these cases.

It is well-accepted today that neurodegenerative disorders based on other pathologies than those characteristic for Alzheimer's disease, nevertheless may appear in a symptomatic pattern mimicking typical Alzheimer's disease [5]. A large prospective trial in the USA, the so-called IDEAS trial provided further evidence supporting this notion. In more than 11,000 patients the clinical value of amyloid imaging has been studied. In approximately 60% of the patients, a change in clinical management resulted. The most frequent reason for change being that Alzheimer's disease has ultimately been excluded

(although clinically suspected) by means of amyloid PET [13].

In summary, amyloid PET imaging may be of great value with regard to detecting amyloid pathology in patients clinically not fulfilling the typical pattern of Alzheimer's disease symptoms. Also, a value can be found to exclude patients with "pseudo"-Alzheimer's disease, i.e., resembling the disorder clinically but not exhibiting the corresponding neuropathology. This may be valuable in differential diagnostic workup, i.e., to distinguish between Alzheimer's disease and other forms of neurodegeneration such as the FTLD disorders and atypical Parkinson's syndromes on the basis of direct assessment of intracerebral pathology rather than clinical signs only.

However, some limitations apply to the value of amyloid imaging in differential diagnosis. For example, amyloid deposition may represent co-pathology, not necessarily driving the symptomatic disease. Particularly with increasing age, it has been demonstrated that amyloid deposition can occur simultaneously with other cerebrovascular or neurodegenerative diseases. Also, it has been shown that amyloid positivity increases with age even in cognitively healthy individuals [29, 32]. In consequence, the presence of amyloid deposition as a co-pathology or the possibility of an interaction of multiple pathologies must be considered in elderly patients. In this context, special consideration must be given to dementia with Lewy bodies (DLB). DLB is characterized by fluctuating cognitive deficits accompanied by Parkinson's disease-like symptomatology and often also visual hallucinations [33]. In DLB, the eponymous synuclein/Lewy body pathology seems to be accompanied rather regularly by amyloid copathology in many patients [34, 35]. However, although frequent, amyloid deposition is not found in all patients, differentiation between amyloid- positive and amyloid-negative cases may potentially be of value with regard to prognosis or novel treatment approaches in the future. At present, however, it must be noted that a reliable differential diagnosis between DLB and AD is not possible by means of amyloid imaging.

Early Diagnosis of Ongoing Alzheimer's Disease

In a clinical setting, reliable diagnosis of patients in the prodromal and dementing phase will represent the dominant issue This, however, may potentially shift toward earlier stages in the future, with the potential introduction of therapies targeting earlier, even asymptomatic stages of disease. As of now, the value for routine application of amyloid PET imaging in asymptomatic individuals is uncertain. There is evidence that amyloid deposition can be identified in a relevant percentage of elderly cognitively healthy subjects [32, 36–38] . Although it has been discussed that this finding may represent early, preclinical Alzheimer's disease [39–41], many questions, e.g., about the possible onset of dementia and the time to onset of symptomatic disease remain unresolved. For this reason, practical consequences of a positive amyloid scan in an otherwise healthy subject remain unclear. Consequently, the amyloid imaging is only recommended in the context of studies in this group (also see appropriate use criteria below). Potentially, a more tangible prognostic value may be found in subjects without objective deficits in neuropsychological tests, but complaining about a subjective cognitive decline (SCD). This question is currently also the matter of ongoing trials (e.g., AMYPAD: the Amyloid imaging for the Prevention of Alzheimer Disease trial) [42]. The clinical value of amyloid-PET in patients with objective mild cognitive impairment (MCI) is more obvious. In these patients, the measurable cognitive deficits are not yet sufficient for the diagnosis of dementia, but conversion to manifest dementia is frequently observed within the near future (2–3 years) in some (but not all) of these patients. Studies on amyloid-PET in MCI were able to demonstrate amyloid-positive findings in approximately half of all cases, already resembling the findings typically observed in AD [43, 44]. The notion that these findings may correspond to early ongoing Alzheimer's disease is supported by longitudinal follow-up studies, demonstrating a higher risk of conversion to

manifest Alzheimer's disease dementia in amyloid-positive MCI patients in a relatively short period of time [43, 45–48]. A prognostic value can also be found in the opposite situation, i.e., in presence of an amyloid negative finding which corresponds to a low risk of conversion to clinical AD.

Value of Amyloid Imaging in Therapy Control and Follow-Up

Amyloid imaging represents an important biomarker for appropriate selection of suitable patients for therapy trials, particularly with regard to novel therapies directed against amyloid deposition. Whereas some trials in the past may have suffered from inclusion of patients without reliable evidence of intracerebral amyloid pathology, more recent anti-amyloid trials regularly employ amyloid imaging as an inclusion criterion to warrant presence of the therapeutic target.

Amyloid imaging is not ideally suited to measure clinical disease progression or advancement of neurodegenerative processes in the brain. Initially, an increase of amyloid deposition can be observed via imaging from healthy amyloid-positive individuals through MCI to mild AD [42]. However, from the stage of manifest AD, studies show a plateau or only a small increase in amyloid deposition [49, 50] despite further increasing symptomatology and neurodegeneration. Consequently, no linear correlation is found between amyloid load and cognitive decline in this stage [51].

There may be a greater value of amyloid-PET imaging with regard to therapy monitoring, i.e., demonstrating removal of existing amyloid pathology/reduction of new build-up. In fact, amyloid imaging has successfully been used to document treatment effects [52, 53]. The first approval of a monoclonal antibody therapy directed against amyloid deposits (Aduhelm™) in 2021 was largely based on results from PET imaging [54]. Some issues with regard to appropriate quantification of therapy effects do arise, however (see below).

Combination with/Comparison to Other Biomarkers

Amyloid imaging can be combined with other imaging biomarkers to allow a comprehensive classification according to the A/T/N scheme. For measuring T, i.e., tau pathology, novel tau PET tracers have become available recently. N representing neuronal injury can be assessed using structural imaging (MRI) and [^{18}F]FDG-PET. In addition to imaging also fluid biomarkers are available, including CSF biomarkers (requiring lumbar puncture) as well as more recently introduced plasma biomarkers (for more details see [55, 56]). The latter, in particular, are being evaluated with great interest as they could represent a low-invasive and possibly low-cost option. However, the information provided by these tests regarding cerebral amyloid pathology are not easily comparable to amyloid PET imaging.

In general, the fluid biomarkers provide an indirect snapshot of ongoing pathological aggregation processes and do not provide information on current localization or extent of pathology. Neither do they allow to quantify changes over time, e.g., in consequence to therapeutic procedures. While being less invasive, the plasma markers of amyloid pathology show only very small effect sizes as compared to CSF-markers and may also be more sensitive to sample handling errors [56, 57]. Nevertheless, particularly the plasma markers may offer a very promising option for screening of candidates for subsequent biomarker examinations. Ideally, in a combination of both types of tests, subjects screening positive on relatively cheap and broadly available plasma markers could be selected for subsequent imaging tests.

Translation of the Theoretical Background into Practical Guidelines

The considerations on the value of amyloid imaging from the existing literature have been translated into corresponding appropriate use criteria for amyloid imaging (AUC) by the Society for Nuclear Medicine and Molecular Imaging and the Alzheimer's Association [58].

The guideline generally considers amyloid PET imaging appropriate in the following situations (for details see [58]):

- Patients with persistent or progressive unexplained mild cognitive impairment.
- Patients fulfilling clinical criteria only for possible (not probable!) Alzheimer's disease because of unclear clinical presentation, either atypical clinical course or etiologically mixed presentation.
- Patients with progressive dementia and atypically early age of onset (usually defined as 65 years or less in age).

In these cases, a positive amyloid scan may indicate ongoing Alzheimer's disease, whereas a negative amyloid scan makes this very unlikely. Amyloid PET imaging is not considered appropriate according to the AUC in the following situations/for the following indications:

- Patients with core clinical criteria for probable Alzheimer's disease with typical age of onset.
- To determine dementia severity.
- Solely based on a positive family history of dementia or presence of APOE4.
- Patients with a cognitive complaint that is unconfirmed on clinical examination.
- In lieu of genotyping for suspected autosomal mutation carriers.
- In asymptomatic individuals.
- Non-medical usage (e.g., legal, insurance coverage, or employment screening).

The AUC also define some general requirements for amyloid PET imaging. These include that Alzheimer's disease represents a possible differential diagnostic option, that cognitive impairment is objectively documented and that knowledge about the presence of amyloid pathology is likely to increase diagnostic confidence and may alter management. To verify these criteria, it is recommended that a dementia expert always sees the affected patients and decides whether amyloid PET is indicated.

The AUC criteria are generally helpful for everyday clinical practice. There is some controversy surrounding some of the positions which may need to be updated in the future. This concerns, e.g., the explicit exclusion of patients with clinically typical Alzheimer's disease from amyloid PET diagnostics. This point raises questions, since it could be shown that patients with clinically typical symptom patterns in quite a few cases do not have pathology typical for Alzheimer's disease. Especially prior to therapeutic decisions, amyloid imaging may therefore considered to be useful in these cases as well. Also, in earlier stages such as SCD, a prognostic benefit of amyloid PET could become apparent in the future [5, 13].

Practical Performance and Interpretation of Amyloid PET Imaging

Commercially Available and Approved Radiotracers for Amyloid Imaging

Today, three ^{18}F-labeled tracers are commercially available. These include ^{18}F-florbetapir (Amyvid™) from Lilly Pharma AG/Avid Radiopharmaceuticals, ^{18}F-flutemetamol (Vizamyl™) from GE Healthcare, and ^{18}F-florbetaben (NeuraCeq™) from Life Molecular Imaging. These tracers obtained FDA/EMA approval only after extensive validation demonstrating a correlation between histopathological assessment of the extent of amyloid pathology in the brain post-mortem and prior in vivo amyloid tracer uptake [59, 60]. Also, the tracers have been evaluated in numerous clinical trials [61–63]. With regard to properties, routine application and interpretation some minor differences apply, however, in general the three tracers compare well with each other. With regard to qualitative (visual) and (semi-)quantitative assessment, comparable results have been reported [63–65].

Basic Principles of Interpreting Amyloid PET Findings

In short, interpretation is based on visual distinction between an amyloid-positive or amyloid-negative scan (Fig. 5.1). Specific training is required for interpretation of all three commercially available amyloid tracers (which can be completed online or in dedicated training sessions). The general principle of interpretation is based on the assessment of tracer uptake in the gray matter of the brain as compared to non-specific white matter uptake.

A scan is considered to be negative if distinctly less tracer accumulation is observed in the cortex than in the white matter, i.e., a clear contrast between gray and white matter is evident. The cerebellum can also serve as a reference in this context, as usually no major amyloid pathology, i.e., no specific uptake is expected in the cerebellar cortex, even in patients with Alzheimer's disease. Thus, contrast between white and gray matter is usually preserved. In contrast, a scan is considered amyloid-positive if the contrast between gray and white matter is noticeably reduced as a consequence of increased specific tracer uptake in cortical brain regions. In patients with amyloid plaque pathology, increased cortical amyloid tracer accumulation is often found predominantly in the frontal and temporoparietal cortex, the posterior cingulate cortex, and the precuneus [61, 62].

Minor differences apply with regard to the official interpretation guidelines for the different tracers, as issued by the manufacturers. This refers to suggested reference regions for intensity normalization/scaling, the color scale or the number of affected regions required for definition of a positive scan. However, a systematic comparison was able to show that the impact of these differences on the assessment can be regarded as small, at least for experienced readers [65]. Interpretation can be hampered by movement artifacts and also by major atrophy (resulting in thinning of the cortex). It has been suggested that comparison with morphological information as derived from CT or MRI scans (if available) can be very helpful in the latter case.

Commercial vendors also offer solutions for standardized automated observer-independent analysis of amyloid PET results. Similar to routines established for FDG-PET imaging, these software solutions are based on stereotactical spatial normalization of the image data followed by voxel-based statistical comparison with a healthy control dataset. As a result, statistically significant deviations can be displayed. Issues such as the high subcortical tracer uptake of amyloid PET imaging data and selection of appropriate spatial templates (different uptake patterns in amyloid-positive and amyloid-negative subjects) need to be considered.

In addition to the basic distinction between amyloid-positive and amyloid-negative scans, semiquantitative assessment of regional uptake is also possible (e.g., by means of measuring regional standardized uptake value ratios (SUVR), again using the cerebellum as a reference region for quantitative normalization of the data). SUVR-values can even be "converted" between the different tracers using the so-called centiloid-scale [63, 64]. Semiquantitive assessment is not usually required with regard to diagnostic purposes, but quantification may gain interest with regard to very early prognosis and also with regard to monitoring of therapeutic effects. It has been discussed that SUVR-values may not represent the ideal tool for this purpose, as perfusion effects asymmetrically affecting target and reference regions may lead to deviations over time [66]. Potentially the acquisition of an early perfusion phase in addition to the specific late phase may be of value for improved quantitative assessment. The perfusion phase may hold additional value as a surrogate for FDG-PET, thus adding the "N"-information to the "A" information as provided by the amyloid scan in a single examination [42, 67].

Reporting

Amyloid imaging provides information about the presence or absence of a specific neuropathology and is therefore not in itself a sufficient test for defining a specific diagnosis. Results of the imaging test need to be considered in the context of other clinical and biomarker information. This also needs to be considered for appropriate reporting of amyloid imaging findings. Reports should conclude if the scan is considered positive/negative, i.e., consistent with presence/absence of ß-amyloid pathology. A negative scan represents lacking or low density of ß-amyloid plaque pathology and, thus, does not support the diagnosis of Alzheimer's disease in a patient with clinically manifest dementia. In patients with objective mild cognitive impairment and a negative amyloid scan, progression to Alzheimer's disease within the near future can also be considered to be unlikely. However, other, amyloid-negative forms of neurodegeneration cannot be excluded.

An amyloid-positive scan is consistent with ongoing Alzheimer's pathology but does not suffice to make the diagnosis of dementia with Alzheimer's disease (which requires clinical and other biomarker confirmation), also because amyloid pathology may occur as a co-pathology of other disorders (as explained above). However, in patients with manifest dementia, a positive amyloid scan is well compatible with the diagnosis of Alzheimer's disease. In patients with MCI a positive scan may indicate ongoing AD-pathology and signify a higher risk of conversion to dementia of the Alzheimer type over time [45–47].

Acknowledgments Content of this article in part derived from previous publications/book chapters including "PET and SPECT Imaging of Neurodegenerative Diseases" in "Molecular Imaging, Principles and Practice, 2nd edition" Editors: Brian Ross, Sanjiv Gambhir as well as "Update Amyloid-Bildgebung in der Diagnostik der Neurodegeneration" in Angewandte Nuklearmedizin 2022, © Georg Thieme Verlag KG Stuttgart, New York.

References

1. Drzezga A. Amyloid-plaque imaging in early and differential diagnosis of dementia. Ann Nucl Med. 2010;24:55–66.
2. Villemagne VL, Klunk WE, Mathis CA, et al. Aβ Imaging: feasible, pertinent, and vital to progress in Alzheimer's disease. Eur J Nucl Med Mol Imaging. 2012;39:209–19.
3. Bonner MF, Ash S, Grossman M. The new classification of primary progressive aphasia into semantic,

logopenic, or nonfluent/agrammatic variants. Curr Neurol Neurosci Rep. 2010;10:484–90.

4. Davies RR, Hodges JR, Kril JJ, et al. The pathological basis of semantic dementia. Brain. 2005;128:1984–95.

5. Salloway S, Sperling R, Fox NC, et al. Two phase 3 trials of bapineuzumab in mild-to-moderate Alzheimer's disease. N Engl J Med. 2014;370:322–33.

6. Johnson JK, Diehl J, Mendez MF, et al. Frontotemporal lobar degeneration: demographic characteristics of 353 patients. Arch Neurol. 2005;62:925–30.

7. Braak E, Griffing K, Arai K, et al. Neuropathology of Alzheimer's disease: what is new since A. Alzheimer? Eur Arch Psychiatry Clin Neurosci. 1999;249:S14–22.

8. Davies L, Wolska B, Hilbich C, et al. A4 amyloid protein deposition and the diagnosis of Alzheimer's disease: prevalence in aged brains determined by immunocytochemistry compared with conventional neuropathologic techniques. Neurology. 1988;38:1688–93.

9. Albert MS, DeKosky ST, Dickson D, et al. The diagnosis of mild cognitive impairment due to Alzheimer's disease: recommendations from the National Institute on Aging-Alzheimer's Association workgroups on diagnostic guidelines for Alzheimer's disease. Alzheimers Dement. 2011;7:270–9.

10. McKhann GM, Knopman DS, Chertkow H, et al. The diagnosis of dementia due to Alzheimer's disease: recommendations from the National Institute on Aging-Alzheimer's Association workgroups on diagnostic guidelines for Alzheimer's disease. Alzheimers Dement. 2011;7:263–9.

11. Sperling RA, Aisen PS, Beckett LA, et al. Toward defining the preclinical stages of Alzheimer's disease: recommendations from the National Institute on Aging-Alzheimer's Association workgroups on diagnostic guidelines for Alzheimer's disease. Alzheimers Dement. 2011;7:280–92.

12. Selkoe DJ. Folding proteins in fatal ways. Nature. 2003;426:900–4.

13. Rabinovici GD, Gatsonis C, Apgar C, et al. Association of amyloid positron emission tomography with subsequent change in clinical management among Medicare beneficiaries with mild cognitive impairment or dementia. JAMA. 2019;321:1286–94.

14. Ceccaldi M, Jonveaux T, Verger A, et al. Added value of 18F-florbetaben amyloid PET in the diagnostic workup of most complex patients with dementia in France: a naturalistic study. Alzheimers Dement. 2018;14:293–305.

15. Decourt B, Boumelhem F, Pope ED, et al. Critical appraisal of amyloid lowering agents in AD. Curr Neurol Neurosci Rep. 2021;21:1–10.

16. Wolk DA. Amyloid imaging in atypical presentations of Alzheimer's disease. Curr Neurol Neurosci Rep. 2013;13:412.

17. Crutch SJ, Lehmann M, Schott JM, et al. Posterior cortical atrophy. Lancet Neurol. 2012;11:170–8.

18. Nestor P, Caine D, Fryer T, et al. The topography of metabolic deficits in posterior cortical atrophy (the visual variant of Alzheimer's disease) with FDG-PET. J Neurol Neurosurg Psychiatry. 2003;74:1521–9.

19. De Souza LC, Corlier F, Habert M-O, et al. Similar amyloid-β burden in posterior cortical atrophy and Alzheimer's disease. Brain. 2011;134:2036–43.

20. Crutch SJ, Schott JM, Rabinovici GD, et al. Consensus classification of posterior cortical atrophy. Alzheimers Dement. 2017;13:870–84.

21. Formaglio M, Costes N, Seguin J, et al. In vivo demonstration of amyloid burden in posterior cortical atrophy: a case series with PET and CSF findings. J Neurol. 2011;258:1841–51.

22. Grossman M. Primary progressive aphasia: clinicopathological correlations. Nat Rev Neurol. 2010;6:88–97.

23. Mesulam M-M, Weintraub S, Rogalski EJ, et al. Asymmetry and heterogeneity of Alzheimer's and frontotemporal pathology in primary progressive aphasia. Brain. 2014;137:1176–92.

24. Mesulam M, Wieneke C, Rogalski E, et al. Quantitative template for subtyping primary progressive aphasia. Arch Neurol. 2009;66:1545–51.

25. Josephs KA, Duffy JR, Strand EA, et al. Progranulin-associated PiB-negative logopenic primary progressive aphasia. J Neurol. 2014;261:604–14.

26. Johnson JK, Head E, Kim R, et al. Clinical and pathological evidence for a frontal variant of Alzheimer disease. Arch Neurol. 1999;56:1233–9.

27. Ossenkoppele R, Pijnenburg YA, Perry DC, et al. The behavioural/dysexecutive variant of Alzheimer's disease: clinical, neuroimaging and pathological features. Brain. 2015;138:2732–49.

28. Rabinovici G, Furst A, O'neil J, et al. 11C-PIB PET imaging in Alzheimer disease and frontotemporal lobar degeneration. Neurology. 2007;68:1205–12.

29. Ossenkoppele R, Jansen WJ, Rabinovici GD, et al. Prevalence of amyloid PET positivity in dementia syndromes: a meta-analysis. JAMA. 2015;313:1939–50.

30. Day GS, Lim TS, Hassenstab J, et al. Differentiating cognitive impairment due to corticobasal degeneration and Alzheimer disease. Neurology. 2017;88:1273–81.

31. Drzezga A, Grimmer T, Henriksen G, et al. Imaging of amyloid plaques and cerebral glucose metabolism in semantic dementia and Alzheimer's disease. NeuroImage. 2008;39:619–33.

32. Jansen WJ, Ossenkoppele R, Knol DL, et al. Prevalence of cerebral amyloid pathology in persons without dementia: a meta-analysis. JAMA. 2015;313:1924–38.

33. McKeith I, Dickson DW, Lowe J, et al. Diagnosis and management of dementia with Lewy bodies: third report of the DLB Consortium. Neurology. 2005;65:1863–72.

34. Rowe CC, Ng S, Ackermann U, et al. Imaging β-amyloid burden in aging and dementia. Neurology. 2007;68:1718–25.

35. Edison P, Rowe CC, Rinne JO, et al. Amyloid load in Parkinson's disease dementia and Lewy body

dementia measured with [11C] PIB positron emission tomography. J Neurol Neurosurg Psychiatry. 2008;79:1331–8.

36. Pike KE, Savage G, Villemagne VL, et al. β-amyloid imaging and memory in non-demented individuals: evidence for preclinical Alzheimer's disease. Brain. 2007;130:2837–44.

37. Mintun M, Larossa G, Sheline Y, et al. [11C] PIB in a nondemented population: potential antecedent marker of Alzheimer disease. Neurology. 2006;67:446–52.

38. Villemagne VL, Pike KE, Darby D, et al. Aβ deposits in older non-demented individuals with cognitive decline are indicative of preclinical Alzheimer's disease. Neuropsychologia. 2008;46:1688–97.

39. Drzezga A, Becker JA, Van Dijk KR, et al. Neuronal dysfunction and disconnection of cortical hubs in non-demented subjects with elevated amyloid burden. Brain. 2011;134:1635–46.

40. Hedden T, Van Dijk KR, Becker JA, et al. Disruption of functional connectivity in clinically normal older adults harboring amyloid burden. J Neurosci. 2009;29:12686–94.

41. Sperling RA, LaViolette PS, O'Keefe K, et al. Amyloid deposition is associated with impaired default network function in older persons without dementia. Neuron. 2009;63:178–88.

42. Frisoni GB, Barkhof F, Altomare D, et al. AMYPAD diagnostic and patient management study: rationale and design. Alzheimers Dement. 2019;15:388–99.

43. Forsberg A, Engler H, Almkvist O, et al. PET imaging of amyloid deposition in patients with mild cognitive impairment. Neurobiol Aging. 2008;29:1456–65.

44. Mormino E, Kluth J, Madison C, et al. Episodic memory loss is related to hippocampal-mediated β-amyloid deposition in elderly subjects. Brain. 2009;132:1310–23.

45. Koivunen J, Scheinin N, Virta J, et al. Amyloid PET imaging in patients with mild cognitive impairment: a 2-year follow-up study. Neurology. 2011;76:1085–90.

46. Okello A, Koivunen J, Edison P, et al. Conversion of amyloid positive and negative MCI to AD over 3 years: an 11C-PIB PET study. Neurology. 2009;73:754–60.

47. Villemagne VL, Pike KE, Chételat G, et al. Longitudinal assessment of Aβ and cognition in aging and Alzheimer disease. Ann Neurol. 2011;69:181–92.

48. Zhang S, Han D, Tan X, et al. Diagnostic accuracy of 18F-FDG and 11C-PIB-PET for prediction of short-term conversion to Alzheimer's disease in subjects with mild cognitive impairment. Int J Clin Pract. 2012;66:185–98.

49. Engler H, Forsberg A, Almkvist O, et al. Two-year follow-up of amyloid deposition in patients with Alzheimer's disease. Brain. 2006;129:2856–66.

50. Grimmer T, Tholen S, Yousefi BH, et al. Progression of cerebral amyloid load is associated with the apolipoprotein E ε4 genotype in Alzheimer's disease. Biol Psychiatry. 2010;68:879–84.

51. Morris GP, Clark IA, Vissel B. Inconsistencies and controversies surrounding the amyloid hypothesis

of Alzheimer's disease. Acta Neuropathol Commun. 2014;2:135.

52. Rinne JO, Brooks DJ, Rossor MN, et al. 11C-PiB PET assessment of change in fibrillar amyloid-β load in patients with Alzheimer's disease treated with bapineuzumab: a phase 2, double-blind, placebo-controlled, ascending-dose study. Lancet Neurol. 2010;9:363–72.

53. Ratner M. Biogen's early Alzheimer's data raise hopes, some eyebrows. Nat Biotechnol. 2015;33:438–9.

54. O'Gorman J, Chiao P, Bussière T, et al. Clinical development of aducanumab, an anti-Aβ human monoclonal antibody being investigated for the treatment of early Alzheimer's disease. J Prev Alzheimers Dis. 2017;4:255–63.

55. Chételat G, Arbizu J, Barthel H, et al. Amyloid-PET and 18F-FDG-PET in the diagnostic investigation of Alzheimer's disease and other dementias. Lancet Neurol. 2020;19:951–62.

56. Leuzy A, Mattsson-Carlgren N, Palmqvist S, et al. Blood-based biomarkers for Alzheimer's disease. EMBO Mol Med. 2022;14:e14408.

57. Rózga M, Bittner T, Batrla R, et al. Preanalytical sample handling recommendations for Alzheimer's disease plasma biomarkers. Alzheimers Dement (Amst). 2019;11:291–300.

58. Johnson KA, Minoshima S, Bohnen NI, et al. Appropriate use criteria for amyloid PET: a report of the amyloid imaging task force, the Society of Nuclear Medicine and Molecular Imaging, and the Alzheimer's Association. J Nucl Med. 2013;54:476–90.

59. Ikonomovic MD, Klunk WE, Abrahamson EE, et al. Post-mortem correlates of in vivo PiB-PET amyloid imaging in a typical case of Alzheimer's disease. Brain. 2008;131:1630–45.

60. Clark CM, Schneider JA, Bedell BJ, et al. Use of florbetapir-PET for imaging β-amyloid pathology. JAMA. 2011;305:275–83.

61. Barthel H, Gertz H-J, Dresel S, et al. Cerebral amyloid-β PET with florbetaben (18F) in patients with Alzheimer's disease and healthy controls: a multicentre phase 2 diagnostic study. Lancet Neurol. 2011;10:424–35.

62. Fleisher AS, Chen K, Liu X, et al. Using positron emission tomography and florbetapir F18 to image cortical amyloid in patients with mild cognitive impairment or dementia due to Alzheimer disease. Arch Neurol. 2011;68:1404–11.

63. Vandenberghe R, Van Laere K, Ivanoiu A, et al. 18F-flutemetamol amyloid imaging in Alzheimer disease and mild cognitive impairment: a phase 2 trial. Ann Neurol. 2010;68:319–29.

64. Klunk WE, Koeppe RA, Price JC, et al. The Centiloid project: standardizing quantitative amyloid plaque estimation by PET. Alzheimers Dement. 2015;11(1–15):e14.

65. Bischof GN, Bartenstein P, Barthel H, et al. Toward a universal readout for 18F-labeled amyloid tracers: the CAPTAINs study. J Nucl Med. 2021;62:999–1005.

66. van Berckel BN, Ossenkoppele R, Tolboom N, et al. Longitudinal amyloid imaging using 11C-PiB: methodologic considerations. J Nucl Med. 2013;54:1570–6.

67. Tiepolt S, Hesse S, Patt M, et al. Early [18F] florbetaben and [11C] PiB PET images are a surrogate biomarker of neuronal injury in Alzheimer's disease. Eur J Nucl Med Mol Imaging. 2016;43:1700–9.

Victor L. Villemagne, Brian J. Lopresti,
Vincent Doré, Davneet Minhas, Alexandra Gogola,
Neelesh Nadkarni, N. Scott Mason,
Pierrick Bourgeat, Oscar Lopez,
Milos D. Ikonomovic, and Ann D. Cohen

Introduction

Tauopathies is the term to define a spectrum of neurodegenerative conditions characterized by the pathological accumulation of tau aggregates in the brain. While Alzheimer's disease (AD) is the most common tauopathy, other neurodegenerative conditions such as chronic traumatic encephalopathy (CTE), corticobasal degeneration (CBD), progressive supranuclear palsy (PSP), and some variants of frontotemporal lobar degeneration (FTLD), are also characterized by the accumulation of tau aggregates [1–4]. While tau lesions do share some immunohistochemical similarities across different tauopathies, they have clear histopathological, biochemical, and ultrastructural distinctions [1], and these differences are associated with distinct clinical phenotypes [1–3] (Fig. 6.1).

Tau is an axonal phosphoprotein that stabilizes microtubules, critical for maintaining the neuron cytoskeleton and axonal transport which are impaired in AD and other neurodegenerative diseases [5]. Some studies propose that Aβ or other stressor promotes tau *uber* phosphorylation which impairs microtubule binding [6] and leads to missorting of tau by retrograde flow and accumulation from the axonal into the somatoden-

V. L. Villemagne (✉)
Department of Psychiatry, University of Pittsburgh, Pittsburgh, PA, USA

Department of Molecular Imaging and Therapy, Austin Health, Melbourne, Australia
e-mail: victor.villemagne@pitt.edu

B. J. Lopresti · D. Minhas · A. Gogola · N. S. Mason
Department of Radiology, University of Pittsburgh, Pittsburgh, PA, USA
e-mail: brianl@pitt.edu; minhasd@upmc.edu; judischal@upmc.edu; masonns@upmc.edu

V. Doré
Department of Molecular Imaging and Therapy, Austin Health, Melbourne, Australia

CSIRO Health and Biosecurity Flagship: The Australian e-Health Research Centre, Melbourne, Australia
e-mail: Vincent.Dore@csiro.au

N. Nadkarni
Department of Geriatric Medicine, University of Pittsburgh, Pittsburgh, PA, USA
e-mail: nadkarnink@upmc.edu

P. Bourgeat
CSIRO The Australian e-Health Research Centre, Brisbane, Australia
e-mail: Pierrick.Bourgeat@csiro.au

O. Lopez
Department of Neurology, University of Pittsburgh, Pittsburgh, PA, USA
e-mail: LopezOL@upmc.edu

M. D. Ikonomovic
Geriatric Research Education and Clinical Center, VA Pittsburgh Healthcare System, Pittsburgh, PA, USA
e-mail: ikonomovicmd@upmc.edu

A. D. Cohen
Department of Psychiatry, University of Pittsburgh, Pittsburgh, PA, USA
e-mail: cohenad@upmc.edu

© The Author(s), under exclusive license to Springer Nature Switzerland AG 2023
D. J. Cross et al. (eds.), *Molecular Imaging of Neurodegenerative Disorders*,
https://doi.org/10.1007/978-3-031-35098-6_6

Isoform	Tauopathy	Histopathology/Ultrastructure		
		light microscope (prevalent lesion)	electron microscope (prevalent ultrastructure)	Cryo-EM

Primary tauopathies

4R	Progressive supranuclear palsy	Globose tangles; Tufted astrocytes	SF (& TF)	PSP
4R	Corticobasal degeneration	Astrocytic plaques	SF (& TF)	CBD
4R	Argyrophilic grain disease	Limbic argyrophilic grains; Oligodendroglial coiled bodies	SF	AGD
				PiD
3R	Pick's disease	Pick's bodies	TF (& SF)	

Secondary tauopathies

3R & 4R	Alzheimer's disease	Neurofibrillary tangles	PHF (& SF)	AD
3R & 4R	Down Syndrome	Neurofibrillary tangles	PHF (& SF)	
3R & 4R	Chronic Traumatic Encephalopathy	Neurofibrillary tangles	PHF (& SF)	CTE
3R & 4R	Niemann-Pick disease type C	Neurofibrillary tangles	PHF (& SF)	

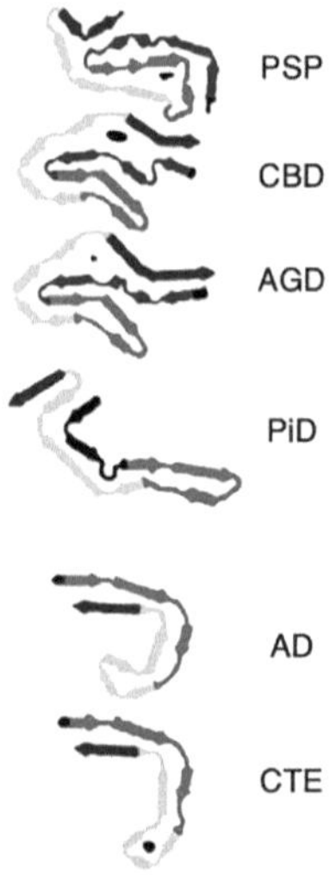

Fig. 6.1 Morphological, ultrastructural conformation, and fibrillar folding of tau isoforms across Primary and Secondary Tauopathies. *3R* three repeats, *4R* four repeats (where R denotes the number of microtubule binding domain repeats), *PHF* paired helical filaments, *SF* straight filaments, *TF* twisted filaments, *PSP* Progressive Supranuclear Palsy, *CBD* corticobasal degeneration, *AGD* argyrophilic grain disease, *PiD* Pick's disease, *AD* Alzheimer's disease, *CTE* chronic traumatic encephalopathy, *Cryo-EM* cryo-electron microscopy. (Adapted from Villemagne et al., Lancet Neurol, 2015; Shi et al., Nature, 2021)

dritic compartment [7]. In humans, six tau isoforms have been described, with distinct N-terminal projection and C-terminus microtubule binding domains [8]. The repeats of the microtubule binding domain have been used to classify the six tau isoforms into two different groups of isoforms, either those with three (3R) or four repeats (4R), respectively [8]. The prevalence of a certain isoform, or their combination is intrinsically associated with their ultrastructural conformation and with specific phenotypes, which can also be classified as primary and secondary tauopathies [4]. Primary tauopathies are characterized by the prevalence of aggregates of a single tau isoform, either 4R, like in PSP, or 3R like in Pick's disease (PiD), while secondary tauopathies are usually characterized by tau aggregates formed by a combination of both 3R and 4R tau isoforms as observed in AD and CTE (for review see [9]).

Tau aggregation into AD tangles is a complex pathobiological process that involves dynamic post-translational modifications in its structure, conformational, and phosphorylation states [10,

11]. As with Aβ, tau fibrils are detectable histologically in hallmark neuropathological lesions of AD, however, prefibrillar forms of soluble oligomeric tau have been considered an early pathological change that is toxic to neurons and their synapses [12, 13]. There is a conformational switch in some parts of the sequence of the unfolded tau protein, leading to a structural transformation from mostly random coil to a fibrillar β-sheet structure, and this transition leads to tau aggregation in the form of filamentous inclusions [14, 15]. Furthermore, newly synthesized tau leads to the breakdown of dendritic microtubules, mitochondria mislocalization, and depletion of dendritic spines [16, 17]. While the mechanisms leading to tau hyperphosphorylation, misfolding, and aggregation have not been fully elucidated, tau pathology tends to evolve in a stereotypical spatiotemporal manner which results in a predictable neuroanatomical distribution in the brain, reflected in the Braak & Braak and Delacourte stages [18–20]. This sequential stereotypical pattern of tau lesions' regional onset and progression has been interpreted recently as a pathogenic propagation of tau [21]. The seeding forms of tau—either normal or abnormal—which initiate and promote pathological tau "transmission" in animal models, the mechanism/s driving the hypothetical release of tau forms into the synapses, and potential roles of exosomes, ectosomes, and tunnelling nanotubes [22] remain to be determined. Relevant to tau imaging, others have proposed that amplification may be more important than propagation of tau [23].

Recent studies using cryo-electron microscopy (CryoEM) characterized the folding patterns of tau aggregates in different tauopathies (for review see [24]) (Fig. 6.1). Combined with molecular dynamics and docking studies, as well as calculations of quantum mechanical fragmentation [25], these studies seek to elucidate specific locations for tau tracers binding on different fibrillar tau aggregates, aiding in the design and development of new and potentially more selective tracers for different tauopathies [25–27].

Besides their pathophysiological significance, the conformation or folding of tau aggregates have important biomarker implications [4, 24]. Moreover, the conformation adopted by these tau fibrils allows phosphorylation of certain epitopes, contributing to the evolution of tau lesions and affecting the degree of seeding, which may be related to different ages of onset and different rates of disease progression [28].

Understanding the mechanisms of tau formation, aggregation, and spreading is important for biomarker development as well as the design of effective anti-tau therapy [29]. Most neurodegenerative conditions are associated with a folded or misfolded aggregated protein. The challenge from a clinical point of view is that a single clinical phenotype can be caused by different aggregated proteins or a single aggregated protein can be the underlying cause of several different clinical phenotypes. Further complicating the issue is that an abnormal protein like tau, undergoes multiple post-translational modifications and can adopt various conformations. Thus, it is imperative to identify pathognomonic tau forms responsible for distinct clinical presentations, in order to design highly disease-specific biomarkers and implement, when available, an appropriate disease-modifying therapy that, in the particular case of progressive neurodegenerative conditions, needs to be implement early, before irreversible neuronal loss occurs.

Selective Tau Imaging Tracers

Tau PET has been the most recent addition to the arsenal of tools for the non-invasive imaging assessment of neurodegenerative proteinopathies. Until recently, postmortem examination of the brain was the only definite way to ascertain the presence and extent of specific pathologies in the brain [30]. Despite the idiosyncratic characteristics of tau pathophysiology which complicate the design of tau imaging ligands (intracellular location, different isoforms, multiple post-translational modifications, heterogeneous ultrastructural conformations, in the case of AD much lower concentrations than co-localized Aβ aggregates (for review see [9])), there has been a tremendous amount of progress in the last few years, with several selective tau tracers being extensively applied to research studies, furthering our understanding of tauopathies as well as the relationship of tau with Aβ and its role in neurodegeneration and cognitive decline in AD [31–38].

Among early-generation selective tau tracers, ^{18}F-flortaucipir (FTP) (a.k.a. Tauvid®, AV1451 or T807) [31, 39] (Fig. 6.2) is approved by the Food and Drug Administration (FDA) for clinical use and has been applied most widely in human research studies. Also among early-generation tau tracers we find the THK tracer series, namely ^{18}F-THK523, ^{18}F-THK5105, ^{18}F-THK5317, and ^{18}F-THK5351 [40–43] (Fig. 6.2), and ^{11}C-PBB3 [32] (Fig. 6.2). This early-generation series was characterized by somewhat low signal-to-noise contrast and noticeable "off-target" binding. Clinical studies with second-generation tracers such as ^{18}F-RO948, ^{18}F-GTP1 (Fig. 6.2) have shown less noticeable "off-target" binding to choroid plexus [35], while others such as ^{18}F-MK6240 or ^{18}F-PI2620 (Fig. 6.2) have shown a different pattern of "off-target" binding to meninges or longitudinal sinuses, respectively [33, 38].

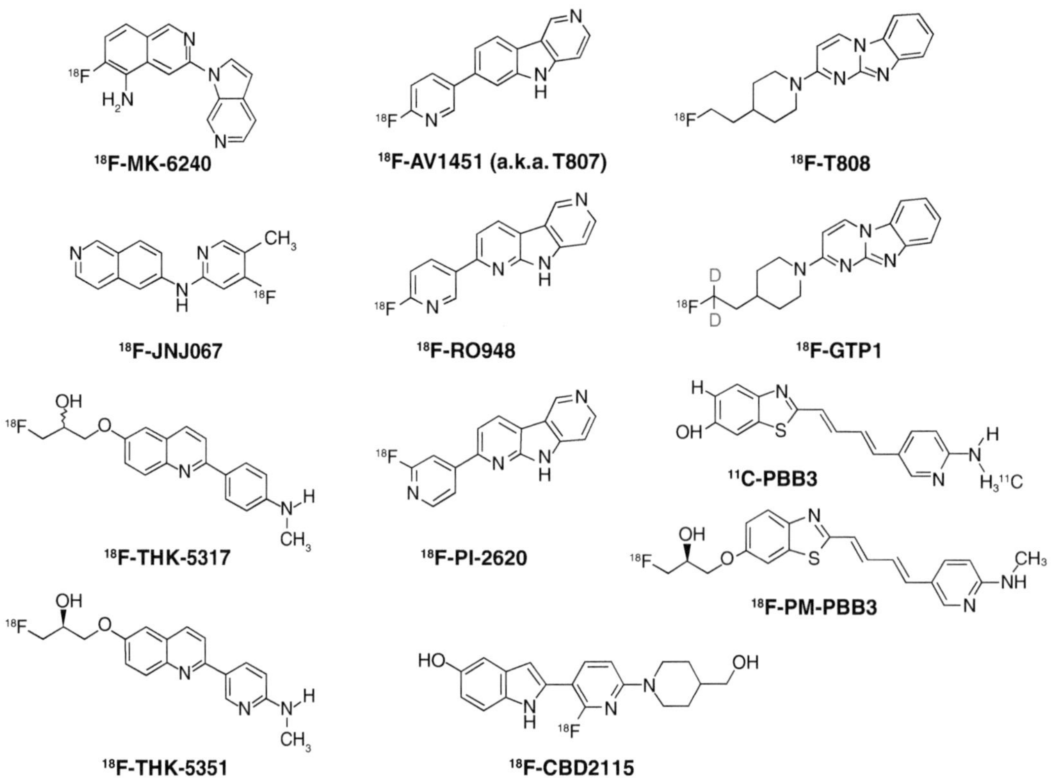

Fig. 6.2 Tau tracers. Chemical structure of several selective tau ligands

The development of selective tau tracers was preceded by many early unsuccessful efforts like those of, for example, Okamura and colleagues [44]. This was followed by the synthesis and characterization of ^{18}F-FDDNP, a radiofluorinated tracer binding non-selectively to both extracellular Aβ plaques and intracellular NFT [45, 46], which, despite its lack of selectivity and limited dynamic range, has been used in the assessment of several neurodegenerative conditions from AD to PSP, from Down syndrome to CTE [47–50].

As confirmed from preclinical in vitro studies, most selective tau tracers were designed to bind the most prevalent isoforms found in AD (3R/4R combination) [51, 52] and have lower of null affinity for the 3R and/or 4R tau isoforms prevalent in primary tauopathies and in marmosets. The combination of lower affinity, a much lower density of tau deposits and a different conformation/folding of the tau fibrils all contribute to the inability of most of these 3R/4R tracers to bind the 4R and 3R tau deposits found in primary

tauopathies like PSP or PiD. A tracer specifically designed to bind 4R tau, ^{18}F-CBD2115 (Fig. 6.2), was not able to cross the blood–brain barrier [53]. On the other hand, there is preclinical and clinical evidence that ^{18}F-PI2620 [54, 55] and ^{18}F-PM-PBB3 [56] bind to 4R tau deposits.

The THK Series: ^{18}F-THK523, ^{18}F-THK5105, ^{18}F-THK5117, and ^{18}F-THK5351

Since 2002, researchers at Tohoku University in Japan have been developing and screening small β-sheet binding molecules targeting misfolded proteins. Several derivatives were identified as potential tau imaging candidates [57, 58]. The first of these derivatives, ^{18}F-THK523, showed low nanomolar affinity to tau fibrils, a 12-fold selectivity for tau over Aβ, and significant in vivo tracer retention in a tau transgenic mouse model, while failing to bind to non-AD tau lesions, or to α-synuclein deposits [59–61]. First-in-human

PET studies showed that while there was a significant higher neocortical ^{18}F-THK523 retention in AD patients than cognitively normal controls, in both groups the non-specific white matter retention was significantly higher than in gray matter, precluding visual inspection of the images [42]. Three novel derivatives, ^{18}F-THK5105, ^{18}F-THK5117, and ^{18}F-THK5351, were developed [58]. Both ^{18}F-THK5105 and ^{18}F-THK5117 showed higher binding affinity than ^{18}F-THK523 to *uber* phosphorylated tau-rich AD brain homogenates [58]. First-in-human ^{18}F-THK5105 and ^{18}F-THK5117 (and its *S* enantiomer, ^{18}F-THK5317) PET studies showed a robust visual and quantitative separation between AD patients and healthy control subjects in those brain areas known to have high burden of tau pathology in AD brains [43]. Furthermore, tracer retention was correlated with dementia severity and brain atrophy [43]. As described for ^{18}F-AV-1451, the tau tracers of the THK series also show "off-target" unexplained high tracer retention in the striatum, even in cognitively unimpaired subjects, while THK5105 and THK5117 also have very high non-specific retention in the midbrain, pons and cerebellar white matter. While the latest addition to the series, ^{18}F-THK-5351 presented a much better kinetic profile, low metabolism, much lower white matter retention and higher signal-to-noise ratios than ^{18}F-THK5105 and ^{18}F-THK-5117 [43], it mainly bound MAO-B, not tau. Recently, this group have developed a new highly selective tau tracer, 18F-SNFT-1, with very high affinity for tau aggregates [62, 63].

[18]F-Flortaucipir (a.k.a. ^{18}F-Tauvid®, ^{18}F-AV1451, ^{18}F-T807)

A benzimidazole-pyrimidines derivative, ^{18}F-T807 [64] (Fig. 6.3) with nanomolar affinity and more than a 25-fold selectivity for PHF-tau over Aβ, was identified by Kolb and colleagues [31, 64, 66]. Initial human ^{18}F-T807 PET studies showed cortical retention that followed the known distribution of PHF-tau in the AD brain (Fig. 6.3) low white matter retention, and a strong association with disease severity [31]. Acquired by Avid Radiophamaceuticals, it was rebranded AV1451, and later flortaucipir. Under the name of

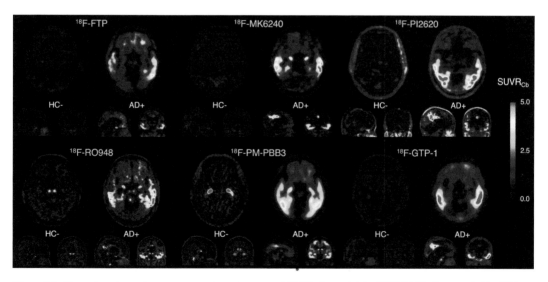

Fig. 6.3 Tau imaging in Alzheimer's disease. Representative sagittal, transaxial, and coronal PET images in healthy elderly controls (HC) and Alzheimer's disease (AD) patients obtained with different tau imaging radiotracers. From left to right, PET images were obtained with ^{18}F-FTP (top left), ^{18}F-MK6240 (top center), ^{18}F-PI2620 (top right), ^{18}F-RO948 (bottom left), ^{18}F-PM-PBB3 (bottom center), and ^{18}F-GTP1 (bottom right). In AD patients, there is marked cortical retention in mesial temporal, temporoparietal and posterior cingulate regions, sometimes extending to the frontal cortex. (Adapted from Doré et al. [65])

Tauvid®, it is the only tau tracer approved by the FDA for clinical use.

Flortaucipir (FTP) is the most widely used tau tracer. Most of this chapter will address studies performed with FTP, from the initial clinical PET studies assessing tau (FTP) and Aβ (PiB) in healthy controls, MCI and AD patients [39, 40, 67] to the pre-mortem PET post-mortem correlation studies [68] that led to the approval by the FDA.

^{11}C-PBB3 and ^{18}F-PM-PBB3

The ^{11}C labeled tau tracer, ^{11}C-PBB3, (Fig. 6.2) was developed by CHIBA which underwent a thorough preclinical evaluation [32, 69]. Although metabolite analysis revealed that only 2% of the parent compound remained at 5 min after injection, 70% of unchanged ^{11}C-PBB3 was found in mice brain homogenates [69]. Clinical studies in cognitively unimpaired participants assessed with both ^{11}C-PBB3 and ^{11}C-PiB showed a different pattern of brain retention between the two tracers suggesting that at high specific activities ^{11}C-PBB3 selectively binds to tau [32]. A ^{11}C-PBB3-PET study in a patient diagnosed with CBD showed tracer retention in the basal ganglia, suggesting ^{11}C-PBB3 might bind other non-AD tau conformations. The problem is that ^{11}C-PBB3 has a lipohillic radiolabeled metabolite that enters the brain [70]. Eventually the tracer was abandoned and a F-18 version was developed [71]. ^{18}F-PM-PBB3 presents a much better dynamic range, much better signal to background contrast although with increased off-target retention in choroid plexus [71] (Fig. 6.3). These PBB3 tracers need to be handled with care because they undergo photoisomerization when exposed to light [69]. PBB3 and ^{18}F-PI2620 are currently the only tau tracers that have also shown binding in primary 4R tauopathies like PSP and CBD.

^{18}F-PI2620

Initially developed by AC Immune and licensed to Life Molecular Imaging [54], ^{18}F-PI2620 showed high cortical tracer retention in AD patients [72–74]. (Fig. 6.3) As described for PBB3, ^{18}F-PI2620 also binds to 4R tauopathies [75] but requires dynamic imaging acquisition and imaging quantification to allow visualizing of the distinct regional distribution of 4R tau in PSP and CBD [55, 76] (Fig. 6.4). ^{18}F-PI2620 has been used to show that potentially tau spreads throughout the brain following functional networks [77], and its binding kinetics allow to distinguish between primary and secondary tauopathies [78].

^{18}F-RO948

Developed by Roche it was initially tested by Wong and colleagues showing high cortical tracer retention in AD patients compared to cognitively normal controls [79], following the known distribution of tau pathology in AD brains (Fig. 6.3) and reaching apparent steady state 3–4 h after injection [80]. ^{18}F-RO948 was adopted by the Biofinder study in Sweden [81]. ^{18}F-RO948 has a similar chemical scaffold as FTP, and in a head-to-head study, ^{18}F-RO948 showed less off-target binding in basal ganglia and choroid plexus, although higher in the scalp [82]. Like FTP, ^{18}F-RO948 has been shown to have high accuracy to distinguish AD from non-AD neurodegeneration [83].

^{18}F-GTP1/^{18}F-T808

Like ^{18}F-T807 (FTP), ^{18}F-T808 was also developed by Kolb and colleagues [66]. While initial human PET studies showed that ^{18}F-T808 presented with faster tracer kinetics than ^{18}F-T807, reaching steady state during the scanning period, substantial defluorination was observed [66]. A PET-autopsy correlation case report in an AD patient who died 5 months after the ^{18}F-T808 PET scan showed high agreement between the in vivo ^{18}F-T808 cortical retention and post-mortem fluorescent PHF-tau staining [84]. Unfortunately, this tracer was abandoned due to defluorination. A deuterized version to prevent defluorination— ^{18}F-GTP1—was developed by Genentech and tested in clinical studies [85] (Fig. 6.3). One particularity of this tracer is that it is probably the

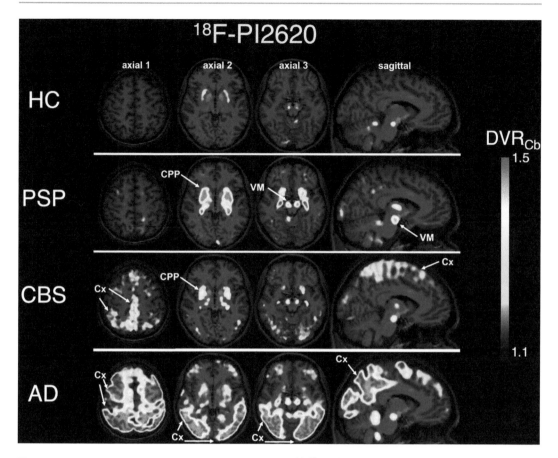

Fig. 6.4 Tau imaging in AD and non-AD tauopathies. Representative sagittal, transaxial, and coronal DVR PET images in a healthy elderly controls (HC, top row) Progressive Supranuclear Palsy (PSP, second row) patient, a Corticobasal syndrome (CBS, third row) patient, and an Alzheimer's disease (AD, bottom row) patient obtained with ^{18}F-PI2620. There is typical cortical and subcortical tracer retention in PSP and CBS 4R tauopathies, which is also much lower that the retention observed in a 3R/4R tauopathy such as AD. (Images courtesy of Dr Matthias Brendel, University Hospital of Munich, LMU Munich, Munich, Germany)

only tau tracer that reaches apparent steady state within 90 min after injection in those with high density of tau pathology in the brain [85]. It has been shown that the degree of ^{18}F-GTP1 retention in the brain is with level of cognitive function, and that it can also predict cognitive decline [86, 87].

^{18}F-MK6240

A recently introduced selective high-affinity 3R/4R tau tracer, ^{18}F-MK6240 [33, 88, 89], has shown high contrast images with low non-specific binding and negligible off-target binding in choroid plexus and basal ganglia [88–93].

^{18}F-MK6240 provides high contrast images with a large dynamic range of SUVR (Fig. 6.3). From a semiquantitative point of view, it has been previously shown that SUVR has a high correlation with BP_{ND} and distribution volume ratio (DVR) [88, 89] and a test-retest variability <7% [94]. While off-target retention in meninges was observed in 8–10% of the cases, there was no off-target binding in choroid plexus and striatum as observed with FTP and PM-PBB3 and, to a lesser degree, with ^{18}F-GTP-1 [85] and ^{18}F-RO948 [95]. The absence of off-target binding in the choroid plexus is important because it allows the examination of MTL structures including the hippocampus without having to account for the potential spill-over from the choroid plexus or, in order to avoid performing complex corrections, discard from the analysis this region that plays a critical role in memory function and is affected early in AD. On the other hand, there are some cases with focal "off-target" accumulation of the tracer in the region of the clivus that might affect assessment of the parahippocampus [89]. As with most tau imaging tracers, there was also off-target retention in anterior midbrain, likely reflecting specific (saturable) binding to melanin [51]. In a head-to-head study with FTP, ^{18}F-MK6240 showed a larger dynamic range and higher contrast, and while there was no off-target binding in basal ganglia and choroid plexus, there was off-target binding to meninges and clivus [89].

^{18}F-MK6240 can detect lower tau levels than earlier tau tracers, crucial for early detection of tau deposition and tracking small tau changes over time. Identification of regional cortical tau deposition has critical diagnostic and prognostic implications and should become a standard tool to identify individuals at risk, and outcome measure, in both anti-Aβ and anti-tau trials.

^{18}F-JNJ-067

Kolb and colleagues developed the most recent entry to the list of selective tau tracers, ^{18}F-JNJ-064326067 (^{18}F-JNJ-067) [96]. Initial clinical studies showed that it can distinguish AD from controls, but presented off-target binding in basal ganglia, midbrain, superior cerebellar gray, and white matter [97, 98]. Initial studies also observed that while it can differentiate AD patients from healthy older controls, that was not the case with MCI or PSP patients suggesting ^{18}F-JNJ-067 may not bind to low levels of AD-related tau pathology or 4R tau aggregates in PSP [98].

Off-Target, Missed Target, and Unclear Binding

With the exception of FTP, current tau tracers have not yet been validated against neuropathology and several case reports have highlighted the

discrepancies between the preclinical in vitro profile of, for example, FTP, the in vivo human PET studies [51, 99], as well as some ante-mortem/post-mortem inconsistencies [100, 101]. As these case reports show, these inconsistencies do not apply to 3R/4R tau paired helical filaments (PHF) found in AD, but mainly to the straight 4R tau filaments found in PSP and CBS. When PET studies in PSP patients are compared at a group level to controls, they show a distinct pattern of tracer retention in the pallidum, midbrain, and dentate nuclei of the cerebellum [102–104], but post-mortem case report studies on some of these patients failed to show binding of the tracer to these structures despite presenting the typical tau lesions [100, 101]. This may be due to a low binding affinity that cannot survive the series of washes required for the in vitro autoradiographic studies.

Another issue to consider is the degree of non-specific binding. For example, in a study by Baker and colleagues [105], it was established that ~60% of the FTP binding in low Aβ controls was non-specific, suggesting that it would be more difficult to detect small levels of early tau accumulation.

There is no tau tracer devoid of off-target binding. Choroid plexus are prominently observed with FTP, PM-PBB3, and GTP-1, tracer retention in basal ganglia is observed in studies with FTP, the longitudinal sinuses are very prominent with PI2620, as skull/meninges with RO948, and retention in the meninges and clivus are frequently observed with MK6240. All tau tracers have some degree of binding to the anterior midbrain that actually seems to be specific (saturable) binding to melanin [51].

Much more problematic is when these tracers bind to a different target as in the case of THK5351. In other words, what we call "off-target" might just be an "alternative" target. In this particular case, it has been shown that an hour after a single oral dose of 5 mg of selegiline there was about a 35% and 50% reduction in the cortical and basal ganglia THK5351 signal, respectively [62], and when a 5 mg selegiline regimen twice daily for 5 days was followed, more than 80% of the signal was lost [106]. This suggests that THK5351 is mainly binding to monoamine oxidase B (MAO-B), clearly indicating that THK5351 is not suitable for selective tau imaging studies.

Another issue is the low hippocampal signal observed with some of these tracers, compounded by the erratic binding to choroid plexus adjacent to the hippocampus. While some have proposed that in the choroid plexus these tracers bind to β-sheet aggregated tau deposits [107] previously described in aged and AD brains as Biondi "ring" tangles [108] or to another β-sheet aggregated protein such as transthyretin, pigments such as lipofuscin, or calcifications [99, 108, 109], in vitro autoradiographic studies failed to detect tracer binding in choroid plexus or striatum [51, 101]. The low signal in the hippocampus in relation to the entorhinal cortex might actually reflect different concentrations of PHF-tau in the two regions, where the reported concentration of PHF-tau in the entorhinal cortex is almost twice the one observed in the hippocampus [110].

Tau Quantification and Sampling

Tau tracers differ in their molecular structures which is reflected in different tau binding affinities, in vivo kinetics, degree of non-specific binding, different regional patterns of "off-target" binding, leading to disparity in PET-derived measurements across tracers. Furthermore, variations in scanning protocols and quantification pipelines even when using the same tau tracer, further increases inconsistencies, decreasing reproducibility. It is important to remember that most of these tau tracers do not reach apparent steady state during the scanning period, and while the use of tissue ratios was adopted early in the implementation of these tracers, kinetic characterization should lead to optimization of scanning protocols [80, 85, 111, 112]. Moreover, the availability of different tau tracers in use by different centers is a challenge for the comparison of the results across sites, which is also a problem when implementing an international multicenter therapeutic trial. In a similar way this problem was addressed with the different Aβ tracers that were

linearly transformed into a universal scale, the Centiloids (CL). We are implementing a similar approach toward a universal tau mask and scale through a multinational collaborative project for the six most commonly used tau radiotracers: FTP, MK6240, PI2620, PM-PBB3, RO948, and GTP-1 (Fig. 6.3). The first step was to construct a universal cortical mask based on the intersection of the subtraction of the signal in Aβ + AD patients and Aβ− controls. This global mask also avoids sampling the different off-target regions idiosyncratic for each tracer [65]. This was followed by the creation of four regional masks—mesial temporal, metatemporal, temporoparietal, and frontal—that were limited to the areas common to all six tau tracers. Then we developed a universal scale—the CenTauR—[113] to be applied both regionally and globally, either adopting a z-score—CenTauR$_Z$—or a linear transformation—CenTauR$_{ES}$—while ensuring a same abnormality threshold value across tracers [114]. Adopting a similar approach, but using Gaussian mixed modeling, we constructed a universal cerebellar cortex refence region that avoids common off-target binding regions like the head of the vermis and the meninges. Head-to-head studies across tracers, and only a few were conducted to date [82, 115], will also help understand and address the differences across tracers.

Another aspect that impacts clinical interpretation is how and what regions of the brain to sample, and what should be considered "high" or clinically meaningful tau signal [116]. Given the low spatial resolution of PET, its counterproductive to impose a neuropathological piecemeal Braak and Braak staging [19], not even a better defined ten stages of Delacourte [18] to the sampling of tau imaging studies [67, 93]. Given the variability of the staging, neuropathologists themselves reduce them to three stages (0–I–II, III–IV, and V–VI). On the other hand, several authors have shown that data driven approaches [77, 117, 118, 119] are better suited to capture the tau distribution, tau levels and tau progression in tau PET studies. Sampling of Braak I, II, and even III will make the partial volume effects more critical. Atypical presentations of tau deposits, and how they relate to the clinical phenotype [120, 121], are missed by the incrementally sequential Braak and Braak staging. Several cognitive domains intimately related to tau deposition do not match the Braak and Braak staging either [122]. Applying the Braak and Braak or Delacourte staging [18, 19] is further complicated by the different neuropathological subtypes of tau deposition [123]. From the pathological subtypes only the typical (reported to be between 55 and 75% in different series) [124–126] fulfills the required sequential Braak and Braak stages. Several reports have shown that a metatemporal region [127] or a temporoparietal (and post-cingulate) AD-signature region [128, 129] outperform the Braak and Braak staging for the early detection of cortical tau, to establish the differential diagnosis of AD vs. non-AD neurodegenerative conditions [130], as well as to capture the longitudinal changes in cortical tau [119, 131]. These regions seems to perform reliably across different centers and using different tracers, and despite these tracers presenting different dynamic ranges, they yielded the same cut-off for abnormality in different cohorts [132]. While the use of tau imaging for disease staging is strongly recommended [133] the use of neuropathological staging should be applied carefully, not as an a priori condition, but as the result of the actual observed pattern of tau deposition on the PET images.

Furthermore, it has been shown that tau imaging, at least with FTP [68], can reliably detect a B3 stage (equivalent to Braak V–VI), so trying to use this tracer for detection of lower Braak stages (I–III) would yield less reliable results.

The AT(N) Research Framework

Neuroimaging studies have shown that about 25% of cognitively unimpaired individuals exhibit evidence of "AD-like" neurodegeneration in the absence of Aβ deposition [134, 135], corroborating the notion that neurodegenerative changes such as hippocampal atrophy, while almost always present in AD, are non-specific of AD, and can be found in other non-AD neurodegenerative conditions such as limbic-predominant age-related TDP-43 encephalopathy (LATE)

with hippocampal sclerosis [136, 137] or in primary age-related tauopathy (PART) [138].

About a decade ago, biochemical and imaging biomarkers were proposed as part of the new diagnostic criteria for Alzheimer's disease [139–141], MCI [142], and preclinical Alzheimer's disease [143].

Along these precise lines, and in a similar way as is routinely applied in oncology [144], it has been proposed to refine the assessment of elderly individuals using biomarkers, ascertaining not only the presence or absence of Aβ pathology with either PET imaging, plasma or CSF, neurodegeneration with cortical or hippocampal atrophy as measured by MRI [145], glucose hypometabolism as measured by FDG PET [146], plasma or CSF Neurofilament Light (NfL) [147]. but also incorporating tau status based on tau imaging or CSF or plasma p-tau [148]. Thus, as the criteria for AD evolves, and is defined by its biology, imaging of protein aggregates of Aβ and tau is likely to play an increasingly crucial role as these techniques are affordably translated into clinical practice [149].

Tau Imaging in Alzheimer's Disease

In AD, a wealth of genetic, cellular and biochemical evidence points at Aβ as being an essential part of a cascade of events preceding and potentially leading to tau deposition, neurodegeneration and dementia [150, 151]. While this supports the value of Aβ as an early biomarker of AD, post-mortem and Aβ imaging studies with PET have clearly demonstrated that Aβ plaque density is poorly associated with cognitive impairment in AD [152, 153]. In contrast, the density of neurofibrillary tangles (NFT) is strongly associated with cognitive impairment and neurodegeneration [152, 154–156]. These patterns could be described by different trajectories of Aβ and tau deposition, with Aβ deposits advancing and reaching a plateau earlier in the disease process than tau pathology which keeps continuously accumulating across clinical disease stages. Furthermore, studies reported that Aβ oligomers are toxic to synapses [157–159] and that Aβ association with cognitive decline in AD is mediated by tau [160–162]. Furthermore, there is a 25–35% prevalence of Aβ deposits in cognitively unimpaired individuals [163–165]. Put together, these studies suggest that Aβ is an early and necessary, though clearly not sufficient, cause for cognitive decline in AD [166], indicating that other mechanisms, such as neuroinflammation, either triggered or not by Aβ, contribute to synaptic failure and eventually neuronal loss.

Initial tau PET imaging studies of AD demonstrated that the regional pattern of tau tracer retention in the brain corresponded to the known distribution of aggregated tau pathology in autopsy brain tissue [18, 19] (Fig. 6.3). PET alterations in tau are intimately associated with cognitive performance [87], and that high tau PET signal in Aβ + individuals can predict cognitive decline in the short term [86, 167, 168], much better than Aβ PET signal alone [169]. Tau tracer retention has a close global and regional relationship with imaging markers of neurodegeneration such as MRI measures of cortical gray matter atrophy or ^{18}F-FDG PET [170–172] while also being highly predictive of changes in gray matter atrophy and glucose metabolism in the short term [173, 174]. Some studies have shown that tau imaging is highly specific and has exquisite differential diagnostic accuracy against other neurodegenerative conditions at the advanced stages of AD dementia, although it is much less accurate at the prodromal (MCI) stage of AD [95, 130]. Tau imaging has even been proposed as a "one-stop shop" for the evaluation of dementing neurodegenerative conditions [175]. To date, all tau PET tracers have present drawbacks such as "off-target" retention areas in the choroid plexus, basal ganglia, longitudinal sinuses or meninges [99] and some show strong binding to monoamine oxidase B (MAO-B) instead of tau [62]. Moreover, some of these tracers' high non-specific binding likely precludes detection of low levels of tau deposition [105]. This might explain why ^{18}F-FTP has very high accuracy in severe AD cases with Braak stages V–VI [68] while it might be much less accurate at detecting earlier stages of tau pathology.

In contrast to CSF or plasma biomarkers, tau imaging provides insight into the regional distribution of tau pathology in the brain (Fig. 6.3). Given the close relationship between tau pathology, cognitive impairment, and neuronal injury, the ability of tau PET to assess both density, extent and regional distribution of tau pathology in the brain can be used for disease staging and to predict clinical progression. While Aβ PET imaging studies have shown that the actual global amount of Aβ in the brain is more relevant than the regional Aβ distribution as an early driver of cognitive decline, post-mortem and initial imaging studies of tau indicate that not only the amount of tau deposition, but also—or mainly—their topographical distribution in the brain [18, 176] might be more relevant and more tightly associated with neurodegeneration and cognitive decline. While most of the research and clinical applications of tau PET imaging are identical to those of Aβ PET imaging (Table 6.1), some potential applications, like disease staging, tracking disease progression, or as surrogate or outcome marker for an anti-Aβ or anti-tau therapeutic trial are better served by assessing tau pathophysiology.

Several groups have reported a robust difference in tau tracer retention between cognitively normal elderly controls and Aβ + AD patients [39, 40, 67, 177–179], as well as in atypical

Table 6.1 Applications of tau imaging

- Accurate and early diagnosis of the underlying pathology
- Assessment of the spatial and temporal pattern of abnormal tau deposition and its relation to age, cognitive performance, disease progression, genotype, and other disease biomarkers
- Validation of new imaging, genetic, cognitive, and fluid biomarkers
  - Disease staging and prognosis
  - Identification of at-risk individuals allows early disease-specific interventions
- Disease-specific trials
  - Patient selection
  - Establish target floor (and ceiling) values for inclusion criteria
  - Proof of target engagement
  - Identification of optimal time window for intervention
  - Monitor effectiveness/surrogate marker/outcome measure

Alzheimer's disease presentations where tau tracer regional retention—not Aβ as assessed by PiB—matched the clinical phenotype [180–182]. Furthermore, ^{18}F-FTP retention, especially in the temporal lobe, correlated with CSF tau levels [183, 184]. Tau PET imaging is helping elucidate the relationship between tau pathology and cognition, where increasing cortical tau levels in Aβ + individuals were associated with increasing impairment in several cognitive domains [67, 184, 185].

Interestingly, most PET imaging studies of AD are showing that while mesial temporal tau signal is high irrespective of neocortical Aβ levels, high tau signal in neocortical regions is in more than 95% of the cases associated with high neocortical Aβ load, suggesting *detectable* (i.e., above PET threshold level) neocortical Aβ precedes *detectable* cortical tau. Moreover, the association between tau levels and age increases in the presence of Aβ [67]. Tau PET imaging studies are showing not only that tau tracer retention follows the known regional evolution of aggregated tau pathology in the brain [19, 186], but also its close relationship with markers of neuronal metabolic and degenerative changes such as FDG PET or cortical gray matter atrophy [172, 173, 187].

In contrast with cortical tau PET signal, postmortem reports from the early 70s [188] reported the presence of tau pathology in the mesial temporal cortex in both demented and non-demented individuals. Similar findings were later reported by Price and Morris [163] and by Delacourte and colleagues [18], the latter stating that "*tauopathy of the hippocampal formation in humans is age-related but not an age-dependent process, also independent of AD, but amplified by APP dysfunctions*" [186]. Amidst some controversy, this almost 50-year old observation [188] has been recently rebranded as PART [138, 189–191]. It is believed that this age-related tau accumulation in the mesial temporal cortex might have mild albeit significant Aβ-independent effects on cognition [192] as well as hippocampal atrophy [191, 193, 194]. If we also consider cortical Aβ, it has been observed that high mesial temporal tau and high diffuse cortical Aβ are both present in some cognitively unimpaired elderly individuals suggesting that these "early" pathologies might not be sufficient to cause significant cognitive impairment, impairment that is only manifest when tau deposits accumulate more substantially in the mesial temporal lobe and also involve cortical polymodal and unimodal association areas of the brain, the point when neocortical Aβ plaque load has already reached high levels [42]. Longitudinal selective tau imaging in combination with Aβ imaging studies are assessing if, how and how much Aβ accelerates and/or triggers the growth of tau deposits outside the mesial temporal cortex, and if this initial dissemination into cortical association areas is manifested as insidious and incipient objective cognitive impairment known as MCI [163, 186]. Post-mortem data suggest that further evolution of tau pathology in the remaining cortical areas is usually observed in individuals with severe cognitive deterioration and dementia [163, 186]. There is emerging evidence of this "neuropathological sequence" of events that will need to be verified by assessing pre-mortem and post-mortem studies, as it is one of the crucial issues being addressed by combining Aβ and tau imaging studies [151].

While the vast majority of AD patients present with both high Aβ and high tau PET levels [39, 67, 181], about 15–20% of subjects diagnosed as probable AD and with high neocortical Aβ in the brain, have subthreshold levels of neocortical tau tracer retention. This might be related to differential regional onset of Aβ (neocortex) and tau (entorhinal cortex/hippocampus) pathologies, as defined by Thal phases [195] and Braak stages [196] respectively. Additionally, it might either reflect a limitation of the currently available tracers (f.e. binding affinity, isoform selectivity, tracer kinetics, and/or metabolism, etc.), differences in the conformation of tau aggregates, as has been observed in some cases of Aβ imaging, low concentration of binding sites or low affinity for pretangle pathology, especially observed at the early stages of cortical tau deposition, concentrations that can be below the threshold of detectability by current PET scanners (which depends on the regional density of binding sites that, compounded with partial volume effects in small or atrophic brain areas, might not be able to yield accurate readout of low-level tau pathology in the brain), or a problem derived from the thresholds used to determine high and low tau (although some of the cases have almost no detectable tau tracer retention). Or a combination or interaction between some or all of the above. Another possible confounder is misdiagnosis, where high Aβ in the brain and an amnestic presentation, which certainly indicates that these patients are on the AD pathway, might not yet be in the dementia stage, stage usually associated with widespread cortical tau deposits. Longitudinal studies of the cognitive trajectories are being conducted in order to elucidate the significance of this phenomenon.

Tau Imaging in Neurodegenerative Dementias and Non-AD Tauopathies

Although most tau these tracers were designed for binding 3R/4R paired helical filaments—the most prevalent tau isoform and conformation in AD—tau imaging is permitting assessment of other neurodegenerative conditions such as DLB where tau tracer retention follows a similar brain distribution than in AD but to a lower degree and a lower prevalence [197, 198]. Tau imaging has also been used to asses participants with Down Syndrome, where the pattern of brain tau tracer retention was very similar to the one observed in AD [199, 200]. Conversely, the brain pattern of tau tracer retention was different in participants with Niemann Pick type C disease [201].

While most of tau tracers do not bind to 3R tau, tau imaging has been somewhat helpful in cases of frontotemporal lobar degeneration with MAPT mutations [202–204], the high tracer retention in cases of the semantic variant of FTLD, which is characterized by the translocation and aggregation of TDP-43 not tau, remains unexplained [205]. Initial studies in primary tauopathies showed little or no binding to 4R

aggregated tau, and a slight difference at a group level, where the typical regional distribution of tau deposits aided in the differential diagnosis of these disorders that might initially present as either aphasia or Parkinsonism [103, 104]. While the search for a selective 3R and/or a 4R tau tracer continues, the introduction of newly developed tau tracers—namely PI-2620 and PM-PBB3—allow imaging and quantification of 4R tau in primary tauopathies. Such as PSP and CBD [55, 76, 206, 207] (Fig. 6.4).

Chronic traumatic encephalopathy (CTE) is, according to neuropathological diagnostic criteria, a neurodegenerative 3R/4R tauopathy associated with a history of repetitive head trauma. Despite being a 3R/4R tauopathy, the folding of the tau fibrils as assessed by Cryo-EM are slightly different from the folding of the tau fibrils in AD [26]. The pattern of tau tracer retention in symptomatic retired football players with a history of repetitive head trauma [208, 209] matches the known distribution of tau aggregates at Stages 3 and 4 of the McKee classification of CTE [210, 211], with high tau in superior frontal and mesial temporal regions, in stark contrast to the predominantly posterior tau deposition observed in patients with AD dementia [185].

When tau pathology accumulates in the mesial temporal lobe in the absence of detectable Aβ pathology, it is usually referred to as primary age-related tauopathy (PART) [138]. Given that there is a high prevalence of some degree of tau pathology in the mesial temporal lobe in individuals cognitively performing within normal limits [67, 212], PART is often regarded as a feature of the aging process [138]. PART is part of the reason why tau tracer retention exclusively in the mesial temporal lobe should not be used to categorize a patient as T+. On the other hand, PART might not be as benign as commonly thought, where Aβ− individuals with high mesial temporal tau, while performing within the normal limits for their age, presented with significant worse cognitive performance that their age-matched Aβ− individuals with low mesial temporal tau [192]. Furthermore, high mesial temporal lobe tau could also be a harbinger of cortical tau [192].

Relationship with Tau Biofluid Biomarkers

While most *uber* phosphorylated tau will accumulate retrogradely into the somatodendritic compartment leading to intracellular ("classic") neurofibrillary tangle formation, soluble tau is also released into the intrasynaptic/interstitial space. There have been tremendous recent advances in the development and implementation of biofluid biomarkers, especially those measured in plasma [213, 214] to the point that appropriate criteria for their use has been recommended [215]. Several plasma p-tau markers has been proposed: p-tau181 [216], p-tau217 [217], and p-tau231 [218] and while they correlate well with tau PET, they tend to correlate even better with Aβ imaging. This is likely related to the progressive conformational changes of tau as it folds and aggregates where different phosphorylated epitopes are exposed in relation to these conformational changes, making different sites accessible to kinases at the different stages of tau aggregation. Further phosphorylation and post-translational modifications lead to further conformational changes making other tau epitopes accessible to kinases. The order of early and late phosphorylation sites is likely the result of conformational changes which are, in turn, influenced by phosphorylation and other post-translational modifications of tau. To better understand these relationships, we need to consider there are at least three major types of AD-relevant tau pathologies: tau aggregates abundant in dystrophic neurites (DN) surrounding neuritic Aβ plaques [219], neurofibrillary tangles (NFTs), and neuropil threads (NTs) [220]. These distinct tau pathologies might have different temporal onsets and functional consequences on neural activity and behavior. Early consolidation of Aβ in plaques leads to DN formation around them, but not all DN have NP tau (especially at the very early stages) [221, 222]. Therefore, it is reasonable to speculate that these early plasma p-tau biomarkers reflect the "neuritization" of plaques. [1] That

would explain why early plasma markers such as p-tau217 and p-tau231 are better related to aggregated Aβ than to aggregated tau as assessed by tau PET.

This will also help explain the discordancy with or time lag between soluble tau in plasma/CSF and imaging insoluble tau becoming abnormal, because, as we observed with Aβ, given the sensitivity of the respective assessing techniques, soluble pools of the protein become detectable earlier than insoluble pools assessed by imaging. Furthermore, the current tau tracers tend not to bind to early stages of tangle formation (pretangle) [99], added to the very low levels of p-tau aggregates in these cells at this stage, and PET requiring a certain density of tau (binding sites) to generate a detectable signal.

Tau Imaging in Therapeutic Trials

Tau imaging has started to be used in therapeutic trials, both as inclusion criteria as well as outcome measure. A small number of participants underwent tau imaging in trials with aducanumab, an Aβ-targeting monoclonal antibody [223]. Despite the small sample size of those who underwent tau imaging, results show a clear significant reduction in the tau signal after aducanumab treatment [224]. It is difficult to explain why insoluble tau *decreases*, after administration of a drug intended to clear (reduce) brain Aβ levels. If Aβ promotes neocortical tau aggregation, we would expect that the anti Aβ treatment can result in slowing or blunting of tau accumulation in the brain. Considering that the PET signal corresponds to post-mortem total tau burden, including tau neurites (threads) and tangles [225], one possible explanation is that part of the tau PET signal also comes from the dystrophic neurites around the plaques and the inflammatory reaction that is triggered by aducanumab—that also leads to amyloid-related imaging abnormalities (ARIA)—may remove dystrophic tau neurites around plaques, therefore leading to a reduction in the tau imaging signal. Post-mortem analyses of brain tissue after aducanumab treatment are required to shed light on this conundrum.

---

[1] As postulated by Zetterberg, H; Hansson, O; and Villemagne, VL.

The best designed anti-Aβ trial to date included tau imaging in the participant selection [226]. Donanemab, like aducanumab [224], gantenerumab [227], and lecanemab [228], lead to robust and significant reductions of insoluble Aβ in the brain. It also leads to a modest cognitive response. What made the donanemab trial different is the inclusion of tau imaging where participants were selected only when they presented moderate levels of cortical tau [226]. The ideal inclusion criteria and/or the optimal window for an anti-Aβ therapy suggests the amount of Aβ in the brain to be between 15 and 50 CL, when there is no or little cortical tau [229]. Certifying that cortical tau is present, even at moderate levels, will likely blunt any cognitive effect of the Aβ reducing therapy. The best design or outcome from an imaging point of view would be to show that the placebo group develops and accumulates cortical tau pathology—and subsequent cognitive decline [167, 168]—while the treated group does not. In a way, this is already illustrated in the donanemab trial [226]. While there were no significant differences in global tau, the figures of regional tau accumulation in Supplementary Materials show a significant effect in reducing or slowing tau accumulation, greatest in the frontal lobe which is one the last regions in the brain that starts accumulating tau. Furthermore, when grouping the participants based on their baseline tau burden, those with the lowest tau burden showed the most significant cognitive response, while those with the highest tau burden in the brain showed none. [2] These findings suggest that, in an anti-Aβ trial, very little or no cortical tau at inclusion will likely translate into a strong cognitive effect.

Concluding Remarks

The neurodegenerative process usually begins decades before clinical symptoms are evident, making early clinical identification difficult. In the absence of sensitive biomarkers, this pre-cluded early intervention with, when available, disease-modifying medications during the pre-symptomatic period, which by preventing neuronal loss would likely achieve the maximum benefits of those therapies [166]. Therefore, a change in the diagnostic paradigm is already happening, with diagnosis moving away from identification of signs and symptoms of neuronal failure—evidence that central compensatory mechanisms have been exhausted and extensive synaptic and neuronal damage is already present—to the non-invasive detection of specific biomarkers for particular traits underlying the pathological process [139, 230, 231] and, as in neuropathology, defining the disease in biological terms [148], where biochemical and neuroimaging biomarkers are ideal for the identification of at-risk individuals before the development of the typical phenotype as well as predictors of cognitive decline. This principle is also guiding the approach to disease-specific therapeutic trials, where the use of biomarkers is allowing shorter trials with a smaller sample size by its use for adequate patient selection, proof of target engagement, as well as outcome measures. It also seems to be a growing consensus that to be effective not only disease-specific therapy needs to be given early in the course of the disease, even before symptoms appear [232], but that downstream mechanisms, co-morbidities as well as lifestyle factors also need to be addressed to successfully prevent the development of AD. We also need to understand that while biomarkers allow to confirm target engagement and efficacy in removing or stopping accumulation of pathological protein aggregates, they cannot replace cognitive or standards of daily living measures. The addition of tau imaging to the biomarker panel for AD allows for more accurate disease staging and prognosis, and will determine if Aβ and/or tau have an independent and/or synergistic effect on cognition, if this effect is sequential or parallel, and if, and at what stage of the disease, one of them becomes—or stops being—the driver of cognitive decline. This knowledge is playing a crucial role In the design of anti-Aβ and/or anti-tau therapeutic trials, allowing the determination of a personalized optimal window

[2]https://www.alzforum.org/news/conference-coverage/donanemab-confirms-clearing-plaques-slows-decline-bit.

for therapeutic intervention. As has been shown in cancer and AIDS therapeutics, it is unlikely that a single disease-modifying agent will be effective in arresting or delay cognitive decline. Therefore, in order to implement a successful therapeutic strategy, it might be necessary to combine disease-specific agents with non-disease-specific therapeutics (e.g., *anti-inflammatories, cholinesterase inhibitors, anti-hypertensives, etc.*) and lifestyle interventions (*focused on diet, exercise, sleep*, etc.), while simultaneously addressing co-morbidities (*diabetes, cardiovascular disease, etc.*).

In vivo imaging of tau allows a deeper insight into the spatial and temporal evolution of AD pathology, facilitating research into the pathophysiology, diagnosis and treatment of those neurodegenerative conditions where tau plays a role.

Tau imaging with PET has come of age. Further studies will continue to define, revise, and refine the role of tau in neurodegenerative conditions.

Acknowledgements This work was supported in part by NIH Grants P01AG025204, AG066468-02, AG073267-01, Aging Mind Foundation DAF2255207, NHMRC IDEAS Grant G1005121.

References

1. Mohorko N, Bresjanac M. Tau protein and human tauopathies: an overview. Zdrav Vestn. 2008;77(Suppl II):35–41.
2. Lee VM, Goedert M, Trojanowski JQ. Neurodegenerative tauopathies. Annu Rev Neurosci. 2001;24:1121–59.
3. McKee AC, et al. Chronic traumatic encephalopathy in athletes: progressive tauopathy after repetitive head injury. J Neuropathol Exp Neurol. 2009;68(7):709–35.
4. Hoglinger GU, Respondek G, Kovacs GG. New classification of tauopathies. Rev Neurol (Paris). 2018;174(9):664–8.
5. Morfini GA, et al. Axonal transport defects in neurodegenerative diseases. J Neurosci. 2009;29(41):12776–86.
6. Maas T, Eidenmuller J, Brandt R. Interaction of tau with the neural membrane cortex is regulated by phosphorylation at sites that are modified in paired helical filaments. J Biol Chem. 2000;275(21):15733–40.
7. Li X, et al. Novel diffusion barrier for axonal retention of Tau in neurons and its failure in neurodegeneration. EMBO J. 2011;30(23):4825–37.
8. Buee L, et al. Tau protein isoforms, phosphorylation and role in neurodegenerative disorders. Brain Res Brain Res Rev. 2000;33(1):95–130.
9. Villemagne VL, et al. Tau imaging: early progress and future directions. Lancet Neurol. 2015;14(1):114–24.
10. Jicha GA, et al. A conformation- and phosphorylation-dependent antibody recognizing the paired helical filaments of Alzheimer's disease. J Neurochem. 1997;69(5):2087–95.
11. Garcia-Sierra F, et al. Conformational changes and truncation of tau protein during tangle evolution in Alzheimer's disease. J Alzheimers Dis. 2003;5(2):65–77.
12. Ward SM, et al. Tau oligomers and tau toxicity in neurodegenerative disease. Biochem Soc Trans. 2012;40(4):667–71.
13. Mufson EJ, Ward S, Binder L. Prefibrillar tau oligomers in mild cognitive impairment and Alzheimer's disease. Neurodegener Dis. 2014;13(2–3):151–3.
14. Hernandez F, Avila J. Tauopathies. Cell Mol Life Sci. 2007;64(17):2219–33.
15. Arima K. Ultrastructural characteristics of tau filaments in tauopathies: immuno-electron microscopic demonstration of tau filaments in tauopathies. Neuropathology. 2006;26(5):475–83.
16. Zempel H, et al. Amyloid-beta oligomers induce synaptic damage via Tau-dependent microtubule severing by TTLL6 and spastin. EMBO J. 2013;32(22):2920–37.
17. Zempel H, et al. Abeta oligomers cause localized Ca(2+) elevation, missorting of endogenous Tau into dendrites, Tau phosphorylation, and destruction of microtubules and spines. J Neurosci. 2010;30(36):11938–50.
18. Delacourte A, et al. The biochemical pathway of neurofibrillary degeneration in aging and Alzheimer's disease. Neurology. 1999;52(6):1158–65.
19. Braak H, Braak E. Frequency of stages of Alzheimer-related lesions in different age categories. Neurobiol Aging. 1997;18(4):351–7.
20. Serrano-Pozo A, et al. Neuropathological alterations in Alzheimer disease. Cold Spring Harb Perspect Med. 2011;1:a006189.
21. Guo JL, Lee VM. Seeding of normal Tau by pathological Tau conformers drives pathogenesis of Alzheimer-like tangles. J Biol Chem. 2011;286(17):15317–31.
22. Zhang H, et al. Possible mechanisms of Tau spread and toxicity in Alzheimer's disease. Front Cell Dev Biol. 2021;9:707268.
23. Meisl G, et al. In vivo rate-determining steps of tau seed accumulation in Alzheimer's disease. Sci Adv. 2021;7(44):eabh1448.
24. Shi Y, et al. Structure-based classification of tauopathies. Nature. 2021;598(7880):359–63.
25. Murugan NA, Nordberg A, Agren H. Cryptic sites in tau fibrils explain the preferential binding of the AV-1451 PET tracer toward Alzheimer's tauopathy. ACS Chem Neurosci. 2021;12(13):2437–47.

26. Shi Y, et al. Cryo-EM structures of tau filaments from Alzheimer's disease with PET ligand APN-1607. Acta Neuropathol. 2021;141(5):697–708.

27. Zhou Y, et al. Dissecting the binding profile of PET tracers to corticobasal degeneration tau fibrils. ACS Chem Neurosci. 2021;12(18):3487–96.

28. Dujardin S, et al. Tau molecular diversity contributes to clinical heterogeneity in Alzheimer's disease. Nat Med. 2020;26(8):1256–63.

29. Imbimbo BP, et al. A critical appraisal of tau-targeting therapies for primary and secondary tauopathies. Alzheimers Dement. 2021;18:1008.

30. O'Brien J, Ames D, Burns A. Dementia. 2nd ed. London: Arnold; 2000.

31. Chien DT, et al. Early clinical PET imaging results with the novel PHF-tau radioligand [F-18]-T807. J Alzheimers Dis. 2013;34(2):457–68.

32. Maruyama M, et al. Imaging of tau pathology in a tauopathy mouse model and in Alzheimer patients compared to normal controls. Neuron. 2013;79:1094–108.

33. Walji AM, et al. Discovery of 6-(Fluoro-(18)F)-3-(1H-pyrrolo[2,3-c]pyridin-1-yl)isoquinolin-5-amine ([(18)F]-MK-6240): a positron emission tomography (PET) imaging agent for quantification of neurofibrillary tangles (NFTs). J Med Chem. 2016;59(10):4778–89.

34. Okamura N, et al. Characterization of [18F]THK-5351, a novel PET tracer for imaging tau pathology in Alzheimer's disease. Eur J Nucl Med Mol Imaging. 2014;41(Suppl 2):S260.

35. Gobbi LC, et al. Identification of three novel radiotracers for imaging aggregated tau in Alzheimer's disease with positron emission tomography. J Med Chem. 2017;60:7350.

36. Declercq L, et al. Preclinical evaluation of 18F-JNJ64349311, a novel PET tracer for tau imaging. J Nucl Med. 2017;58(6):975–81.

37. Fawaz MV, et al. High affinity radiopharmaceuticals based upon lansoprazole for PET imaging of aggregated tau in Alzheimer's disease and progressive supranuclear palsy: synthesis, preclinical evaluation, and lead selection. ACS Chem Neurosci. 2014;5(8):718–30.

38. Stephens A, et al. Characterization of novel PET tracers for the assessment of tau pathology in Alzheimer's disease and other tauopathies. In: AD/PD. Vienna: Krager AG; 2017.

39. Johnson KA, et al. Tau positron emission tomographic imaging in aging and early Alzheimer disease. Ann Neurol. 2016;79(1):110–9.

40. Lockhart SN, et al. Dynamic PET measures of tau accumulation in cognitively Normal older adults and Alzheimer's disease patients measured using [18F] THK-5351. pLoS One. 2016;11(6):e0158460.

41. Chiotis K, et al. Imaging in-vivo tau pathology in Alzheimer's disease with THK5317 PET in a multimodal paradigm. Eur J Nucl Med Mol Imaging. 2016;43:1686.

42. Villemagne VL, et al. In vivo evaluation of a novel tau imaging tracer for Alzheimer's disease. Eur J Nucl Med Mol Imaging. 2014;41(5):816–26.

43. Okamura N, et al. Non-invasive assessment of Alzheimer's disease neurofibrillary pathology using 18F-THK5105 PET. Brain. 2014;137(Pt 6):1762–71.

44. Kudo Y, et al. Quinoline derivative as diagnostic probe for disease with tau protein accumulation. U.S. Patent 7,118,730; 2006.

45. Shoghi-Jadid K, et al. Localization of neurofibrillary tangles and beta-amyloid plaques in the brains of living patients with Alzheimer disease. Am J Geriatr Psychiatry. 2002;10(1):24–35.

46. Smid LM, et al. Postmortem 3-D brain hemisphere cortical tau and amyloid-beta pathology mapping and quantification as a validation method of neuropathology imaging. J Alzheimers Dis. 2013;36(2):261–74.

47. Small GW, et al. PET of brain amyloid and tau in mild cognitive impairment. N Engl J Med. 2006;355(25):2652–63.

48. Nelson LD, et al. Positron emission tomography of brain beta-amyloid and tau levels in adults with Down syndrome. Arch Neurol. 2011;68(6):768–74.

49. Small GW, et al. PET scanning of brain tau in retired National Football League Players: preliminary findings. Am J Geriatr Psychiatry. 2013;21(2):138–44.

50. Kepe V, et al. PET imaging of neuropathology in tauopathies: progressive supranuclear palsy. J Alzheimers Dis. 2013;36(1):145–53.

51. Marquie M, et al. Validating novel tau positron emission tomography tracer [F-18]-AV-1451 (T807) on postmortem brain tissue. Ann Neurol. 2015;78(5):787–800.

52. Aguero C, et al. Autoradiography validation of novel tau PET tracer [F-18]-MK-6240 on human postmortem brain tissue. Acta Neuropathol Commun. 2019;7(1):37.

53. Lindberg A, et al. Radiosynthesis, in vitro and in vivo evaluation of [(18)F]CBD-2115 as a first-in-class radiotracer for imaging 4R-tauopathies. ACS Chem Neurosci. 2021;12(4):596–602.

54. Kroth H, et al. Discovery and preclinical characterization of [(18)F]PI-2620, a next-generation tau PET tracer for the assessment of tau pathology in Alzheimer's disease and other tauopathies. Eur J Nucl Med Mol Imaging. 2019;46(10):2178–89.

55. Brendel M, et al. Assessment of 18F-PI-2620 as a biomarker in progressive supranuclear palsy. JAMA Neurol. 2020;77(11):1408–19.

56. Endo H, et al. In vivo binding of a tau imaging probe, [(11)C]PBB3, in patients with progressive supranuclear palsy. Mov Disord. 2019;34(5):744–54.

57. Okamura N, et al. Quinoline and benzimidazole derivatives: candidate probes for in vivo imaging of tau pathology in Alzheimer's disease. J Neurosci. 2005;25(47):10857–62.

58. Okamura N, et al. Novel 18F-labeled arylquinoline derivatives for noninvasive imaging of tau pathology in Alzheimer disease. J Nucl Med. 2013;54(8):1420–7.

59. Fodero-Tavoletti MT, et al. 18F-THK523: a novel in vivo tau imaging ligand for Alzheimer's disease. Brain. 2011;134(Pt 4):1089–100.

60. Harada R, et al. Comparison of the binding characteristics of [18F]THK-523 and other amyloid imaging tracers to Alzheimer's disease pathology. Eur J Nucl Med Mol Imaging. 2013;40(1):125–32.

61. Fodero-Tavoletti MT, et al. Assessing THK523 selectivity for tau deposits in Alzheimer's disease and non-Alzheimer's disease tauopathies. Alzheimers Res Ther. 2014;6(1):11.

62. Ng KP, et al. Monoamine oxidase B inhibitor, selegiline, reduces 18F-THK5351 uptake in the human brain. Alzheimers Res Ther. 2017;9(1):25.

63. Harada R, Lerdsirisuk P, Shimizu Y, Yokoyama Y, Du Y, Kudo K, Ezura M, Ishikawa Y, Iwata R, Shidahara M, Ishiki A, Kikuchi A, Hatano Y, Ishihara T, Onodera O, Iwasaki Y, Yoshida M, Taki Y, Arai H, Kudo Y, Yanai K, Furumoto S, Okamura N. Preclinical Characterization of the Tau PET Tracer [18F]SNFT-1: Comparison of Tau PET Tracers. J Nucl Med. 2023. https://doi.org/10.2967/jnumed.123.265593.

64. Xia CF, et al. [(18)F]T807, a novel tau positron emission tomography imaging agent for Alzheimer's disease. Alzheimers Dement. 2013;9:666–76.

65. Dore V, et al. Towards a universal cortical tau sampling mask. Alzheimers Dement. 2021;17:e055816.

66. Chien DT, et al. Early clinical PET imaging results with the novel PHF-tau radioligand [F18]-T808. J Alzheimers Dis. 2014;38:171–84.

67. Scholl M, et al. PET imaging of tau deposition in the aging human brain. Neuron. 2016;89(5):971–82.

68. Fleisher AS, et al. Positron emission tomography Imaging With [18F]flortaucipir and postmortem assessment of Alzheimer disease Neuropathologic changes, vol. 77. JAMA Neurol; 2020. p. 829.

69. Hashimoto H, et al. Radiosynthesis, photoisomerization, biodistribution, and metabolite analysis of 11C-PBB3 as a clinically useful PET probe for imaging of tau pathology. J Nucl Med. 2014;55(9):1532–8.

70. Hashimoto H, et al. Identification of a major radiometabolite of [11C]PBB3. Nucl Med Biol. 2015;42(12):905–10.

71. Kawamura K, et al. Radiosynthesis and quality control testing of the tau imaging positron emission tomography tracer [(18) F]PM-PBB3 for clinical applications. J Labelled Comp Radiopharm. 2021;64(3):109–19.

72. Mueller A, et al. Tau PET imaging with (18)F-PI-2620 in patients with Alzheimer disease and healthy controls: a first-in-humans study. J Nucl Med. 2020;61(6):911–9.

73. Mormino EC, et al. Tau PET imaging with (18)F-PI-2620 in aging and neurodegenerative diseases. Eur J Nucl Med Mol Imaging. 2020;48:2233.

74. Bullich S, et al. Evaluation of dosimetry, quantitative methods, and test-retest variability of (18)F-PI-2620 PET for the assessment of tau deposits in the human brain. J Nucl Med. 2020;61(6):920–7.

75. Malarte ML, et al. Discriminative binding of tau PET tracers PI2620, MK6240 and RO948 in Alzheimer's disease, corticobasal degeneration and progressive supranuclear palsy brains. Mol Psychiatry. 2023;28:1272.

76. Palleis C, et al. Cortical [(18) F]PI-2620 binding differentiates corticobasal syndrome subtypes. Mov Disord. 2021;36(9):2104–15.

77. Franzmeier N, et al. Tau deposition patterns are associated with functional connectivity in primary tauopathies. Nat Commun. 2022;13(1):1362.

78. Song M, et al. Binding characteristics of [(18)F] PI-2620 distinguish the clinically predicted tau isoform in different tauopathies by PET. J Cereb Blood Flow Metab. 2021;41:2957.

79. Wong DF, et al. Characterization of 3 novel tau radiopharmaceuticals, (11)C-RO-963, (11)C-RO-643, and (18)F-RO-948, in healthy controls and in Alzheimer subjects. J Nucl Med. 2018;59(12):1869–76.

80. Kuwabara H, et al. Evaluation of (18)F-RO-948 PET for quantitative assessment of tau accumulation in the human brain. J Nucl Med. 2018;59(12):1877–84.

81. Palmqvist S, et al. Detailed comparison of amyloid PET and CSF biomarkers for identifying early Alzheimer disease. Neurology. 2015;85(14):1240–9.

82. Smith R, et al. Head-to-head comparison of tau positron emission tomography tracers [(18)F]flortaucipir and [(18)F]RO948. Eur J Nucl Med Mol Imaging. 2020;47(2):342–54.

83. Leuzy A, et al. Diagnostic performance of RO948 F 18 tau positron emission tomography in the differentiation of Alzheimer disease From other neurodegenerative disorders. JAMA Neurol. 2020;77(8):955–65.

84. Kolb H, et al. First case report: image to autopsy correlation for tau imaging with [18F]-T808 (AV-680). Alzheimers Dement. 2013;9(Suppl):P844–5.

85. Sanabria Bohorquez S, et al. [(18)F]GTP1 (Genentech tau probe 1), a radioligand for detecting neurofibrillary tangle tau pathology in Alzheimer's disease. Eur J Nucl Med Mol Imaging. 2019;46(10):2077–89.

86. Teng E, et al. Baseline [(18)F]GTP1 tau PET imaging is associated with subsequent cognitive decline in Alzheimer's disease. Alzheimers Res Ther. 2021;13(1):196.

87. Teng E, et al. Cross-sectional associations between [(18)F]GTP1 tau PET and cognition in Alzheimer's disease. Neurobiol Aging. 2019;81:138–45.

88. Pascoal TA, et al. In vivo quantification of neurofibrillary tangles with [(18)F]MK-6240. Alzheimers Res Ther. 2018;10(1):74.

89. Betthauser TJ, et al. In vivo characterization and quantification of neurofibrillary tau PET radioligand (18)F-MK-6240 in humans from Alzheimer disease dementia to young controls. J Nucl Med. 2019;60(1):93–9.

90. Villemagne VL, et al. Imaging tau and amyloid-beta proteinopathies in Alzheimer disease and other conditions. Nat Rev Neurol. 2018;14(4):225–36.

91. Kreisl WC, et al. Patterns of tau pathology identified with 18F-MK-6240 PET imaging. Alzheimers Dementer's. 2021;18:272.

92. Pascoal TA, et al. Longitudinal 18F-MK-6240 tau tangles accumulation follows Braak stages. Brain. 2021;144(11):3517–28.

93. Pascoal TA, et al. 18F-MK-6240 PET for early and late detection of neurofibrillary tangles. Brain. 2020;143(9):2818–30.

94. Salinas C, et al. Test-retest characterization and pharmacokinetic properties of [18F]MK-6240. In: Human amyloid imaging, Miami; 2018.

95. Leuzy A, et al. Diagnostic performance of RO948 F 18 tau positron emission tomography in the differentiation of Alzheimer disease From Other neurodegenerative disorders, vol. 77. JAMA Neurol; 2020. p. 955.

96. Rombouts FJR, et al. Discovery of N-(4-[(18)F]Fluoro-5-methylpyridin-2-yl)isoquinolin-6-amine (JNJ-64326067), a new promising tau positron emission tomography imaging tracer. J Med Chem. 2019;62(6):2974–87.

97. Schmidt ME, et al. Clinical evaluation of [(18)F]JNJ-64326067, a novel candidate PET tracer for the detection of tau pathology in Alzheimer's disease. Eur J Nucl Med Mol Imaging. 2020;47(13):3176–85.

98. Baker SL, et al. Evaluation of [(18)F]-JNJ-64326067-AAA tau PET tracer in humans. J Cereb Blood Flow Metab. 2021;41(12):3302–13.

99. Lowe VJ, et al. An autoradiographic evaluation of AV-1451 tau PET in dementia. Acta Neuropathol Commun. 2016;4(1):58.

100. Marquie M, et al. [F-18]-AV-1451 binding correlates with postmortem neurofibrillary tangle Braak staging. Acta Neuropathol. 2017;134:619. https://doi.org/10.1007/s00401-017-1740-8.

101. Marquie M, et al. Pathological correlations of [F-18]-AV-1451 imaging in non-Alzheimer tauopathies. Ann Neurol. 2017;81(1):117–28.

102. Ishiki A, et al. Tau imaging with [18 F]THK-5351 in progressive supranuclear palsy. Eur J Neurol. 2017;24(1):130–6.

103. Perez-Soriano A, Stoessl AJ. Tau imaging in progressive supranuclear palsy. Mov Disord. 2017;32(1):91–3.

104. Schonhaut DR, et al. 18 F-flortaucipir tau positron emission tomography distinguishes established progressive supranuclear palsy from controls and Parkinson disease: a multicenter study. Ann Neurol. 2017;82(4):622–34.

105. Baker SL, et al. Effect of off-target binding on (18) F-flortaucipir variability in healthy controls across the life span. J Nucl Med. 2019;60(10):1444–51.

106. Villemagne VL, et al. First-in-humans evaluation of (18)F-SMBT-1, a novel (18)F-labeled monoamine oxidase-B PET tracer for imaging reactive astrogliosis. J Nucl Med. 2022;63(10):1551–9.

107. Ikonomovic MD, et al. [F-18]AV-1451 positron emission tomography retention in choroid plexus: More than "off-target" binding. Ann Neurol. 2016;80(2):307–8.

108. Wen GY, Wisniewski HM, Kascsak RJ. Biondi ring tangles in the choroid plexus of Alzheimer's disease and normal aging brains: a quantitative study. Brain Res. 1999;832(1–2):40–6.

109. Chen R, Chen CP, Preston JE. Effects of transthyretin on thyroxine and beta-amyloid removal from cerebrospinal fluid in mice. Clin Exp Pharmacol Physiol. 2016;43(9):844–50.

110. Mukaetova-Ladinska EB, et al. Biochemical and anatomical redistribution of tau protein in Alzheimer's disease. Am J Pathol. 1993;143(2):565–78.

111. Barret O, et al. Kinetic modeling of the tau PET tracer (18)F-AV-1451 in human healthy volunteers and Alzheimer disease subjects. J Nucl Med. 2017;58(7):1124–31.

112. Guehl NJ, et al. Evaluation of pharmacokinetic modeling strategies for in-vivo quantification of tau with the radiotracer [(18)F]MK6240 in human subjects. Eur J Nucl Med Mol Imaging. 2019;46(10):2099–111.

113. Villemagne VL, Leuzy A, Sanabria Bohorquez S, Bullich S, Shimada H, Rowe CC, Bourgeat P, Lopresti BJ, Huang K, Krishnadas N, Fripp J, Takado Y, Gogola A, Minhas D, Weimer R, Higuchi M, Stephens A, Oskar Hansson O, Doré D. medRxiv. https://doi.org/10.1101/2023.03.22.23287009. 2023.

114. Dore V, et al. Towards a CenTauR cortical mask. In: 14th human amyloid imaging, Miami; 2020.

115. Gogola A, et al. Direct comparison of the tau PET tracers (18)F-flortaucipir and (18) F-MK-6240 in human subjects. J Nucl Med. 2022;63(1):108–16.

116. Villemagne VL, et al. What is T+? A Gordian knot of tracers, thresholds, and topographies. J Nucl Med. 2021;62(5):614–9.

117. Vogel JW, et al. Data-driven approaches for tau-PET imaging biomarkers in Alzheimer's disease. Hum Brain Mapp. 2019;40(2):638–51.

118. Vogel JW, et al. Four distinct trajectories of tau deposition identified in Alzheimer's disease. Nat Med. 2021;27(5):871–81.

119. Leuzy A, Binette AP, Vogel JW, Klein G, Borroni E, Tonietto M, Strandberg O, Mattsson-Carlgren N, Palmqvist S, Pontecorvo MJ, Iaccarino L, Stomrud E, Ossenkoppele R, Smith R, Hansson O. Comparison of Group-Level and Individualized Brain Regions for Measuring Change in Longitudinal Tau Positron Emission Tomography in Alzheimer Disease. JAMA Neurol. 2023;80(6):614–23.

120. Ossenkoppele R, et al. Tau PET patterns mirror clinical and neuroanatomical variability in Alzheimer's disease. Brain. 2016;139(Pt 5):1551–67.

121. La Joie R, et al. Association of APOE4 and clinical variability in Alzheimer disease With the pattern of tau- and amyloid-PET. Neurology. 2021;96(5):e650–61.

122. Devous MD Sr, et al. Relationships between cognition and neuropathological tau in Alzheimer's disease assessed by 18F flortaucipir PET. J Alzheimers Dis. 2021;80(3):1091–104.

123. Murray ME, et al. Neuropathologically defined subtypes of Alzheimer's disease with distinct clinical characteristics: a retrospective study. Lancet Neurol. 2011;10(9):785–96.

124. Whitwell JL, et al. Neuroimaging correlates of pathologically defined subtypes of Alzheimer's disease: a case-control study. Lancet Neurol. 2012;11(10):868–77.

125. Ferreira D, Nordberg A, Westman E. Biological subtypes of Alzheimer disease: a systematic review and meta-analysis. Neurology. 2020;94(10):436–48.

126. Charil A, et al. Tau subtypes of Alzheimer's disease determined in vivo using flortaucipir PET imaging. J Alzheimers Dis. 2019;71(3):1037–48.

127. Jack CR Jr, et al. Longitudinal tau PET in ageing and Alzheimer's disease. Brain. 2018;141(5):1517–28.

128. Villemagne VL, et al. The tau MeTeR composites for the generation of continuous and categorical measures of tau deposits in the brain. J Mol Med Ther. 2017;1(1):25–9.

129. Wang L, et al. Evaluation of tau imaging in staging Alzheimer disease and revealing interactions between beta-amyloid and tauopathy. JAMA Neurol. 2016;73(9):1070–7.

130. Ossenkoppele R, et al. Discriminative accuracy of [18F]flortaucipir positron emission tomography for Alzheimer disease vs other neurodegenerative disorders. JAMA. 2018;320(11):1151–62.

131. Krishnadas N, Doré V, Robertson JS, Ward L, Fowler C, Masters CL, Bourgeat P, Fripp J, Villemagne VL, Rowe CC. Rates of regional tau accumulation in ageing and across the Alzheimer's disease continuum: an AIBL 18F-MK6240 PET study. EBioMedicine. 2023;88:104450.

132. Leuzy A, et al. A multicenter comparison of [(18)F]flortaucipir, [(18)F]RO948, and [(18)F]MK6240 tau PET tracers to detect a common target ROI for differential diagnosis. Eur J Nucl Med Mol Imaging. 2021;48(7):2295–305.

133. Del Tredici K, Braak H. To stage, or not to stage. Curr Opin Neurobiol. 2020;61:10–22.

134. Jack CR Jr, et al. Tracking pathophysiological processes in Alzheimer's disease: an updated hypothetical model of dynamic biomarkers. Lancet Neurol. 2013;12(2):207–16.

135. Jack CR Jr, et al. An operational approach to National Institute on Aging-Alzheimer's Association criteria for preclinical Alzheimer disease. Ann Neurol. 2012;71(6):765–75.

136. Dutra JR, Cortes EP, Vonsattel JP. Update on hippocampal sclerosis. Curr Neurol Neurosci Rep. 2015;15(10):592.

137. Nelson PT, et al. Limbic-predominant age-related TDP-43 encephalopathy (LATE): consensus working group report. Brain. 2019;142(6):1503–27.

138. Crary JF, et al. Primary age-related tauopathy (PART): a common pathology associated with human aging. Acta Neuropathol. 2014;128(6):755–66.

139. Sperling R, Johnson K. Pro: Can biomarkers be gold standards in Alzheimer's disease? Alzheimers Res Ther. 2010;2(3):17.

140. Dubois B, et al. Revising the definition of Alzheimer's disease: a new lexicon. Lancet Neurol. 2010;9(11):1118–27.

141. McKhann GM, et al. The diagnosis of dementia due to Alzheimer's disease: recommendations from the National Institute on Aging-Alzheimer's Association workgroups on diagnostic guidelines for Alzheimer's disease. Alzheimers Dement. 2011;7(3):263–9.

142. Albert MS, et al. The diagnosis of mild cognitive impairment due to Alzheimer's disease: recommendations from the National Institute on Aging-Alzheimer's Association workgroups on diagnostic guidelines for Alzheimer's disease. Alzheimers Dement. 2011;7(3):270–9.

143. Sperling RA, et al. Toward defining the preclinical stages of Alzheimer's disease: recommendations from the National Institute on Aging-Alzheimer's Association workgroups on diagnostic guidelines for Alzheimer's disease. Alzheimers Dement. 2011;7(3):280–92.

144. Webber C, et al. Improving the TNM classification: findings from a 10-year continuous literature review. Int J Cancer. 2014;135(2):371–8.

145. Frisoni GB, et al. The clinical use of structural MRI in Alzheimer disease. Nat Rev Neurol. 2010;6(2):67–77.

146. Minoshima S, et al. Brain [F-18]FDG PET for clinical dementia workup: differential diagnosis of Alzheimer's disease and other types of dementing disorders. Semin Nucl Med. 2021;51(3):230–40.

147. Dittrich A, et al. Plasma and CSF NfL are differentially associated with biomarker evidence of neurodegeneration in a community-based sample of 70-year-olds. Alzheimers Dement. 2022;14(1):e12295.

148. Jack CR Jr, et al. A/T/N: an unbiased descriptive classification scheme for Alzheimer disease biomarkers. Neurology. 2016;87(5):539–47.

149. Villemagne VL, Rowe CC. Amyloid ligands for dementia. PET Clin. 2010;5:33–53.

150. Masters CL, Selkoe DJ. Biochemistry of amyloid beta-protein and amyloid deposits in Alzheimer disease. Cold Spring Harb Perspect Med. 2012;2(6):a006262.

151. Hanseeuw BJ, et al. Association of Amyloid and Tau With cognition in preclinical Alzheimer disease: a longitudinal study, vol. 76. JAMA Neurol; 2019. p. 915.

152. Arriagada PV, et al. Neurofibrillary tangles but not senile plaques parallel duration and severity of Alzheimer's disease. Neurology. 1992;42(3 Pt 1):631–9.

153. Rowe CC, et al. Imaging beta-amyloid burden in aging and dementia. Neurology. 2007;68(20):1718–25.
154. Nelson PT, et al. Correlation of Alzheimer disease neuropathologic changes with cognitive status: a review of the literature. J Neuropathol Exp Neurol. 2012;71(5):362–81.
155. Giannakopoulos P, et al. Tangle and neuron numbers, but not amyloid load, predict cognitive status in Alzheimer's disease. Neurology. 2003;60(9):1495–500.
156. Bierer LM, et al. Neocortical neurofibrillary tangles correlate with dementia severity in Alzheimer's disease. Arch Neurol. 1995;52(1):81–8.
157. Walsh DM, et al. Naturally secreted oligomers of amyloid beta protein potently inhibit hippocampal long-term potentiation in vivo. Nature. 2002;416(6880):535–9.
158. Lacor PN, et al. Synaptic targeting by Alzheimer's-related amyloid beta oligomers. J Neurosci. 2004;24(45):10191–200.
159. Lacor PN, et al. Abeta oligomer-induced aberrations in synapse composition, shape, and density provide a molecular basis for loss of connectivity in Alzheimer's disease. J Neurosci. 2007;27(4):796–807.
160. Zempel H, Mandelkow EM. Linking amyloid-beta and tau: amyloid-beta induced synaptic dysfunction via local wreckage of the neuronal cytoskeleton. Neurodegener Dis. 2012;10(1–4):64–72.
161. Ittner LM, Ke YD, Gotz J. Phosphorylated tau interacts with c-Jun N-terminal kinase-interacting protein 1 (JIP1) in Alzheimer disease. J Biol Chem. 2009;284(31):20909–16.
162. Bennett DA, et al. Neurofibrillary tangles mediate the association of amyloid load with clinical Alzheimer disease and level of cognitive function. Arch Neurol. 2004;61(3):378–84.
163. Price JL, Morris JC. Tangles and plaques in nondemented aging and "preclinical" Alzheimer's disease. Ann Neurol. 1999;45(3):358–68.
164. Mintun MA, et al. [11C]PIB in a nondemented population: potential antecedent marker of Alzheimer disease. Neurology. 2006;67(3):446–52.
165. Villemagne VL, et al. Aβ deposits in older nondemented individuals with cognitive decline are indicative of preclinical Alzheimer's disease. Neuropsychologia. 2008;46(6):1688–97.
166. Villemagne VL, et al. The ART of loss: Aβ imaging in the evaluation of Alzheimer's disease and other dementias. Mol Neurobiol. 2008;38(1):1–15.
167. Strikwerda-Brown C, et al. Association of Elevated Amyloid and Tau Positron Emission Tomography Signal With near-term development of Alzheimer disease symptoms in older adults without cognitive impairment. JAMA Neurol. 2022;79(10):975–85.
168. Ossenkoppele R, et al. Amyloid and tau PET-positive cognitively unimpaired individuals are at high risk for future cognitive decline. Nat Med. 2022;28(11):2381–7.
169. Ossenkoppele R, et al. Accuracy of tau positron emission tomography as a prognostic marker in preclinical and prodromal Alzheimer disease: a head-to-head comparison against amyloid positron emission tomography and magnetic resonance imaging. JAMA Neurol. 2021;78(8):961–71.
170. Ossenkoppele R, et al. Distinct tau PET patterns in atrophy-defined subtypes of Alzheimer's disease. Alzheimers Dement. 2020;16(2):335–44.
171. van Eimeren T, Bischof GN, Drzezga A. Is tau Imaging More Than Just upside-down (18)F-FDG imaging? J Nucl Med. 2017;58(9):1357–9.
172. Xia C, et al. Association of in vivo [18F]AV-1451 tau PET imaging results with cortical atrophy and symptoms in typical and atypical Alzheimer disease. JAMA Neurol. 2017;74(4):427–36.
173. Chiotis K, et al. Longitudinal changes of tau PET imaging in relation to hypometabolism in prodromal and Alzheimer's disease dementia. Mol Psychiatry. 2018;23:1666. https://doi.org/10.1038/mp.2017.108.
174. La Joie R, et al. Prospective longitudinal atrophy in Alzheimer's disease correlates with the intensity and topography of baseline tau-PET. Sci Transl Med. 2020;12(524):eaau5732.
175. Hammes J, et al. One-stop shop: (18)F-flortaucipir PET differentiates amyloid-positive and -negative forms of neurodegenerative diseases. J Nucl Med. 2021;62(2):240–6.
176. Royall DR. Location, location, location! Neurobiol Aging. 2007;28(10):1481–2.
177. Sarazin M, Lagarde J, Bottlaender M. Distinct tau PET imaging patterns in typical and atypical Alzheimer's disease. Brain. 2016;139(Pt 5):1321–4.
178. Wang L, et al. Evaluation of tau imaging in staging Alzheimer disease and revealing interactions between beta-amyloid and tauopathy, vol. 73. JAMA Neurol; 2016. p. 1070.
179. Cho H, et al. Tau PET in Alzheimer disease and mild cognitive impairment. Neurology. 2016;87(4):375–83.
180. Ossenkoppele R, et al. Atrophy patterns in early clinical stages across distinct phenotypes of Alzheimer's disease. Hum Brain Mapp. 2015;36(11):4421–37.
181. Ossenkoppele R, et al. The behavioural/dysexecutive variant of Alzheimer's disease: clinical, neuroimaging and pathological features. Brain. 2015;138(Pt 9):2732–49.
182. Ossenkoppele R, et al. Tau, amyloid, and hypometabolism in a patient with posterior cortical atrophy. Ann Neurol. 2015;77(2):338–42.
183. Gordon BA, et al. The relationship between cerebrospinal fluid markers of Alzheimer pathology and positron emission tomography tau imaging. Brain. 2016;139(Pt 8):2249–60.
184. Brier MR, et al. Tau and Abeta imaging, CSF measures, and cognition in Alzheimer's disease. Sci Transl Med. 2016;8(338):338ra66.

185. Pontecorvo MJ, et al. Relationships between flortaucipir PET tau binding and amyloid burden, clinical diagnosis, age and cognition. Brain. 2017;140(3):748–63.

186. Delacourte A, et al. Tau aggregation in the hippocampal formation: an ageing or a pathological process? Exp Gerontol. 2002;37(10–11):1291–6.

187. van Eimeren T, Bischof GN, Drzezga AE. Is tau imaging more than just "upside-down" FDG imaging? J Nucl Med. 2017;58:1357.

188. Tomlinson BE, Blessed G, Roth M. Observations on the brains of demented old people. J Neurol Sci. 1970;11(3):205–42.

189. Jellinger KA, et al. PART, a distinct tauopathy, different from classical sporadic Alzheimer disease. Acta Neuropathol. 2015;129:757.

190. Duyckaerts C, et al. PART is part of Alzheimer disease. Acta Neuropathol. 2015;129(5):749–56.

191. Jack CR Jr. PART and SNAP. Acta Neuropathol. 2014;128(6):773–6.

192. Groot C, et al. Mesial temporal tau is related to worse cognitive performance and greater neocortical tau load in amyloid-beta-negative cognitively normal individuals. Neurobiol Aging. 2021;97:41–8.

193. Josephs KA, et al. Tau aggregation influences cognition and hippocampal atrophy in the absence of beta-amyloid: a clinico-imaging-pathological study of primary age-related tauopathy (PART). Acta Neuropathol. 2017;133(5):705–15.

194. Jack CR Jr, Holtzman DM. Biomarker modeling of Alzheimer's disease. Neuron. 2013;80(6):1347–58.

195. Thal DR, et al. Phases of a beta-deposition in the human brain and its relevance for the development of AD. Neurology. 2002;58:1791–800.

196. Braak H, Braak E. Neuropathological staging of Alzheimer-related changes. Acta Neuropathol. 1991;82(4):239–59.

197. Kantarci K, et al. AV-1451 tau and beta-amyloid positron emission tomography imaging in dementia with Lewy bodies. Ann Neurol. 2017;81(1):58–67.

198. Mak E, et al. Imaging tau burden in dementia with Lewy bodies using [(18)F]-AV1451 positron emission tomography. Neurobiol Aging. 2021;101:172–80.

199. Rafii MS. Tau PET imaging for staging of Alzheimer's disease in down syndrome. Dev Neurobiol. 2019;79(7):711–5.

200. Rafii MS, et al. PET imaging of tau pathology and relationship to amyloid, longitudinal MRI, and cognitive change in down syndrome: results from the Down Syndrome Biomarker Initiative (DSBI). J Alzheimers Dis. 2017;60(2):439–50.

201. Villemagne VL, et al. Imaging of tau deposits in adults with Niemann-Pick type C disease: a case-control study. Eur J Nucl Med Mol Imaging. 2019;46(5):1132–8.

202. Smith R, et al. 18F-AV-1451 tau PET imaging correlates strongly with tau neuropathology in MAPT mutation carriers. Brain. 2016;139(Pt 9):2372–9.

203. Su Y, et al. Tau PET imaging with [18F]PM-PBB3 in frontotemporal dementia with MAPT mutation. J Alzheimers Dis. 2020;76(1):149–57.

204. Zhou XY, et al. In vivo (18) F-APN-1607 tau positron emission tomography imaging in MAPT mutations: cross-sectional and longitudinal findings. Mov Disord. 2022;37(3):525–34.

205. Makaretz SJ, et al. Flortaucipir tau PET imaging in semantic variant primary progressive aphasia. J Neurol Neurosurg Psychiatry. 2018;89(10):1024–31.

206. Messerschmidt K, et al. (18)F-PI-2620 tau PET improves the imaging diagnosis of progressive supranuclear palsy. J Nucl Med. 2022;63:1754.

207. Ishizuchi K, et al. A case of progressive supranuclear palsy with predominant cerebellar ataxia diagnosed by [(18)F]PM-PBB3 tau PET. J Neurol Sci. 2021;425:117440.

208. Stern RA, et al. Tau positron-emission tomography in former National Football League Players. N Engl J Med. 2019;380(18):1716–25.

209. Krishnadas N, et al. Case report: (18)F-MK6240 tau positron emission tomography pattern resembling chronic traumatic encephalopathy in a retired Australian rules football player. Front Neurol. 2020;11:598980.

210. Montenigro PH, et al. Chronic traumatic encephalopathy: historical origins and current perspective. Annu Rev Clin Psychol. 2015;11:309–30.

211. McKee AC, et al. The spectrum of disease in chronic traumatic encephalopathy. Brain. 2013;136(Pt 1):43–64.

212. Bennett DA, et al. Neuropathology of older persons without cognitive impairment from two community-based studies. Neurology. 2006;66(12):1837–44.

213. Cullen NC, et al. Plasma biomarkers of Alzheimer's disease improve prediction of cognitive decline in cognitively unimpaired elderly populations. Nat Commun. 2021;12(1):3555.

214. Chatterjee P, et al. Diagnostic and prognostic plasma biomarkers for preclinical Alzheimer's disease. Alzheimers Dement. 2022;18(6):1141–54.

215. Hansson O, et al. The Alzheimer's Association appropriate use recommendations for blood biomarkers in Alzheimer's disease. Alzheimers Dement. 2022;18:2669.

216. Janelidze S, et al. Plasma P-tau181 in Alzheimer's disease: relationship to other biomarkers, differential diagnosis, neuropathology and longitudinal progression to Alzheimer's dementia. Nat Med. 2020;26(3):379–86.

217. Dore V, et al. Plasma p217+tau versus NAV4694 amyloid and MK6240 tau PET across the Alzheimer's continuum. Alzheimers Dement. 2022;14(1):e12307.

218. Ashton NJ, et al. Plasma p-tau231: a new biomarker for incipient Alzheimer's disease pathology. Acta Neuropathol. 2021;141:709.

219. Schmidt ML, et al. An extensive network of PHF tau-rich dystrophic neurites permeates neocortex

and nearly all neuritic and diffuse amyloid plaques in Alzheimer disease. FEBS Lett. 1994;344(1):69–73.

220. Mandelkow EM, Mandelkow E. Tau in Alzheimer's disease. Trends Cell Biol. 1998;8(11):425–7.

221. Vickers JC, et al. Dystrophic neurite formation associated with age-related beta amyloid deposition in the neocortex: clues to the genesis of neurofibrillary pathology. Exp Neurol. 1996;141(1):1–11.

222. Dickson TC, et al. Neurochemical diversity of dystrophic neurites in the early and late stages of Alzheimer's disease. Exp Neurol. 1999;156(1):100–10.

223. Sevigny J, et al. The antibody aducanumab reduces Abeta plaques in Alzheimer's disease. Nature. 2016;537(7618):50–6.

224. Budd Haeberlein S, et al. Two randomized phase 3 studies of Aducanumab in early Alzheimer's disease. J Prev Alzheimers Dis. 2022;9(2):197–210.

225. Smith R, et al. Correlation of in vivo [18F] Flortaucipir With Postmortem Alzheimer disease tau pathology. JAMA Neurol. 2019;76(3):310–7.

226. Mintun MA, et al. Donanemab in early Alzheimer's disease. N Engl J Med. 2021;384(18):1691–704.

227. Ostrowitzki S, et al. A phase III randomized trial of gantenerumab in prodromal Alzheimer's disease. Alzheimers Res Ther. 2017;9(1):95.

228. Swanson CJ, et al. A randomized, double-blind, phase 2b proof-of-concept clinical trial in early Alzheimer's disease with lecanemab, an anti-Abeta protofibril antibody. Alzheimers Res Ther. 2021;13(1):80.

229. Dore V, et al. Relationship between amyloid and tau levels and its impact on tau spreading. Eur J Nucl Med Mol Imaging. 2021;48(7):2225–32.

230. Clark CM, et al. Biomarkers for early detection of Alzheimer pathology. Neurosignals. 2008;16(1):11–8.

231. Sperling R, Johnson K. Biomarkers of Alzheimer disease: current and future applications to diagnostic criteria. Continuum. 2013;19(2 Dementia):325–38.

232. Sperling RA, Jack CR Jr, Aisen PS. Testing the right target and right drug at the right stage. Sci Transl Med. 2011;3(111):111cm33.

Dopaminergic Nerve Terminal Imaging Across the Spectrum of Aging, Idiopathic Rapid Eye Movement (REM) Sleep Behavior Disorder, Parkinsonism and Dementia

Yoshiaki Ota, Prabesh Kanel, Jaimie Barr, C. Chauncey Spears, and Nico Bohnen

Introduction

Recently, various neuroimaging techniques such as structural MRI, functional neuroimaging using DTI and fMRI, and metabolic neuroimaging using PET and SPECT have been widely used for visualizing the brain's regional pathologic features, assessing disease progression, and monitoring treatment effects for movement disorders, such as Parkinson's disease (PD), atypical Parkinsonian syndromes (APS), and other neurodegenerative diseases [1]. This chapter will summarize the key mechanisms of each neuroimaging technique with a particular emphasis on presynaptic nerve terminal dopaminergic molecular imaging, and the clinical application of these

Y. Ota
The Division of Neuroradiology, Department of Radiology, University of Michigan, Ann Arbor, MI, USA

The Division of Nuclear Medicine, Department of Radiology, University of Michigan, Ann Arbor, MI, USA
e-mail: yoshiako@med.umich.edu

P. Kanel · J. Barr
The Division of Nuclear Medicine, Department of Radiology, University of Michigan, Ann Arbor, MI, USA

Morris K. Udall Center of Excellence for Parkinson's Disease Research, University of Michigan, Ann Arbor, MI, USA

University of Michigan Parkinson's Foundation Research Center of Excellence, Ann Arbor, MI, USA
e-mail: prabeshk@umich.edu; jaimieba@med.umich.edu

C. C. Spears
Morris K. Udall Center of Excellence for Parkinson's Disease Research, University of Michigan, Ann Arbor, MI, USA

Department of Neurology, University of Michigan, Ann Arbor, MI, USA
e-mail: spearscc@med.umich.edu

N. Bohnen (✉)
The Division of Nuclear Medicine, Department of Radiology, University of Michigan, Ann Arbor, MI, USA

Morris K. Udall Center of Excellence for Parkinson's Disease Research, University of Michigan, Ann Arbor, MI, USA

University of Michigan Parkinson's Foundation Research Center of Excellence, Ann Arbor, MI, USA

Department of Neurology, University of Michigan, Ann Arbor, MI, USA

GRECC and Neurology Service, VAAAHS, Ann Arbor, MI, USA
e-mail: nbohnen@umich.edu

imaging techniques across the spectrum of aging, parkinsonism, and dementia.

Dopaminergic (DA) Targets/ Ligands: DAT, DA Synthesis, VMAT2, DA Receptors

Dopamine (DA) is an important neurotransmitter responsible for control of movement. Axonal projections from the substantia nigra dopaminergic neurons give rise to an extensive network of axonal processes that innervate the basal ganglia. Lower nigrostriatal availability of DA is a hallmark of neurodegenerative parkinsonism. Dopaminergic projections from the ventral tegmental area (VTA) innervate the anteroventral striatum (nucleus accumbens) and the mesolimbic and mesofrontal cortices. In this section, we will review dopaminergic targets and ligands of molecular imaging.

Dopamine Transporter (DAT)

DAT is a transmembrane sodium chloride dependent protein that is expressed in presynaptic dopaminergic cells. Reduction of DAT is caused by loss of the nigral neuron cell bodies, axons, or nerve terminals, which is characteristic in PD [2, 3]. DAT is responsible for DA reuptake from the synaptic cleft and has a critical role in the spatial and temporal buffering of DA levels in the synaptic cleft [4]. [^{123}I]-FP-CIT [^{123}I]-ioflupane is the most commonly used radiotracer of the DAT ligand in clinical settings and can show significantly reduced striatal uptake of the radiotracer in specific posterior-to-anterior and asymmetric striatal denervation patters in PD. Early reduction of uptake progresses from the dorsal and posterior putamen correlates with disease severity and duration in PD [5]. There are other DAT ligands of SPECT such as [^{99m}]Tc-TRODAT [6], [^{123}I]-β-CIT [7], and [^{123}I]-IPT [8], and [^{18}F]-FP-CIT [9], which may have different kinetic and more advantageous imaging properties [10]. DAT-

SPECT and PET allows us to reveal the integrity of the nigrostriatal and ventral tegmental dopaminergic pathways and provide robust biomarkers of dopaminergic neuronal degeneration in PD [11].

Dopamine (DA) Synthesis

DA is a neurotransmitter produced by dopaminergic neurons and is synthesized from the amino acid tyrosine [12]. Tyrosine hydroxylase enzymes transform tyrosine ammino acids into L-DOPA, the precursor of the neurotransmitter dopamine [12]. The degree of accumulation of the L-6-[^{18}F] fluoro-3,4-dihydroxyphenylalanine ([^{18}F]-DOPA) PET ligand, which is an analog of L-DOPA, can measure the functional integrity of presynaptic dopaminergic synthesis and visualize the activity of aromatic amino acid decarboxylase (AADC), which converts [^{18}F]-DOPA to [^{18}F]-dopamine [13].

Vesicular Monoamine Transporter Type 2 (VMAT2)

After DA synthesis, VMAT2, which is an integral protein located in the presynaptic vesicular membrane, translocates DA from the cytoplasm into vesicles that then release DA into the synaptic cleft [12]. [^{11}C]-dihydrotetrabenazine ([^{11}C]-DTBZ) and [^{18}F]-FP-DTBZ PET ligands both have high affinity toward VMAT2 and allow for the assessment of the integrity of the presynaptic dopaminergic in the nigra, VTA or at the level of the striatum [14].

Dopamine (DA) Receptors

After release into the synaptic cleft, DA binds to and activates both presynaptic and postsynaptic DA receptors. DA binding to D1-like receptors in the postsynaptic terminal can potentiate α-amino-3-hydroxy-5-methyl-4-isoxazolepropionic acid

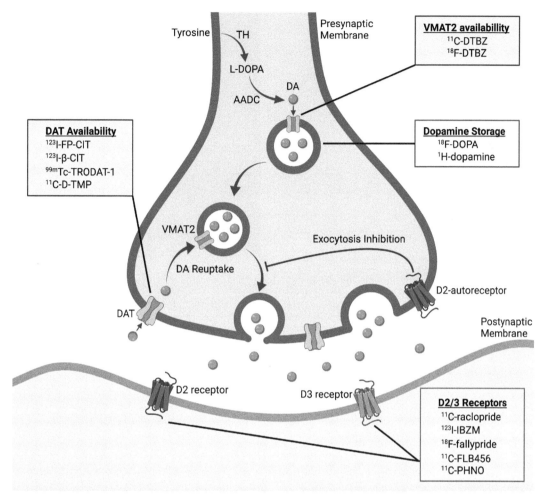

Fig. 7.1 A scheme of dopamine synthesis pathway and radiotracers for dopaminergic molecular imaging. Tyrosine hydroxylase (TH) converts tyrosine to L-DOPA, which is then converted to dopamine (DA) by aromatic L-amino acid decarboxylase (AAAD). Dopamine is stored in vesicles and its release is triggered by action potentials. Dopamine transmits signals from the pre- to the postsynaptic neuron by binding to postsynaptic receptors (D_2 and D_3) and activating a cascade of events in the postsynaptic neuron. Dopamine reuptake is performed by dopamine transporters (DAT) into the presynaptic neuron, and then dopamine is transported back into the vesicle by vesicular monoamine transporter type 2 (VMAT2). The available tracers for each domain are listed in the scheme. *^{11}C-DTBZ* ^{11}C-dihydrotetrabenazine, *^{18}F-DTBZ* ^{11}C-dihydrotetrabenazine, *^{18}F-DOPA* ^{18}F-fluorodeoxyphenylalanine, *^{123}I-FP-CIT* ^{123}I-ioflupane, *^{123}I-β-CIT* ^{123}I-2β-carbomethoxy-3 beta-(4-iodophenyl) tropane, *^{99m}Tc-TRODAT-1* ^{99m}Tc-tropane for imaging dopamine transporter, *$11C$-D-TMP* ^{11}C-trimethoprim, *^{123}I-IBZM* ^{123}I-iodobenzamide, *^{11}C-PHNO* ^{11}C-4-propyl-9-hydroxynaphthoxazine

(AMDA) and N-methyl-D-aspartate (NMDA) currents, while DA binding to D2-like receptors in the postsynaptic terminal can reduce these currents. These opposite mechanisms modulate the synaptic plasticity [12]. Figure 7.1 demonstrates dopamine synthesis pathway and available radiotracers for imaging of the dopaminergic systems.

Normal Aging and Age-Accelerated Striatal Dopaminergic Degeneration (AASDD)

Dopaminergic nigrostriatal losses shown using DAT and VMAT2 ligands have been associated with normal aging (Fig. 7.2) [15, 16]. DAT losses between 5 and 8% per decade of life since young

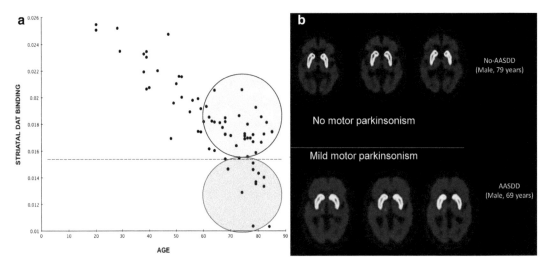

Fig. 7.2 DAT PET ([^{11}]C-βCFT) and normal aging: Age-Accelerated Striatal Dopaminergic Degeneration (AASDD) and motor effects in non-PD persons. Age-accelerated striatal DA losses and presence of mild clinical parkinsonism in non-PD older adults (modified from reference (15)). (**a**) Scatter plot showing striatal DAT binding for normal aging and age-associated dopaminergic degeneration. (**b**) Vesicular monoamine trans-porter type 2 [^{11}C] dihydrotetrabenazine (DTBZ) parametric PET scans of the basal ganglia showing striatum DTBZ binding for AASDD (lower case) versus no-AASDD (upper case) patients. The AASDD patients show lower diffuse striatal DTBZ binding compared to those with no AASSD. Note the absence of a specific posterior-to-anterior and/or asymmetric denervation gradient in AASDD

adulthood may manifest as minimally symptomatic parkinsonism in older adults in the absence of a typical posterior-to-anterior striatal denervation gradient [15]. A recent study showed that white matter vascular lesions in the presence of age-associated nigrostriatal losses may result in more symptomatic parkinsonism, and this may be one of the potential mechanisms of VaP [17]. There is substantial heterogeneity of age-associated nigrostriatal losses in older adults that corresponds to the severity of parkinsonian motor ratings [15]. It is unclear whether this reflects non-resilience of DA nerve terminals due to genetic, systemic medical comorbidities or the prodromal presence of an α-synucleinopathy, such as DLB. Interestingly, DAT-SPECT studies have shown evidence of lower putaminal DAT binding in older non-PD diabetics compared to non-diabetics [18]. Furthermore, the presence of diabetes mellitus in non-PD older adults has also been associated higher CSF tau and α-synucleinopathy levels compared to non-diabetic controls [18]. Interestingly, FDOPA PET studies have not shown conclusive evidence of age-associated striatal losses [19–21]. This may

be due to possible differential vulnerability of the distal nerve terminal (DAT, VMAT2) versus the soma of the dopaminergic neurons. Alternatively, early upregulation of AADC as a possible compensatory mechanism in aging may also play a role. Although striatal FDOPA synthesis may not decline with age per se, there is also evidence of substantially increased washout across the brain reflecting impaired vesicular storage capacity and resulting in enhanced exposure of cytosolic FDOPA to monoamine oxidase [20].

Idiopathic Rapid Eye Movement (REM) Behavior Disorder (iRBD)

Idiopathic rapid eye movement (REM) behavior disorder (iRBD) is classified as a REM sleep parasomnia and is characterized by the loss of muscular atonia present during REM sleep, which results in patients acting out their dreams with vigorous and often violent behaviors [22–24]. Isolated (idiopathic) RBD is defined when it occurs in the absence of any other medical conditions and is considered one of the more robust prodromal clinical markers of α-synucleinopathies: PD, DLB, and MSA [22, 25–27]. Early recognition of α-synucleinopathy could contribute to early treatment induction at a phase when therapies might be most effective. Recently, novel neuroimaging techniques have been developed to investigate iRBD pathological processes and to provide diagnostic and prognostic markers. DAT-SPECT as dopaminergic imaging is the most investigated functional neuroimaging technique and is a well-established method for the assessment of iRBD that can provide a semiquantitative assessment of altered nigrostriatal dopaminergic nerve terminal functions. In semiquantitative assessments, a region of interest is placed in the striatum, the caudate, and the anterior and posterior putamen, as well as in the occipital cortex or the cerebellar hemisphere, which shows non-specific radiotracer uptake. Uptake ratios of radiotracer in striatal regions of interest can be quantified relative to the non-specific uptake in the occipital cortex or cerebellar hemisphere, both of which are areas with minimal or no specific dopaminergic binding [28, 29].

Studies using DAT-SPECT have shown reduced uptake in the nigrostriatal system in approximately 50% of iRBD patients [26, 30]. Reduced uptake in DAT-SPECT as observed in iRBD is generally less severe than that seen in established PD [31, 32]. A recent study has shown that a cut-off of 48% uptake reduction of DAT specific binding ratios (SBR) within the putamen at baseline can predict phenoconversion to PD after a mean of 4.8 years follow-up [33]. Additionally, a greater 25% uptake reduction of putamen DAT SBR compared to that of the occipital cortex at baseline can predict α-synucleinopathy phenoconversion after 3 years follow-up with a likelihood ratio of 1.54 [34].

There is a wide variety of semiquantitative definitions of nigrostriatal dopaminergic losses to define DAT scan abnormalcy for being used as a predictor for phenoconversion in iRBD patients. Examples of these varying abnormalcy definition may include requiring the presence of a putamen-to-caudate nucleus denervation gradient versus absolute quantification cut-offs of global striatal, putamen or caudate nucleus ligand

binding, preferably based on age and gender adjusted Z-score changes using a normative database [30, 35]. It is plausible that early striatal DA losses may be (more) global before developing a denervation gradient. However, a reverse denervation gradient with vulnerability of the caudate nucleus has also been used as a DAT scan abnormalcy definition being used as DAT biomarkers to predict phenoconversion in iRBD.

Parkinson's Disease (PD)

PD is the second most common age-related neurodegenerative disease and has an increasing prevalence with age [36]. PD is characterized by progressive degeneration of the dopaminergic neurons in the substantia nigra pars compacta (SNpc), typically observed in the ventrolateral tier. Decreased dopaminergic input to striatum along the nigrostriatal pathway is responsible for most of the classical motor manifestations in PD (Fig. 7.3) [37]. Presynaptic DA nerve terminal studies, such as DAT-SPECT or PET, VMAT2 or FDOPA PET, are used for assessing PD severity and progression. Nigrostriatal losses are often asymmetric in PD, especially during early disease phase at the level of the dorsal and posterior putamen. More symmetric and progressive losses in the putamen and subsequent reductions in the caudate nuclei are seen with disease progression when end-stage disease residual uptake can be seen mainly in the anteroventral striatum (nucleus accumbens region; Fig. 7.4), which is innervated mostly by DA projections originating in the VTA. The clinical relevance of the VTA versus nigral DA losses remains poorly studied to this date but may play an early role in AD. DAT PET studies have also shown DA losses in the thalamus that may contribute to the clinical phenotype in PD [38]. A three-ligand presynaptic dopaminergic (FDOPA, DAT, VMAT2) PET study showed greatest striatal reduction for DAT, intermediate ranges for VMATA2 and the lowest reductions for FDOPA [39]. These observations suggest that the activity of aromatic L-amino acid decarboxylase (AADC) is up-regulated, whereas the plasma membrane DA transporter is down-regulated in the striatum of patients with PD.

Nigrastriatal DA losses in PD result from both normal aging and PD-specific losses

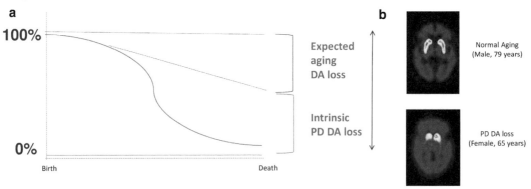

Fig. 7.3 Cumulative nigrostriatal DA losses in PD result from both normal aging and PD-specific losses. PD and age-associated losses (**a**) charting the course of expected nigrostriatal dopamine losses in healthy aging and intrinsic losses seen in Parkinson's disease. (**b**) Vesicular mono- amine transporter type 2 [^{11}C]dihydrotetrabenazine (DTBZ) parametric PET scans of the basal ganglia show- ing striatum DTBZ binding in a normal aging patient and a PD patient, with the PD patient showing dopamine losses in the typical posterior-to-anterior denervation gradient

Fig. 7.4 Vesicular monoamine transporter type 2 [^{11}C] dihydrotetrabenazine (DTBZ) parametric PET scans of the basal ganglia showing striatum DTBZ binding in three patients with PD of varying severity. With disease progression, greater losses of striatal uptake are seen in moderate and severe PD patients which affect both sides of the striatum. End-stage PD shows mild residual uptake seen mainly in the nucleus accumbens regions (anteroventral striatum)

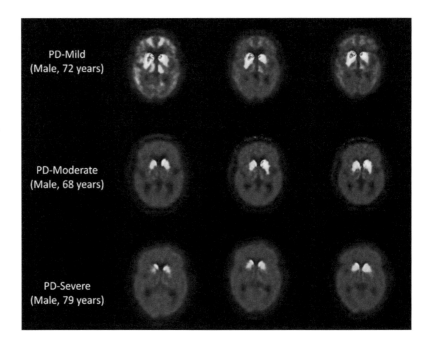

Atypical Parkinsonian Syndromes (APS)

While DAT-SPECT has been widely accepted for its clinical utility in detecting a presynaptic dopa- minergic deficit, its use has largely served to separate conditions such as PD and the atypical parkinsonian syndromes (APS) from the likes of essential tremor, vascular parkinsonism (VaP), and drug-induced parkinsonism (DIP) [3]. However, investigations into the use of presynap- tic nerve terminal dopaminergic imaging to dif- ferentiate between PD and APS (PSP, MSA or corticobasal syndrome, CBS) has been equivo- cal, at least when based on traditional visual scan interpretation. Some findings have sound theo- retical reasoning, such as attempting to match clinical phenotype to imaging characteristics. To this extent, several studies have found a general trend toward asymmetry of the dopamine deficit in PD when compared to the more symmetric deficits found in MSA and PSP. However, when comparing PD to MSA at autopsy the opposite was also found to be true [40, 41]. Other studies have taken to parcellating the striatum into smaller subregions for analysis, leading to findings of preferential dopamine transporter loss in the anterior caudate and ventral putamen subregions in MSA and PSP when compared to PD, however, attempts at using this technique to further discriminate between MSA and PSP have failed to do so [42–44]. Most consistent in differentiating MSA-P (MSA-parkinsonian type) and PSP from PD has been the use of postsynaptic D2 receptor imaging, such as [^{123}I]-123iodobenzamide IBZM SPECT]. These methods have shown reduced uptake in MSA-P and PD when compared to drug-naïve PD subjects, but this too comes with caveats as such inconsistencies seen in imaging findings of medicated subjects [45–49]. As of recently, imaging of striatal D$_{2/3}$ receptors is no longer recommended for the differential diagnosis of parkinsonian disorders in clinical practice [50].

CBS is a more rare APS that has proved to be a challenge to effectively apply the tool of dopaminergic imaging to, with speculation that this is largely due to the conditions underlying pathologic heterogeneity. While most cases do demonstrate a dopamine deficit, at times more than that seen in PD, there are also recorded instances of normal scans [51–53]. [^{18}F]-Fluorodeoxyglucose (FDG) PET imaging may have clinical utility for the diagnosis and differential diagnosis of CBS [49].

A comprehensive review on dopaminergic imaging in parkinsonian diseases by Nicastro and colleagues eloquently reviews much of the above and beyond [54].

Dopaminergic Imaging in Vascular Parkinsonism (VaP)

Most studies have found the use of presynaptic dopaminergic imaging, such as DAT-SPECT, helpful in the differentiation of PD from VaP, as

those with VaP can generally be expected to have normal or near-normal imaging [55]. Inquiries into whether those who have a dopamine deficit on a scan have a higher likelihood of response to levodopa or dopamine replacement therapies have failed to show consistent response. Focal areas of signal loss in those with VaP can sometimes be misleading, thus correlation with CT or MRI is preferred. It should be noted that vascular gray or white matter changes commonly accompany nigrostriatal losses in patients with neurodegenerative parkinsonism. More recently, a diagnostic approach toward a subtyping definition of VaP has been proposed that allows for identification of mixed and more pure subtypes of VaP based on nigrostriatal nerve terminal and cardiac sympathetic innervation radionuclide imaging techniques [56].

Dementia with Lewy Bodies (DLB)

DLB is behind only AD as the leading cause of neurodegenerative dementia [57]. It is defined as a syndrome with progressive cognitive impairment accompanied by at least two out of four core clinical features (visual hallucination, cognitive fluctuation, REM sleep behavior disorder, spontaneous parkinsonism) [57]. Intracellular inclusions of Lewy bodies are present in areas such as the olfactory bulb, brainstem, limbic, and cortex [58]. The spread of these proteins made predominately of alpha-synuclein is thought to play a central role in progressive cognitive impairment due to neuronal cell death in the cortex and subcortex [59]. In the latest diagnostic consensus criteria [57], reduced striatal dopamine transporter and abnormal [^{123}I]-MIBG cardiac scintigraphy were added as supportive biomarkers to help differentiate DLB from prototypical AD. Using molecular imaging SPECT or PET, previous studies have observed reduced presynaptic dopamine uptake [44, 54, 60–63] and preserved postsynaptic D$_2$ receptors uptake in DLB [64]. A recent study has found decreased striatal dopamine in DLB associated with glucose hypometabolism in the occipital, lateral parietal, and lateral frontal cortices that contribute to the cognitive impairment syndrome in DLB [65]. Another study found striatal dopamine depletion with hypermetabolic activities in the basal ganglia and limbic system at an early stage of dopamine depletion [66]. The study also found a significant correlation between putamen dopamine depletion and bilateral striatal hypermetabolism compared to healthy controls. This finding suggests a compensatory response to the decreasing signal input in the dopamine-depleted basal ganglia with increased striatal and limbic glucose metabolism at an early stage of disease [66]. As the disease progresses, the nigrostriatal dopaminergic degeneration advances with decreased metabolic connectivity between the basal ganglia and the limbic system, and switch from hyper- to hypometabolism in the associated areas [66]. In a study that looked at the relationship between β-amyloid load and striatal dopamine depletion in autopsy confirmed DLB, the presence of elevated neocortical β-amyloid depositions, as shown in amyloid imaging with the [^{11}C]-Pittsburgh compound B, also had decreased DAT concentration in DAT imaging using [^{11}C] Altropane PET [67]. Another study found that amyloid-positive DLB subjects, when compared with amyloid-negative DLB subjects, had a higher amyloid load in the cortex and the striatum with lower DAT activity in the anterior putamen and ventral striatum [68]. Amyloid-positive DLB subjects were of younger age at diagnosis, had greater cognitive deficit, and higher neuropsychiatric burden with reduced ventral striatum DAT activity. This might explain neurobehavioral changes, such as anxiety in DLB [68]. The finding is consistent with observations in PD patients at risk of cognitive decline, where striatal β-amyloid deposition closely relates with their apathy scores [69]. Possible interactive effects between regional β-amyloid deposition, intra-striatal dopaminergic losses, and glucose metabolism in striatal and extra-striatal regions deserve further study.

Alzheimer's Disease (AD)

AD is a progressive neurodegenerative disorder characterized by complex etiology. Multiple factors are known to cause damage to the brain in AD, including the presence of extracellular β-amyloid protein in senile plaques and intracellular neurofibrillary tangles. These factors are responsible for progressive neuronal cell dysfunction, degeneration, and impaired neurotransmission. An early post-mortem study of confirmed patients with AD found a decrease in [^{3}H]-spiroperidol DA$_2$ receptor binding in the caudate nucleus [70]. Subsequent pathological studies found alternations in the substantia nigra [71–75], the ventral tegmental area (VTA) [72] and their pre- [76–79] and postsynaptic [74, 80–82] dopaminergic targets. Belbin et al. suggested that the AD pathophysiology progression might be associated with a dopamine β-hydroxylase (DBH) polymorphism [83]. However, dopamine loss occurs during the neurological aging process, and it is not clear whether the dopamine loss in AD patients is the cause or the effect of aging or disease [84, 85]. Previous in vivo and post-mortem studies focused on dopaminergic projection arising from ventral VTA dopaminergic neurons to the cerebral cortex, nucleus accumbent, and hippocampus found evidence of dopaminergic neuron loss and dopaminergic degeneration in the VTA well before the "preplaque" stage in the hippocampus [71, 76, 86, 87]. A recent study by Sala et al. [88] confirms those findings using [^{123}I]-FP-CIT-SPECT. They found reduced binding of [^{123}I]-FP-CIT in both amyloid-positive mild cognitive impairment due to AD (AD-MCI) and patients with probable AD (AD-D) when compared with neurologically intact older adults in the areas associated with the targets of ventrotegmental-mesocorticolimbic pathways, namely the hippocampus and the ventral striatum. A similar reduction was found in the cingulate gyrus but only in the AD-D group. Reduced dorsal caudate nucleus [^{123}I] FP-CIT binding was observed in both AD-MCI and AD-D groups in nigrostriatal pathways. A previous post-mortem study found that unlike PD ventral portion of SNpc involvement, presynaptic dopaminergic functions were seen mainly in the dorsal tier of the SNpc in AD [71]. This finding could explain why the caudate nuclei that receives the dopamine input from the dorsomedial portion of the SNpc showed

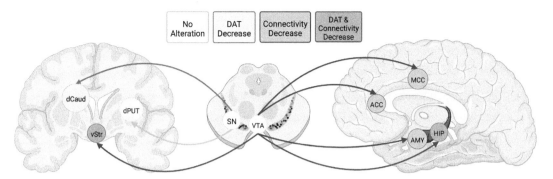

Fig. 7.5 A summary of dopamine vulnerability in prodromal AD (modified from reference [88]). The rendered figure showing prodromal AD having a decreased DAT activity in dopaminergic target (blue color), loss of connectivity (brown color), or both (purple color). *dCaud* dorsal caudate nucleus, *dPUT* dorsal putamen, *vStr* ventral striatum, *SN* substantia nigra, *VTA* ventral tegmental area, *ACC* anterior cingulate cortex, *MCC* middle cingulate cortex, *AMY* amygdala, *HIP* hippocampus

decreased [123]FP-CIT binding in AD. Although, the finding suggests evidence of nigrostriatal pathways vulnerability in AD, the degree and topography are quite different than that seen in PD [88]. In the same study, a molecular connectivity assessment using multivariate analysis found widespread dopaminergic loss in cortical and subcortical targets of the mesocorticolimbic pathways, but no alteration found in caudate and putamen inter-connections within the nigrostriatal pathways in both AD-MCI and AD-D groups. The overall finding from the Sala et al. study is described in Fig. 7.5. These findings may suggest differential vulnerability of the VTA vs. SN projections in AD and may also have relevance for DLB. VTA vulnerability has also been linked to impairments in a neural network resembling the default mode network.

MRI Sequences: Free Water/ DA-Dependent Neural Networks

Diffusion imaging is a MRI technique sensitive to the mean displacement of water molecules along a specified direction [89]. The most commonly used method for estimating tissue macroscopic geometry from water displacement is diffusion tensor imaging (DTI) [90]. DTI is a non-invasive imaging technique for characterizing the structural integrity of anatomical connections and provides a quantitative assessment of the brain's white matter microstructure by detecting the amount and direction of myelin water movement in extracellular and intracellular white matter spaces [91, 92]. Free water is defined as water molecules found in cerebrospinal fluid (CSF) spaces, such as the ventricles and around the brain parenchyma, and may also accumulate within the brain parenchyma in the extracellular space due to processes such as tumors, brain trauma, or inflammation that cause a breach the blood–brain barrier [93–95]. DTI can identify and assess free water based on its isotropic diffusion, which is almost four times higher than the brain parenchyma [96]. The DTI indices may be regarded as tissue-specific as long as image voxels contain a single type of tissue. However, edema and CSF can cause partial volume of different diffusion compartments, which degrades markers derived from DTI as non-specific. In order to minimize the effect of contamination from edema and CSF, Pierpaoli and Jones proposed a bi-tensor model [89, 97, 98], which assumes two compartments: a free water compartment characterized by isotropic tensor with diffusivity of free water, and a tissue compartment modeled by a diffusion tensor. Recently, DTI technique using a bi-tensor model have been used for evaluating neurodegenerative diseases such as PD and assessing its disease progression [99–102].

Previous studies have found that free water is elevated in the posterior SN (pSN) in PD patients compared to healthy controls [102]. This suggests that free water can provide an indirect measure of dopaminergic degeneration within the SN. Furthermore, longitudinal studies have shown that free water in the pSN in PD patients increase over a 1-year period of time and that free water in pSN continues to increase over 4 years in PD [99, 100].

In extracellular spaces, fluid diffuses between fibers, while in intracellular spaces, fluid diffuses in the axoplasm [92]. DTI can detect the amount and direction of myelin water movement in these extracellular and intracellular components, which allows for evaluation of the brain's white matter microstructure and neural network's structural integrity. DTI is sensitive for detecting white matter's linear structures, principally composed of axons. Disruption of white matter microstructure detectable with DTI can reflect the breakdown of myelin, certain constituents of the cytoskeleton, and axon density [92]. Fractional anisotropy (FA), mean diffusivity (MD), axial diffusivity (AD), and radial diffusivity (RD) are all commonly used to detect alteration of microscopic changes in white matter tissue integrity. Decreases in FA and AD and increases in MD and RD are interpreted as an alteration in white matter microstructure integrity. DTI has been utilized in Alzheimer's disease (AD) [103–105] and PD [106, 107]. For example, studies in AD patients have shown that there is a reduction of FA and an increase of MD in corpus callosum, medial and lateral temporal lobes, as well as in the fornix, cingulate gyrus, pre- cuneus, and prefrontal lobe white matter [105]. Gray matter atrophy was most pronounced in medial and lateral temporal lobe as well as parietal and prefrontal association cortex [105]. In PD, FA, and MD within the corpus callosum, the cingulate and the temporal cortices are reported to be lower than in normal controls, while these values are reported to be invertedly increased in the corticospinal tracts when compared to normal controls [106]. A more recent and emerging technique is neuromelanin-sensitive MRI to detect nigral signal changes in PD [50].

Approaches to Augment the Research and Clinical Utility of DA Nerve Terminal Molecular Imaging Ligands: Correlational Tractography, Radiomics, and Machine Vector Learning

There is an increasing interest in taking advantage of the complementary information captured not only in DAT or SPECT DA scans but also from MRI sequences. Correlational tractography is an example of one such multimodal imaging analysis technique that has been applied in PD. For example, we recently published a study where we defined the nigrostriatal pathways using MRI tractography and then incorporated information from DA (VMAT2) PET scans resulting in greater DA-specific definition of this pathway (Fig. 7.6) [108, 109].

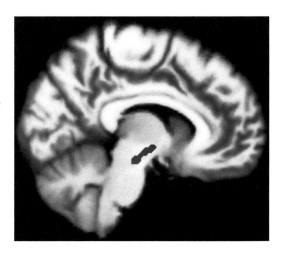

Fig. 7.6 Example of nigrostriatal tract visualization using [¹¹C]-DTBZ-PET and MRI correlational tractography (sagittal)

Similarly, deep learning architectures have recently gained popularity due to their tremendous potential in image segmentation, reconstruction, recognition, and classification. With the development of machine learning algorithms and deep learning architecture, the field of radiomics and their use in extracting features from medical images for quantitative image analysis and then converting them to medical imaging information for clinical and biological endpoints is gaining popularity. A recent study used a 3D convolution neural network to learn to distinguish features (like deep learning guided binding ratio) from DAT PET images ($[^{11}C]$-CFT PET). The neural network was able to distinguish idiopathic PD, MSA, and PSP and improved the previous conventional volume-of-interest method of using putamen and caudate binding ratio that failed to distinguish iPD from MSA [110]. Multiple studies have used radiomics on DAT-SPECT to detect PD and have tried to understand the progression of the disease [111–113]. Adams et al. improved on the previous method to by including non-imaging clinical measures to predict UPDRS-III motor scores at year 4 [114]. The radiomics method has enormous potential in clinical image analysis and decision-making. A necessary future step is the construction of generalized prognostic and predictive models using a careful selection of features, which could be achieved through the standardization of methods and made available to the clinical community as a valuable tool.

Fluid and Skin Biomarkers

In both PD and atypical parkinsonian syndromes there has long been a need for improved biomarkers for any number of purposes: predictive, susceptibility risk, diagnostic, monitoring or prognostic [115]. Considerable effort has already taken place in surveying imaging (some of which reviewed herein), blood, CSF, and additional nuanced measures (e.g., autonomic testing). While partly encouraging, these have fallen flat in finding the biomarker that is needed. In both serum and CSF, various forms of the proteins α-synuclein (total, oligomeric, and phosphorylated), tau (total, isoforms, phosphorylated), and neurofilament light chain have been studied (Fig. 7.7). There has been some evidence that the independent presence, ratio or combination of such proteins can have importance in differentiating between such conditions as PD and PSP, however, none have become validated biomarkers for monitoring in clinical trials yet. Brain biopsy have been honored as the most definitive source of biomarkers, however, for obvious reasons it is of course relegated as a post-mortem evaluation. Newer approaches that have garnered interest and investigation include biopsy of more accessible tissues including skin, secretory tissues, salivary glands or nerves. Skin biopsy has shown the most promise for specificity in antemortem differentiation of the α-synucleinopathies (PD, DLB, MSA) from other neurodegenerative conditions, including real-time quaking-induced conversion (RT-QuIC) and protein misfolding cyclic amplification (PMCA) assays, however, recent results from the Systemic Synuclein Sampling Study showcase its low sensitivity [116, 117]. While an independent and readily accessible biomarker remains a goal of the [near] future, current evidence directs toward utilization of a combination of biomarkers and/or correlation with dopaminergic imaging studies as best practice.

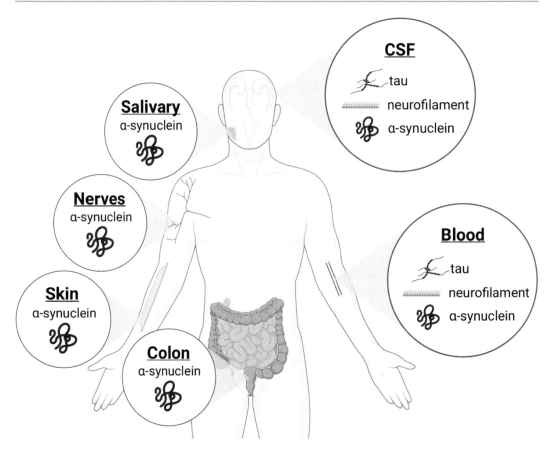

Fig. 7.7 A figure showing biomarkers under investigation for parkinsonian disorders. Blood biomarker, α-synuclein, tau neurofilament light chain; CSF bio-marker, α-synuclein, tau neurofilament light chain, skin, peripheral nerves, salivary gland, secretory glands (colon), α-synuclein

Future Directions: Novel Alpha-Synuclein Ligands

Although molecular imaging of dopaminergic systems has been used for early detection of neurodegenerative diseases causing movement disorders with synucleinopathy, such as PD, MSA, and PSP, and the monitoring of the effects of investigational disease-modifying treatments, degeneration of dopaminergic neurons is a downstream effect of α-synuclein deposition, which has been thought to be initiate α-synucleinopathy. This can currently only be detected by the histological examination of post-mortem brain tissue. There is great interest in imaging α-synuclein deposition for detecting very early stage of neurodegenerative diseases and monitoring disease progression accurately. PET is a non-invasive

in vivo imaging technique that can quantify target expression with high-resolution images, especially when combined with MRI and novel α-synuclein PET tracers and are thus highly sought. However, the development of α-synuclein PET tracers face several challenges. First, the low abundance of α-synuclein within the brain tissue necessitates the development of a high-affinity ligand. Second, α-synuclein depositions occur predominantly intracellularly, which limits the tracer accessibility. Lastly, there is the issue of ligand selectivity over structurally similar amyloids such as beta-amyloid or tau, which are often co-localized with α-synuclein pathology. Imaging of α-synuclein deposition could be a game-changer [118] and could facilitate the development of effective treatments [118]. Recently, [^{11}C]-MODAG-001, a PET tracer targeting α-synuclein aggregates, has shown a high-affinity and selectivity in α-synuclein aggregates with suitable pharmacokinetics and biodistribution properties, which can be utilized as a lead structure for future compound development [119]. Availability of tissue or fluid biomarkers for α-synuclein may become a first-line screening test for α-synucleinopathy in clinical practice but it may require a brain α-synuclein molecular imaging scan for confirmation and/or treatment response assessments.

Discussion/Summary

Movement disorders are caused by Lewy body parkinsonism, such as PD or DLB, or atypical parkinsonian syndromes including MSA, PSP, VaP. These disorders can also be accompanied by AD β-amyloid or tau pathology to variable degrees. Idiopathic RBD may predate or accompany PD, DLB or MSA. Molecular DA imaging techniques have played a large role in studying the underlying pathophysiology of these disorders at a neurotransmitter level and are being used for differential diagnostic purposes in the clinical setting. Furthermore, DAT imaging may play a role in prediction phenoconversion in patient with iRBD. There is increasing recognition of the effects of age-accelerated nigrostriatal dopaminergic losses that may in part reflect the presence of medical comorbidities, such as diabetes, or perhaps prodromal DLB or PD in the absence of iRBD. Elucidation of underlying mechanisms may hold therapeutic promise for patients with altered nigrostriatal nerve terminals across the spectrum of aging, parkinsonism and dementia. Differential vulnerability of VTA dopaminergic projections in AD may shine a new light on the phenotypic presentation of this dementia and its overlap with DLB. Diffusion tensor "free water" MRI is a promising tool with not only clinically diagnostic capabilities but it may also provide valuable prognostic information. Integrated PET/SPECT and MRI analyses, such as radiomics, correlation tractography and data-driven approaches (e.g., machine vector learning) may augment not only research but also

the clinical utility of DA nerve terminal imaging in patients across the spectrum of aging, age-accelerated striatal dopaminergic loss, parkinsonism, and dementia. Development of α-synuclein PET or SPECT imaging has proven to be challenging but recent candidate ligands show promise for the near future.

References

1. Eckert T, Eidelberg D. Neuroimaging and therapeutics in movement disorders. NeuroRx. 2005;2(2):361–71.
2. Carvey PM, Punati A, Newman MB. Progressive dopamine neuron loss in Parkinson's disease: the multiple hit hypothesis. Cell Transplant. 2006;15(3):239–50.
3. Palermo G, Ceravolo R. Molecular imaging of the dopamine transporter. Cell. 2019;8(8):872.
4. Uhl GR. Dopamine transporter: basic science and human variation of a key molecule for dopaminergic function, locomotion, and parkinsonism. Mov Disord. 2003;18(Suppl 7):S71–80.
5. Benamer HT, Patterson J, Wyper DJ, Hadley DM, Macphee GJ, Grosset DG. Correlation of Parkinson's disease severity and duration with 123I-FP-CIT SPECT striatal uptake. Mov Disord. 2000;15(4):692–8.
6. Mozley PD, Schneider JS, Acton PD, Plossl K, Stern MB, Siderowf A, et al. Binding of [99mTc] TRODAT-1 to dopamine transporters in patients with Parkinson's disease and in healthy volunteers. J Nucl Med. 2000;41(4):584–9.
7. Marek K, Innis R, van Dyck C, Fussell B, Early M, Eberly S, et al. [123I]beta-CIT SPECT imaging assessment of the rate of Parkinson's disease progression. Neurology. 2001;57(11):2089–94.
8. Kim HJ, Im JH, Yang SO, Moon DH, Ryu JS, Bong JK, et al. Imaging and quantitation of dopamine transporters with iodine-123-IPT in normal and Parkinson's disease subjects. J Nucl Med. 1997;38(11):1703–11.
9. Yang Y, Cheon M, Kwak YT. 18F-FP-CIT positron emission tomography for correlating motor and cognitive symptoms of Parkinson's disease. Dement Neurocogn Disord. 2017;16(3):57–63.
10. Tatsch K, Poepperl G. Nigrostriatal dopamine terminal imaging with dopamine transporter SPECT: an update. J Nucl Med. 2013;54(8):1331–8.
11. Saeed U, Compagnone J, Aviv RI, Strafella AP, Black SE, Lang AE, et al. Imaging biomarkers in Parkinson's disease and parkinsonian syndromes: current and emerging concepts. Transl Neurodegener. 2017;6:8.
12. Speranza L, di Porzio U, Viggiano D, de Donato A, Volpicelli F. Dopamine: the neuromodulator of long-

term synaptic plasticity, reward and movement control. Cell. 2021;10(4):735.

13. Ibrahim N, Kusmirek J, Struck AF, Floberg JM, Perlman SB, Gallagher C, et al. The sensitivity and specificity of F-DOPA PET in a movement disorder clinic. Am J Nucl Med Mol Imaging. 2016;6(1):102–9.

14. Nag S, Jahan M, Toth M, Nakao R, Varrone A, Halldin C. PET imaging of VMAT2 with the novel radioligand [(18)F]FE-DTBZ-d4 in nonhuman primates: comparison with [(11)C]DTBZ and [(18)F]FE-DTBZ. ACS Chem Neurosci. 2021;12(24):4580–6.

15. Bohnen NI, Muller ML, Kuwabara H, Cham R, Constantine GM, Studenski SA. Age-associated striatal dopaminergic denervation and falls in community-dwelling subjects. J Rehabil Res Dev. 2009;46(8):1045–52.

16. Bohnen NI, Albin RL, Koeppe RA, Wernette KA, Kilbourn MR, Minoshima S, et al. Positron emission tomography of monoaminergic vesicular binding in aging and Parkinson disease. J Cereb Blood Flow Metab. 2006;26(9):1198–212.

17. Rosano C, Metti AL, Rosso AL, Studenski S, Bohnen NI. Influence of striatal dopamine, cerebral small vessel disease, and other risk factors on age-related parkinsonian motor signs. J Gerontol A Biol Sci Med Sci. 2020;75(4):696–701.

18. Pagano G, Polychronis S, Wilson H, Giordano B, Ferrara N, Niccolini F, et al. Diabetes mellitus and Parkinson disease. Neurology. 2018;90(19):e1654–e62.

19. Chiaravalloti A, Barbagallo G, Ricci M, Sannino P, Karalis G, Ursini F, et al. Ageing effect on 18F-DOPA and 123I-MIBG uptake: a cross-sectional study. Nucl Med Commun. 2018;39(6):539–44.

20. Kumakura Y, Vernaleken I, Buchholz HG, Borghammer P, Danielsen E, Grunder G, et al. Age-dependent decline of steady state dopamine storage capacity of human brain: an FDOPA PET study. Neurobiol Aging. 2010;31(3):447–63.

21. Eidelberg D, Takikawa S, Dhawan V, Chaly T, Robeson W, Dahl R, et al. Striatal 18F-dopa uptake: absence of an aging effect. J Cereb Blood Flow Metab. 1993;13(5):881–8.

22. Ferini-Strambi L, Fasiello E, Sforza M, Salsone M, Galbiati A. Neuropsychological, electrophysiological, and neuroimaging biomarkers for REM behavior disorder. Expert Rev Neurother. 2019;19(11):1069–87.

23. Sakurai H, Hanyu H, Inoue Y, Kanetaka H, Nakamura M, Miyamoto T, et al. Longitudinal study of regional cerebral blood flow in elderly patients with idiopathic rapid eye movement sleep behavior disorder. Geriatr Gerontol Int. 2014;14(1):115–20.

24. Ota Y, Kanel P, Bohnen N. Imaging of sleep disorders in pre-Parkinsonian syndromes. Curr Opin Neurol. 2022;35(4):443–52.

25. Hustad E, Aasly JO. Clinical and imaging markers of prodromal Parkinson's disease. Front Neurol. 2020;11:395.

26. Meles SK, Oertel WH, Leenders KL. Circuit imaging biomarkers in preclinical and prodromal Parkinson's disease. Mol Med. 2021;27(1):111.

27. Miglis MG, Adler CH, Antelmi E, Arnaldi D, Baldelli L, Boeve BF, et al. Biomarkers of conversion to α-synucleinopathy in isolated rapid-eye-movement sleep behaviour disorder. Lancet Neurol. 2021;20(8):671–84.

28. Rolinski M, Griffanti L, Piccini P, Roussakis AA, Szewczyk-Krolikowski K, Menke RA, et al. Basal ganglia dysfunction in idiopathic REM sleep behaviour disorder parallels that in early Parkinson's disease. Brain. 2016;139(Pt 8):2224–34.

29. Wasserman D, Bindman D, Nesbitt AD, Cash D, Milosevic M, Francis PT, et al. Striatal dopaminergic deficit and sleep in idiopathic rapid eye movement behaviour disorder: an explorative study. Nat Sci Sleep. 2021;13:1–9.

30. Kim YK, Yoon IY, Kim JM, Jeong SH, Kim KW, Shin YK, et al. The implication of nigrostriatal dopaminergic degeneration in the pathogenesis of REM sleep behavior disorder. Eur J Neurol. 2010;17(3):487–92.

31. Bauckneht M, Chincarini A, De Carli F, Terzaghi M, Morbelli S, Nobili F, et al. Presynaptic dopaminergic neuroimaging in REM sleep behavior disorder: a systematic review and meta-analysis. Sleep Med Rev. 2018;41:266–74.

32. Iranzo A, Valldeoriola F, Lomeña F, Molinuevo JL, Serradell M, Salamero M, et al. Serial dopamine transporter imaging of nigrostriatal function in patients with idiopathic rapid-eye-movement sleep behaviour disorder: a prospective study. Lancet Neurol. 2011;10(9):797–805.

33. Chahine LM, Brumm MC, Caspell-Garcia C, Oertel W, Mollenhauer B, Amara A, et al. Dopamine transporter imaging predicts clinically-defined alpha-synucleinopathy in REM sleep behavior disorder. Ann Clin Transl Neurol. 2021;8(1):201–12.

34. Iranzo A, Santamaria J, Valldeoriola F, Serradell M, Salamero M, Gaig C, et al. Dopamine transporter imaging deficit predicts early transition to synucleinopathy in idiopathic rapid eye movement sleep behavior disorder. Ann Neurol. 2017;82(3):419–28.

35. Li Y, Kang W, Yang Q, Zhang L, Zhang L, Dong F, et al. Predictive markers for early conversion of iRBD to neurodegenerative synucleinopathy diseases. Neurology. 2017;88(16):1493–500.

36. Pringsheim T, Jette N, Frolkis A, Steeves TD. The prevalence of Parkinson's disease: a systematic review and meta-analysis. Mov Disord. 2014;29(13):1583–90.

37. Kalia LV, Lang AE. Parkinson's disease. Lancet. 2015;386(9996):896–912.

38. Muller M, Albin RL, Bohnen NI. Association of cardinal motor symptoms with region-specific dopamine transporter activity in mild to moderate Parkinson's disease. Eur Neurol J. 2013;4(2):1–7.

39. Lee CS, Samii A, Sossi V, Ruth TJ, Schulzer M, Holden JE, et al. In vivo positron emission tomographic evidence for compensatory changes in pre-

synaptic dopaminergic nerve terminals in Parkinson's disease. Ann Neurol. 2000;47(4):493–503.

40. Knudsen GM, Karlsborg M, Thomsen G, Krabbe K, Regeur L, Nygaard T, et al. Imaging of dopamine transporters and D2 receptors in patients with Parkinson's disease and multiple system atrophy. Eur J Nucl Med Mol Imaging. 2004;31(12):1631–8.

41. Perju-Dumbrava LD, Kovacs GG, Pirker S, Jellinger K, Hoffmann M, Asenbaum S, et al. Dopamine transporter imaging in autopsy-confirmed Parkinson's disease and multiple system atrophy. Mov Disord. 2012;27(1):65–71.

42. Oh M, Kim JS, Kim JY, Shin KH, Park SH, Kim HO, et al. Subregional patterns of preferential striatal dopamine transporter loss differ in Parkinson disease, progressive supranuclear palsy, and multiple-system atrophy. J Nucl Med. 2012;53(3):399–406.

43. Filippi L, Manni C, Pierantozzi M, Brusa L, Danieli R, Stanzione P, et al. 123I-FP-CIT in progressive supranuclear palsy and in Parkinson's disease: a SPECT semiquantitative study. Nucl Med Commun. 2006;27(4):381–6.

44. Badoud S, Van De Ville D, Nicastro N, Garibotto V, Burkhard PR, Haller S. Discriminating among degenerative parkinsonisms using advanced (123) I-ioflupane SPECT analyses. Neuroimage Clin. 2016;12:234–40.

45. Antonini A, Leenders KL, Vontobel P, Maguire RP, Missimer J, Psylla M, et al. Complementary PET studies of striatal neuronal function in the differential diagnosis between multiple system atrophy and Parkinson's disease. Brain. 1997;120(Pt 12):2187–95.

46. Ghaemi M, Hilker R, Rudolf J, Sobesky J, Heiss WD. Differentiating multiple system atrophy from Parkinson's disease: contribution of striatal and midbrain MRI volumetry and multi-tracer PET imaging. J Neurol Neurosurg Psychiatry. 2002;73(5):517–23.

47. van Royen E, Verhoeff NF, Speelman JD, Wolters EC, Kuiper MA, Janssen AG. Multiple system atrophy and progressive supranuclear palsy. Diminished striatal D2 dopamine receptor activity demonstrated by 123I-IBZM single photon emission computed tomography. Arch Neurol. 1993;50(5):513–6.

48. Kim YJ, Ichise M, Ballinger JR, Vines D, Erami SS, Tatschida T, et al. Combination of dopamine transporter and D2 receptor SPECT in the diagnostic evaluation of PD, MSA, and PSP. Mov Disord. 2002;17(2):303–12.

49. Hellwig S, Amtage F, Kreft A, Buchert R, Winz OH, Vach W, et al. [(1)(8)F]FDG-PET is superior to [(1)(2)(3)I]IBZM-SPECT for the differential diagnosis of parkinsonism. Neurology. 2012;79(13):1314–22.

50. Wallert ED, van de Giessen E, Knol RJJ, Beudel M, de Bie RMA, Booij J. Imaging dopaminergic neurotransmission in neurodegenerative disorders. J Nucl Med. 2022;63(Suppl 1):27S–32S.

51. Cilia R, Rossi C, Frosini D, Volterrani D, Siri C, Pagni C, et al. Dopamine transporter SPECT imaging in Corticobasal syndrome. PLoS One. 2011;6(5):e18301.

52. Kaasinen V, Gardberg M, Roytta M, Seppanen M, Paivarinta M. Normal dopamine transporter SPECT in neuropathologically confirmed corticobasal degeneration. J Neurol. 2013;260(5):1410–1.

53. O'Sullivan SS, Burn DJ, Holton JL, Lees AJ. Normal dopamine transporter single photon-emission CT scan in corticobasal degeneration. Mov Disord. 2008;23(16):2424–6.

54. Nicastro N, Nencha U, Burkhard PR, Garibotto V. Dopaminergic imaging in degenerative parkinsonisms, an established clinical diagnostic tool. J Neurochem. 2021;164:346.

55. Gerschlager W, Bencsits G, Pirker W, Bloem BR, Asenbaum S, Prayer D, et al. [123I]beta-CIT SPECT distinguishes vascular parkinsonism from Parkinson's disease. Mov Disord. 2002;17(3):518–23.

56. Rektor I, Bohnen NI, Korczyn AD, Gryb V, Kumar H, Kramberger MG, et al. An updated diagnostic approach to subtype definition of vascular parkinsonism—recommendations from an expert working group. Parkinsonism Relat Disord. 2018;49:9–16.

57. McKeith IG, Boeve BF, Dickson DW, Halliday G, Taylor JP, Weintraub D, et al. Diagnosis and management of dementia with Lewy bodies: fourth consensus report of the DLB consortium. Neurology. 2017;89(1):88–100.

58. Spillantini MG, Crowther RA, Jakes R, Hasegawa M, Goedert M. Alpha-synuclein in filamentous inclusions of Lewy bodies from Parkinson's disease and dementia with Lewy bodies. Proc Natl Acad Sci U S A. 1998;95(11):6469–73.

59. Lashuel HA, Overk CR, Oueslati A, Masliah E. The many faces of alpha-synuclein: from structure and toxicity to therapeutic target. Nat Rev Neurosci. 2013;14(1):38–48.

60. O'Brien JT, Colloby S, Fenwick J, Williams ED, Firbank M, Burn D, et al. Dopamine transporter loss visualized with FP-CIT SPECT in the differential diagnosis of dementia with Lewy bodies. Arch Neurol. 2004;61(6):919–25.

61. Brigo F, Turri G, Tinazzi M. 123I-FP-CIT SPECT in the differential diagnosis between dementia with Lewy bodies and other dementias. J Neurol Sci. 2015;359(1–2):161–71.

62. Jin S, Oh M, Oh SJ, Oh JS, Lee SJ, Chung SJ, et al. Differential diagnosis of parkinsonism using dual-phase F-18 FP-CIT PET imaging. Nucl Med Mol Imaging. 2013;47(1):44–51.

63. Thomas AJ, Attems J, Colloby SJ, O'Brien JT, McKeith I, Walker R, et al. Autopsy validation of 123I-FP-CIT dopaminergic neuroimaging for the diagnosis of DLB. Neurology. 2017;88(3):276–83.

64. Plotkin M, Amthauer H, Klaffke S, Kuhn A, Ludemann L, Arnold G, et al. Combined 123I-FP-CIT and 123I-IBZM SPECT for the diagnosis of parkinsonian syndromes: study on 72 patients. J Neural Transm (Vienna). 2005;112(5):677–92.

65. Yoo HS, Jeong SH, Oh KT, Lee S, Sohn YH, Ye BS, et al. Interrelation of striatal dopamine, brain metabolism and cognition in dementia with Lewy bodies. Brain. 2022;145:4448.

66. Huber M, Beyer L, Prix C, Schonecker S, Palleis C, Rauchmann BS, et al. Metabolic correlates of dopaminergic loss in dementia with Lewy bodies. Mov Disord. 2020;35(4):595–605.

67. Shirvan J, Clement N, Ye R, Katz S, Schultz A, Johnson KA, et al. Neuropathologic correlates of amyloid and dopamine transporter imaging in Lewy body disease. Neurology. 2019;93(5):e476–e84.

68. Yoo HS, Lee S, Chung SJ, Lee YH, Ye BS, Sohn YH, et al. Clinical and striatal dopamine transporter predictors of beta-amyloid in dementia with Lewy bodies. Neurology. 2020;94(13):e1344–e52.

69. Zhou Z, Muller M, Kanel P, Chua J, Kotagal V, Kaufer DI, et al. Apathy rating scores and beta-amyloidopathy in patients with Parkinson disease at risk for cognitive decline. Neurology. 2020;94(4):e376–e83.

70. Reisine TD, Yamamura HI, Bird ED, Spokes E, Enna SJ. Pre- and postsynaptic neurochemical alterations in Alzheimer's disease. Brain Res. 1978;159(2):477–81.

71. Joyce JN, Smutzer G, Whitty CJ, Myers A, Bannon MJ. Differential modification of dopamine transporter and tyrosine hydroxylase mRNAs in midbrain of subjects with Parkinson's, Alzheimer's with parkinsonism, and Alzheimer's disease. Mov Disord. 1997;12(6):885–97.

72. Gibb WR, Mountjoy CQ, Mann DM, Lees AJ. The substantia nigra and ventral tegmental area in Alzheimer's disease and Down's syndrome. J Neurol Neurosurg Psychiatry. 1989;52(2):193–200.

73. Mann DM, Yates PO, Marcyniuk B. Monoaminergic neurotransmitter systems in presenile Alzheimer's disease and in senile dementia of Alzheimer type. Clin Neuropathol. 1984;3(5):199–205.

74. Rinne JO, Sako E, Paljarvi L, Molsa PK, Rinne UK. Brain dopamine D-1 receptors in senile dementia. J Neurol Sci. 1986;73(2):219–30.

75. Attems J, Quass M, Jellinger KA. Tau and alpha-synuclein brainstem pathology in Alzheimer disease: relation with extrapyramidal signs. Acta Neuropathol. 2007;113(1):53–62.

76. Gottfries CG, Adolfsson R, Aquilonius SM, Carlsson A, Eckernas SA, Nordberg A, et al. Biochemical changes in dementia disorders of Alzheimer type (AD/SDAT). Neurobiol Aging. 1983;4(4):261–71.

77. Arai H, Kosaka K, Iizuka R. Changes of biogenic amines and their metabolites in postmortem brains from patients with Alzheimer-type dementia. J Neurochem. 1984;43(2):388–93.

78. Murray AM, Weihmueller FB, Marshall JF, Hurtig HI, Gottlieb GL, Joyce JN. Damage to dopamine systems differs between Parkinson's disease and Alzheimer's disease with parkinsonism. Ann Neurol. 1995;37(3):300–12.

79. Storga D, Vrecko K, Birkmayer JG, Reibnegger G. Monoaminergic neurotransmitters, their precursors and metabolites in brains of Alzheimer patients. Neurosci Lett. 1996;203(1):29–32.

80. Seeman P, Bzowej NH, Guan HC, Bergeron C, Reynolds GP, Bird ED, et al. Human brain D1 and D2 dopamine receptors in schizophrenia, Alzheimer's, Parkinson's, and Huntington's diseases. Neuropsychopharmacology. 1987;1(1):5–15.

81. Kumar U, Patel SC. Immunohistochemical localization of dopamine receptor subtypes (D1R-D5R) in Alzheimer's disease brain. Brain Res. 2007;1131(1):187–96.

82. Rinne JO, Sahlberg N, Ruottinen H, Nagren K, Lehikoinen P. Striatal uptake of the dopamine reuptake ligand [11C]beta-CFT is reduced in Alzheimer's disease assessed by positron emission tomography. Neurology. 1998;50(1):152–6.

83. Belbin O, Morgan K, Medway C, Warden D, Cortina-Borja M, van Duijn CM, et al. The epistasis project: a multi-cohort study of the effects of BDNF, DBH, and SORT1 epistasis on Alzheimer's disease risk. J Alzheimers Dis. 2019;68(4):1535–47.

84. Backman L, Farde L. Dopamine and cognitive functioning: brain imaging findings in Huntington's disease and normal aging. Scand J Psychol. 2001;42(3):287–96.

85. Li SC, Lindenberger U, Backman L. Dopaminergic modulation of cognition across the life span. Neurosci Biobehav Rev. 2010;34(5):625–30.

86. Karrer TM, Josef AK, Mata R, Morris ED, Samanez-Larkin GR. Reduced dopamine receptors and transporters but not synthesis capacity in normal aging adults: a meta-analysis. Neurobiol Aging. 2017;57:36–46.

87. Nam E, Derrick JS, Lee S, Kang J, Han J, Lee SJC, et al. Regulatory activities of dopamine and its derivatives toward metal-free and metal-induced amyloid-beta aggregation, oxidative stress, and inflammation in Alzheimer's disease. ACS Chem Neurosci. 2018;9(11):2655–66.

88. Sala A, Caminiti SP, Presotto L, Pilotto A, Liguori C, Chiaravalloti A, et al. In vivo human molecular neuroimaging of dopaminergic vulnerability along the Alzheimer's disease phases. Alzheimers Res Ther. 2021;13(1):187.

89. Pasternak O, Sochen N, Gur Y, Intrator N, Assaf Y. Free water elimination and mapping from diffusion MRI. Magn Reson Med. 2009;62(3):717–30.

90. Basser PJ, Mattiello J, LeBihan D. MR diffusion tensor spectroscopy and imaging. Biophys J. 1994;66(1):259–67.

91. Blinkouskaya Y, Cacoilo A, Gollamudi T, Jalalian S, Weickenmeier J. Brain aging mechanisms with mechanical manifestations. Mech Ageing Dev. 2021;200:111575.

92. Sullivan EV, Pfefferbaum A. Diffusion tensor imaging and aging. Neurosci Biobehav Rev. 2006;30(6):749–61.

93. Papadopoulos MC, Saadoun S, Binder DK, Manley GT, Krishna S, Verkman AS. Molecular mechanisms of brain tumor edema. Neuroscience. 2004;129(4):1011–20.

94. Unterberg AW, Stover J, Kress B, Kiening KL. Edema and brain trauma. Neuroscience. 2004;129(4):1021–9.

95. Ota Y, Srinivasan A, Capizzano AA, Bapuraj JR, Kim J, Kurokawa R, et al. Central nervous system systemic lupus erythematosus: pathophysiologic, clinical, and imaging features. Radiographics. 2022;42(1):212–32.

96. Pierpaoli C, Basser PJ. Toward a quantitative assessment of diffusion anisotropy. Magn Reson Med. 1996;36(6):893–906.

97. Alexander AL, Hasan KM, Lazar M, Tsuruda JS, Parker DL. Analysis of partial volume effects in diffusion-tensor MRI. Magn Reson Med. 2001;45(5):770–80.

98. Behrens TE, Woolrich MW, Jenkinson M, Johansen-Berg H, Nunes RG, Clare S, et al. Characterization and propagation of uncertainty in diffusion-weighted MR imaging. Magn Reson Med. 2003;50(5):1077–88.

99. Burciu RG, Ofori E, Archer DB, Wu SS, Pasternak O, McFarland NR, et al. Progression marker of Parkinson's disease: a 4-year multi-site imaging study. Brain. 2017;140(8):2183–92.

100. Ofori E, Pasternak O, Planetta PJ, Li H, Burciu RG, Snyder AF, et al. Longitudinal changes in free-water within the substantia nigra of Parkinson's disease. Brain. 2015;138(Pt 8):2322–31.

101. Yang J, Archer DB, Burciu RG, Muller M, Roy A, Ofori E, et al. Multimodal dopaminergic and free-water imaging in Parkinson's disease. Parkinsonism Relat Disord. 2019;62:10–5.

102. Ofori E, Pasternak O, Planetta PJ, Burciu R, Snyder A, Febo M, et al. Increased free water in the substantia nigra of Parkinson's disease: a single-site and multi-site study. Neurobiol Aging. 2015;36(2):1097–104.

103. Clerx L, Visser PJ, Verhey F, Aalten P. New MRI markers for Alzheimer's disease: a meta-analysis of diffusion tensor imaging and a comparison with medial temporal lobe measurements. J Alzheimers Dis. 2012;29(2):405–29.

104. Sexton CE, Kalu UG, Filippini N, Mackay CE, Ebmeier KP. A meta-analysis of diffusion tensor imaging in mild cognitive impairment and Alzheimer's disease. Neurobiol Aging. 2011;32(12):2322.e5–e18.

105. Teipel SJ, Wegrzyn M, Meindl T, Frisoni G, Bokde AL, Fellgiebel A, et al. Anatomical MRI and DTI in the diagnosis of Alzheimer's disease: a European multicenter study. J Alzheimers Dis. 2012;31(Suppl 3):S33–47.

106. Atkinson-Clement C, Pinto S, Eusebio A, Coulon O. Diffusion tensor imaging in Parkinson's disease: review and meta-analysis. Neuroimage Clin. 2017;16:98–110.

107. Cochrane CJ, Ebmeier KP. Diffusion tensor imaging in parkinsonian syndromes: a systematic review and meta-analysis. Neurology. 2013;80(9):857–64.

108. Sanchez-Catasus CA, Bohnen NI, Yeh FC, D'Cruz N, Kanel P, Muller M. Dopaminergic nigrostriatal connectivity in early Parkinson disease: in vivo neuroimaging study of (11)C-DTBZ PET combined with correlational tractography. J Nucl Med. 2021;62(4):545–52.

109. Sanchez-Catasus CA, Bohnen NI, D'Cruz N, Muller M. Striatal acetylcholine-dopamine imbalance in Parkinson disease: In vivo neuroimaging study with dual-tracer PET and dopaminergic PET-informed correlational tractography. J Nucl Med. 2022;63(3):438–45.

110. Zhao Y, Wu P, Wu J, Brendel M, Lu J, Ge J, et al. Decoding the dopamine transporter imaging for the differential diagnosis of parkinsonism using deep learning. Eur J Nucl Med Mol Imaging. 2022;49(8):2798–811.

111. Salmanpour MR, Shamsaei M, Hajianfar G, Soltanian-Zadeh H, Rahmim A. Longitudinal clustering analysis and prediction of Parkinson's disease progression using radiomics and hybrid machine learning. Quant Imaging Med Surg. 2022;12(2):906–19.

112. Rahmim A, Huang P, Shenkov N, Fotouhi S, Davoodi-Bojd E, Lu L, et al. Improved prediction of outcome in Parkinson's disease using radiomics analysis of longitudinal DAT SPECT images. Neuroimage Clin. 2017;16:539–44.

113. Shiiba T, Arimura Y, Nagano M, Takahashi T, Takaki A. Improvement of classification performance of Parkinson's disease using shape features for machine learning on dopamine transporter single photon emission computed tomography. PLoS One. 2020;15(1):e0228289.

114. Adams MP, Rahmim A, Tang J. Improved motor outcome prediction in Parkinson's disease applying deep learning to DaTscan SPECT images. Comput Biol Med. 2021;132:104312.

115. Parnetti L, Gaetani L, Eusebi P, Paciotti S, Hansson O, El-Agnaf O, et al. CSF and blood biomarkers for Parkinson's disease. Lancet Neurol. 2019;18(6):573–86.

116. Wang Z, Becker K, Donadio V, Siedlak S, Yuan J, Rezaee M, et al. Skin alpha-synuclein aggregation seeding activity as a novel biomarker for Parkinson disease. JAMA Neurol. 2020;78:30.

117. Chahine LM, Beach TG, Brumm MC, Adler CH, Coffey CS, Mosovsky S, et al. In vivo distribution of alpha-synuclein in multiple tissues and biofluids in Parkinson disease. Neurology. 2020;95(9):e1267–e84.

118. Korat S, Bidesi NSR, Bonanno F, Di Nanni A, Hoang ANN, Herfert K, et al. Alpha-synuclein PET tracer development-an overview about current efforts. Pharmaceuticals (Basel). 2021;14(9):847.

119. Kuebler L, Buss S, Leonov A, Ryazanov S, Schmidt F, Maurer A, et al. [(11)C]MODAG-001-towards a PET tracer targeting alpha-synuclein aggregates. Eur J Nucl Med Mol Imaging. 2021;48(6):1759–72.

Niels Okkels, Jacob Horsager, Nicola Pavese,
David J. Brooks, and Per Borghammer

Key Points

- Cholinergic molecular imaging can detect abnormalities in early disease stages of dementia and follow progression over time.
- The cholinergic system is implicated in a myriad of functions of the central and peripheral nervous systems, several of which are affected in dementia.
- In Alzheimer's disease and a significant proportion of patients Lewy body disease, early changes may occur in cholinergic axons or cell bodies of the basal forebrain.
- In another group of patients with Lewy body disease, the earliest changes most likely occur in cholinergic parasympathetic neurons innervating internal organs.

Cholinergic neurons, so called because they release the neurotransmitter acetylcholine, are found in several locations of the human body. Somatic motor neurons in the spinal cord and brainstem transmit acetylcholine to activate striated muscle tissue. Parasympathetic neurons in the brain stem and spinal cord release acetylcholine to smooth muscles in glands and organs. The interneurons of the striatum and preganglionic sympathetic neurons also transmit acetylcholine, as do the enteric neurons of the gastrointestinal tract. From a dementia research point of view, perhaps the most interesting group of cholinergic neurons are located in the poorly defined nuclei of the upper brainstem and basal forebrain. From here, the cholinergic neurons project their axons to almost all areas of the brain.

N. Okkels (✉)
Department of Nuclear Medicine and PET, Aarhus University Hospital, Aarhus, Denmark

Department of Clinical Medicine, Aarhus University, Aarhus, Denmark

Department of Neurology, Aarhus University Hospital, Aarhus, Denmark
e-mail: niels.okkels@clin.au.dk

J. Horsager
Department of Nuclear Medicine and PET, Aarhus University Hospital, Aarhus, Denmark

Department of Clinical Medicine, Aarhus University, Aarhus, Denmark
e-mail: jacobhorsager@clin.au.dk

N. Pavese
Department of Nuclear Medicine and PET, Aarhus University Hospital, Aarhus, Denmark

Clinical Ageing Research Unit, Newcastle University, Newcastle upon Tyne, UK
e-mail: npavese@clin.au.dk

D. J. Brooks
Department of Nuclear Medicine and PET, Aarhus University Hospital, Aarhus, Denmark

Positron Emission Tomography Centre, Newcastle University, Newcastle upon Tyne, UK
e-mail: dbrooks@clin.au.dk

P. Borghammer
Department of Nuclear Medicine and PET, Aarhus University Hospital, Aarhus, Denmark
e-mail: borghammer@clin.au.dk

© The Author(s), under exclusive license to Springer Nature Switzerland AG 2023
D. J. Cross et al. (eds.), *Molecular Imaging of Neurodegenerative Disorders*,
https://doi.org/10.1007/978-3-031-35098-6_8

For decades, the cholinergic system has been a cornerstone in dementia research. There are at least three plausible reasons. First, important cognitive functions are heavily dependent on a well-functioning cholinergic system [1, 2]. Second, the cortical cholinergic activity is decreased in manifest dementia, particularly in Alzheimer's disease dementia, Parkinson's disease dementia, and dementia with Lewy bodies [3–6]. This has been demonstrated consistently in both post-mortem and in vivo studies. Third, cognitive symptoms of dementia improve when treated with inhibitors of acetylcholinesterase (AChE), the enzyme responsible for the breakdown of acetylcholine.

Today, acetylcholine is acknowledged to be involved in many functions other than cognition. Correspondingly, it is increasingly acknowledged that neurodegenerative disorders affect multiple functions. For example, cholinergic dysfunction in Parkinson's disease is implicated in falls and freezing of gait, abnormal movements during REM sleep, hyposmia, depression, visual hallucinations, autonomic dysfunction, and psychosis [7, 8].

The cholinergic system can be visualized with both single-photon emission computed tomography (SPECT) and positron emission tomography (PET) using radiotracers engaging various molecular targets involved in the synthesis, storage, reception, and hydrolysis of acetylcholine. Cholinergic molecular imaging in dementia has proved to have multiple interesting applications (Fig. 8.1).

One example is proof of mechanism of drugs. A study used PET to measure the cerebral activity of AChE in patients with mild cognitive impairment due to Alzheimer's disease. The authors found that the efficacy of an AChE-inhibitor depended on the activity of AChE [9]. At clinically tolerated doses, it emerged only around 25% of AChE sites were being occupied by the inhibitor donepezil.

Fig. 8.1 Cholinergic imaging in dementia research. A graphic illustration of the many applications of cholinergic molecular imaging in dementia research

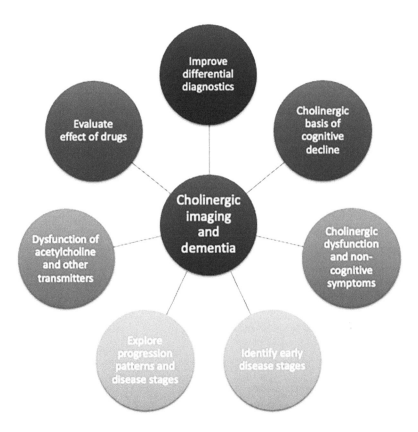

Another application of cholinergic imaging focuses on understanding the neuropathological basis of symptoms and signs. For example, studies have looked at the role of cholinergic dysfunction in visual hallucinations, hyposmia, gait disturbances, and of course; cognition [7]. The contribution of cholinergic dysfunction to symptoms and signs, however, can be difficult to disentangle, as the processes occur on a background of pathology involving multiple transmitter systems and cell types.

A third example on how cholinergic imaging is used in research is to understand cholinergic changes in relation to other pathological markers such as metabolic activity [10], inflammation [11], amyloid [12], and structural atrophy [13]. Unfortunately, there is not yet a tracer that specifically binds to aggregated alpha-synuclein, the pathological substrate of Lewy body diseases. So far, cholinergic imaging is not routinely used in the clinic to diagnose or differentiate disorders. This chapter will focus on cholinergic imaging in dementia *research* [14].

In the first part of this chapter, we will introduce the cholinergic neuron. To understand PET-images, it is crucial to know where the different PET-tracers bind and the function of these target-molecules. Then we present the organization of the cholinergic system on a macroscopic level. The second part of the chapter will focus on the role of cholinergic imaging in identifying preclinical or prodromal disease stages of Alzheimer's disease dementia, Parkinson's disease dementia, and dementia with Lewy bodies [15]. From a clinical perspective, patients at very early stages represent optimal candidates for evaluating disease modifying therapies and possibly curative treatments while the disease remains rather localized. From a basic scientific perspective, studying early disease stages can shed light on fundamental questions about when and where the pathology begins and how it spreads. Cholinergic imaging may be a very important tool for exploring these questions.

Cholinergic Neurons and Tracer Molecules

Acetylcholine is synthesized in the nerve terminal by choline acetyltransferase (ChAT) and loaded into vesicles by the vesicular acetylcholine transporter (VAChT) (Fig. 8.2). Even small decreases of VAChT may have large effects on the release of acetylcholine by reducing the amount of acetylcholine release by vesicles [16]. [^{18}F]FEOBV is a PET-tracer for VAChT and a very specific marker of cholinergic terminals (Fig. 8.3) [12, 17, 18]. [^{123}I]IBVM is the corresponding tracer for SPECT.

In the synaptic cleft, acetylcholine is hydrolyzed by acetylcholinesterase (AChE). PET-tracers targeting AChE are among the most used in dementia research. The activity of AChE can be measured by substrate-tracers that are metabolized by AChE, such as [^{11}C]MP4A and [^{11}C]MP4P ([^{11}C]PMP). These are lipophilic and pass the blood–brain barrier but become hydrophilic when metabolized and trapped inside the brain [19]. Another group of radioligands for AChE act as ligands that bind to AChE, such as [^{11}C]donepezil. In the CNS, AChE is expressed by cholinergic as well as cholinoceptive non-cholinergic neurons.

Upon release from the cholinergic neuron, acetylcholine can bind to metabotropic muscarinic receptors or ionotropic nicotinic receptors [20, 21]. These receptors comprise several subtypes that are located on dendrites, cell bodies, and axons, on pre-terminal and post-terminal membranes of cholinergic and non-cholinergic cells. In general, presynaptic and preterminal nicotinic receptors enhance release of neurotransmitter, whereas post-synaptic and non-synaptic nicotinic receptors mediate excitation. The PET-tracers [^{18}F]flubatine and [^{18}F]FA have been implemented in clinical research and bind the alpha 4 beta 2 nicotinic acetylcholine receptor [22, 23]. The PET-tracer [^{11}C]nicotine is a non-selective agonist to nicotinic receptor subtypes [24]. [^{11}C]NMBP binds to all muscarinic receptor subtypes [25].

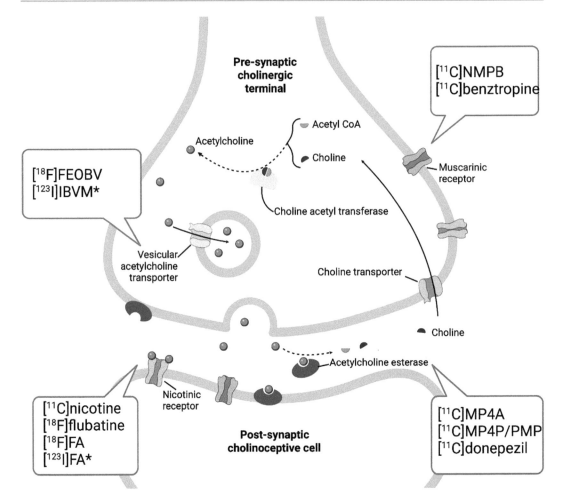

Fig. 8.2 Acetylcholine metabolism in cholinergic nerve terminals and relevant positron emission tomography (PET) tracers. Acetylcholine is synthesized from acetyl coenzyme A and choline by choline acetyl transferase in the cholinergic terminal. The vesicular acetylcholine transporter loads acetylcholine into pre-synaptic vesicles. Upon release, acetylcholine can engage its receptors. Acetylcholine esterase hydrolyses acetylcholine into acetic acid and choline. Tracers marked by an asterisk are used in single photon emission computed tomography (SPECT)

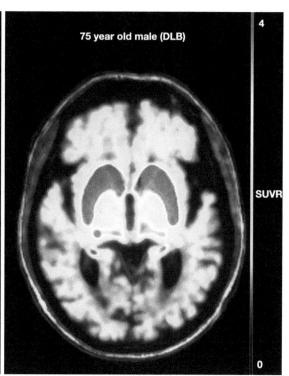

Fig. 8.3 [^{18}F]fluroetoxybenzovesamicol (FEOBV) positron emission tomography (PET) of healthy control and patient with dementia with Lewy bodies. A 75-year-old man with DLB (right side) and lower uptake of [^{18}F] FEOBV, a PET-ligand for the vesicular acetylcholine transporter, compared to a non-demented age- and sex-matched control (left). The images are sliced axially on the AC-PC line and present an [^{18}F]FEOBV-PET superimposed on a T1-MRI scan. The colorbar is scaled to a standard uptake value ratio (SUVR) of 0 to 4 where red colors indicate high uptake of tracer, and blue colors low uptake. *SUVR* standard uptake value ratio

In summary, the cholinergic molecules and their corresponding tracers are markers of different aspects of the cholinergic system.

Cholinergic Neurons in the Human Organism

Cholinergic neurons in the basal forebrain provide the principal source of acetylcholine to the cortex and limbic structures (Fig. 8.4). They can be divided into four overlapping groups of cell bodies [26]. The cholinergic neurons located on the medial septum and horizontal band project to the hippocampus and hypothalamus. The neurons associated with the diagonal band project to the olfactory tubercle. The largest group of cholinergic cell bodies is associated with the nucleus basalis of Meynert (NBM) and project to the cortex and amygdala [27]. From the NBM the fiber tracts bundle in a lateral and a medial pathway before they fan out to the cortex [28]. The long and unmyelinated axons pass close to the lateral ventricles and reach the cortex through the underlying white matter. Interestingly, recent studies have documented that periventricular white mat-

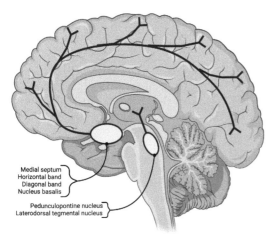

Medial septum
Horizontal band
Diagonal band
Nucleus basalis

Pedunculopontine nucleus
Laterodorsal tegmental nucleus

Fig. 8.4 Main cholinergic projecting neurons of the central nervous system. The basal forebrain is composed of four overlapping cell groups and provide the principal source of acetylcholine to the cortex and limbic structures. The pedunculopontine nucleus and laterodorsal tegmental nucleus provide the main cholinergic innervation of the thalamus. The cholinergic projecting neurons of the medial habenula and parabigeminal nucleus are not presented on this figure. Neither are the cholinergic interneurons of the striatum or the motor neurons of the brainstem

ter lesions correlate with decreased cognition and decreased cortical cholinergic activity. Thus, periventricular white matter lesions may disrupt the cholinergic projections from the NBM to the cortex [29].

When reaching the cortex, the projecting neurons from the NBM arborize extensively and each cover an area of about 1–1.5 mm^2. Along the thin axons there are multiple varicosities. These represent sites for transmitter release, and some make direct contact with other neurons to form a synapse. Other varicosities release their transmitter molecules into the extracellular space to signal multiple cells simultaneously. The NBM innervates the entire cortex, but only limbic areas project back to the NBM. These limbic areas assign relevance to sensory stimuli and thereby modulate the response by the NBM [27]. If stimuli have high salience, acetylcholine is released to augment or amplify the signal in relevant cortical areas. For example, acetylcholine increases the responsiveness of neurons in the visual cortex to inputs from the lateral geniculate nucleus [2].

There is another significant group of cholinergic neurons on the junction of the pons and mesencephalon. The neurons are dispersed around the pedunculopontine and laterodorsal tegmental nuclei (PPN/LDT), and project their axons mainly to the thalamus.

Alzheimer's Disease and Lewy Body Disease

Alzheimer's disease (AD) is characterized by the accumulation of beta amyloid and tau tangles. The aggregation of these misfolded proteins is closely linked with neuronal dysfunction and degeneration. Over years, AD pathology can lead to Alzheimer's disease dementia (ADD), the most common cause of dementia worldwide. The second most common cause of neurodegenerative dementia is Lewy body disease. Lewy bodies are pathological aggregates that are formed in neurons and defined by their content of phosphorylated alpha synuclein. Lewy body disease can lead to several clinical syndromes including Parkinson's disease (PD), Parkinson's disease dementia (PDD), dementia with Lewy bodies (DLB), pure autonomic failure, and REM sleep behavior disorder (RBD), a sleep disorder characterized by abnormal movements during REM sleep. These are collectively referred to as Lewy body disorders (LBD). The related disorder multiple system atrophy is also caused by aggregated alpha synuclein, but these aggregates do not form Lewy bodies and the patients rarely become demented, so this disease will not be dealt with in this chapter. Up to 95% of patients with isolated RBD (iRBD) will eventually develop either PD or DLB, and more than 80% of patients with PD will eventually develop PDD [30, 31]. Thus, the end-stages of Lewy body diseases converge on dementia. Therefore, in this chapter, we will consider LBD in general, and not only the manifest dementia stages.

The natural history of AD and LBD can be illustrated on a timeline (Fig. 8.5). In the beginning, there is no pathology. An individual's risk of dementia is defined by genetic predisposition and environmental exposure. Some genetic traits

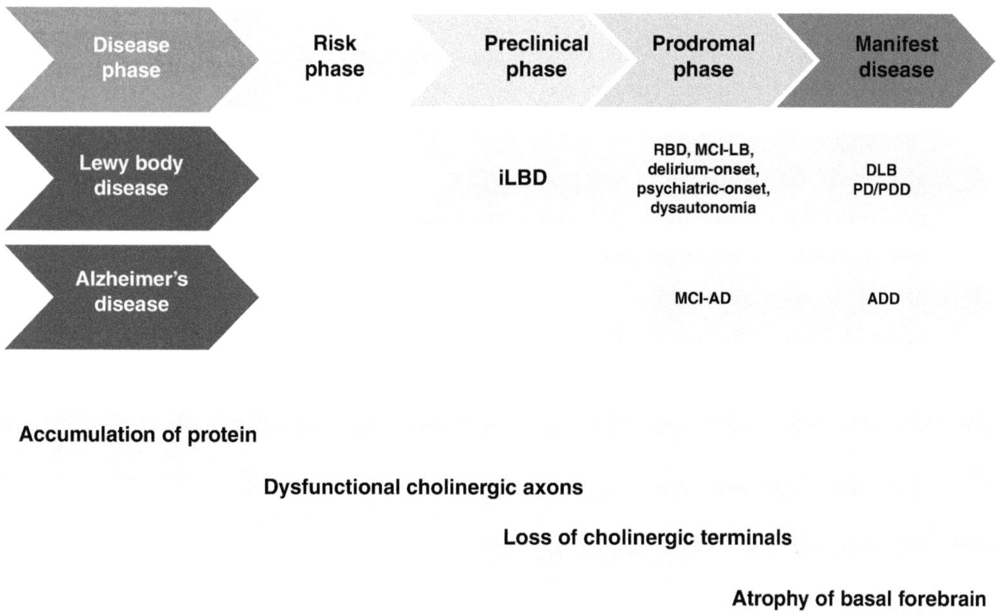

| Disease phase | Risk phase | Preclinical phase | Prodromal phase | Manifest disease |

Lewy body disease — iLBD — RBD, MCI-LB, delirium-onset, psychiatric-onset, dysautonomia — DLB PD/PDD

Alzheimer's disease — MCI-AD — ADD

Accumulation of protein

Dysfunctional cholinergic axons

Loss of cholinergic terminals

Atrophy of basal forebrain

Fig. 8.5 Timeline of early disease stages of Alzheimer's disease dementia and Lewy body disorders. The stages in Alzheimer's disease and Lewy body disorders depicted on a timeline. The figure should be read from left to right. In the beginning (left), there is no pathology. The balance of genetic traits and environmental factors determine the likelihood of developing neurodegenerative disease (risk phase). In the preclinical phase pathology has developed, but there are not yet any signs or symptoms. Then follows the prodromal phase with emergence of signs and symptoms, and finally manifest dementia when cognitive difficulties begin to interfere with daily life functions

and environmental factors increase the risk of disease, others protect against disease. This stage can be referred to as the *risk phase*. Then follows the *preclinical phase* where pathology is present, at least at a cellular level, but there are not yet any symptoms or detectable signs. These *incidental cases* are asymptomatic with signs of pathology on post-mortem examination or PET scans. During the *prodromal stage* the pathological processes evolve to a degree where symptoms and signs develop. An example is mild cognitive impairment (MCI) where subjects have cognitive difficulties that are not yet severe enough to cause loss of independence. Another example is iRBD which is considered a prodromal stage of PD and DLB. The final step to *manifest dementia* occurs when the cognitive difficulties are severe enough to interfere with daily life functions.

MCI can be diagnosed when there is concern about a decline in cognition and evidence of impairment in one or more cognitive domains in combination with preserved independence in activities of daily living [32]. MCI with affected memory increases the likelihood that the cause of MCI is AD (MCI-AD). Biomarkers showing brain beta-amyloid aggregation and neuronal injury can further increase the likelihood of MCI due to AD. These markers include PET amyloid imaging and low β-amyloid 42 in the cerebrospinal fluid. Markers of neuronal injury include high tau in the cerebrospinal fluid, atrophy on structural imaging, and decreased perfusion or glucose metabolism on PET.

Cholinergic Molecular Imaging in Alzheimer's Disease and Lewy Body Disorders

The first molecular imaging studies using cholinergic markers in vivo with ADD, PD, and PDD were performed in the mid 1990s. Studies on

DLB appeared a few years later, as formal diagnostic criteria for DLB were defined in 1996. These in vivo studies confirmed decades of post-mortem studies showing cortical cholinergic depletion in *manifest dementia* [10, 33]. They also confirmed the general tendency of a severe and indistinguishable cortical depletion in PDD and DLB, milder cholinergic involvement in cases at early stages, and more severe depletion in PDD and DLB compared to ADD [23, 34–36]. Overall, the cortical cholinergic integrity correlates with disease severity and dementia. We will focus initially on studies that investigated early disease stages using cholinergic imaging.

A study used the AChE substrate-tracer [11C] MP4A to investigate the cholinergic system of patients with MCI-AD. Apart from MCI, the patients were characterized by memory impairment, atrophy of the medial temporal lobe, and lowered amyloid in the CSF. The authors found decreased cortical activity of AChE, particularly in the temporal, parietal, and occipital lobes [29]. A similar pattern of reduced AChE activity was reported in a group of MCI characterized by memory decline [37]. Again, the activity of AChE was reduced in several cortical regions, but mostly in the temporal cortex. A third study using the same tracer on a comparable MCI population came to similar results, except that they found the hippocampus to be the structure most severely affected [38]. These findings suggest that cholinergic dysfunction in the temporal lobe may be a sign of early AD.

Another study followed a group of patients with MCI and affected memory and decreased performance in at least one other cognitive domain. They found that individuals with MCI who progressed to ADD had widespread reductions of cortical AChE activity, particularly in the parietotemporal regions. Activity in the hippocampus and thalamus was preserved among MCI who did not progress [39]. The cholinergic projections to the hippocampus come from the rostral sectors of the basal forebrain, and the cholinergic projections to the thalamus come from the PPN/LDT complex in the brainstem. This suggests that more rostral sectors of the basal forebrain are affected later and marks the

transition to dementia. A similar sequential involvement could be true for the PPN/LDT, although evidence of thalamic reductions in cholinergic signal in ADD is less convincing.

[18F]FA binds to the alpha 4 beta 2 nicotinic receptor and has been used to image MCI with PET. On follow up, those MCI cases who progressed to dementia had significant baseline reductions in [18F]FA binding in several cortical areas, most pronounced in the temporal cortex and caudate [40]. Another study used the same tracer to study amnestic MCI and reported significant decreases in signal in all investigated cortical regions in addition to the hippocampus and caudate. The most severe reductions were found in those patients who progressed to ADD. Overall, the reductions among patients with MCI who progressed were almost as severe as those seen in fully developed ADD. This suggests that marked cholinergic dysfunction occurs at an early disease stage of AD [41].

Another more recent study used [18F]FA to investigate patients with MCI and impairment in the memory domain. They found that the level of change in nicotinic cholinergic receptor binding was between that of healthy controls and manifest ADD [23]. This supports the view that AD-MCI represents a stage on the spectrum to fulminant dementia. Furthermore, it seems that the density of nicotinic cholinergic receptors declines initially in the entorhinal cortex and other limbic structures suggesting that the cholinergic projections from the NBM to the entorhinal cortex are affected at a very early stage. Interestingly, the study found [18F]FA uptake in the hippocampus to be almost normal in AD-MCI, but severely decreased in ADD. This implies that the cholinergic cell bodies in the medial septum and horizontal limb are affected later than those in the NBM, in line with AD-pathology spreading through the basal forebrain in a rostral direction [42]. Another possible explanation for preserved hippocampal uptake in AD-MCI could be a compensatory upregulation in the density of receptors.

Overall, PET imaging has shown that there is impaired cholinergic integrity in MCI-AD that is more severe in limbic and medial temporal structures. Also, impairment is more severe in MCI cases who are close to converting to dementia [43]. While *early-stage* MCI patients also have impaired cholinergic integrity, their reductions often fall short of statistical significance, probably due to small study sample sizes. It is likely that the cholinergic system is affected from the beginning of the MCI-stage and possibly before the onset of MCI. This is supported by longitudinal data showing that the cognitive decline in MCI can be detected 4–6 years before MCI is diagnosed, implying a long-term temporal window of Alzheimer progression before MCI diagnosis [44]. Molecular cholinergic imaging in preclinical stages of AD has not yet been performed.

Magnetic resonance imaging (MRI) can be used to measure the size of the basal forebrain [45]. Decreases in grey matter volume detected with MRI-based volumetry can be used to measure rates of neurodegeneration. A study found an association between atrophy in the basal forebrain measured using MRI and amyloid deposition measured using PET in preclinical and prodromal stages of AD [46]. Moreover, among MCI cases, lower volumes of the basal forebrain were found to be associated with impaired cognition and cortical hypometabolism assessed using PET [47]. A study using MRI to investigate patients with MCI-AD found that atrophy of the NBM precedes atrophy of the entorhinal cortex, which is then followed by memory impairment. Interestingly, pathology of the NBM alone does not lead to memory impairment. Rather, the memory impairments of early AD arise when there is degeneration of the projections from the NBM to the entorhinal cortex. Thus, a subcortical to cortical spread of pathology may be a very early stage in AD pathology [48].

iRBD

Isolated RBD (iRBD) is characterized by accumulation of Lewy bodies in neurons and abnormal movement and behavior during REM sleep. The vast majority of patients with iRBD will develop either PD or DLB, and the majority of

patients with PD progress to dementia (PDD) [30, 31]. This makes iRBD an excellent disorder for studying prodromal stages of DLB and PDD. Surprisingly, very little research has yet been carried out on the cholinergic system in iRBD. A study investigated patients with iRBD using PET and [^{11}C]donepezil, a tracer that binds to AChE. Although the patients did not have any symptoms or signs of cognitive decline or motor disturbances, the authors found decreased uptake of tracer in the cortex of patients with iRBD compared to controls [49]. The cortical levels of [^{11}C]donepezil were lower in the superior temporal cortex, the cingulum, dorsolateral prefrontal, and occipital cortices. Interestingly, this pattern of dysfunction resembles that seen in manifest Lewy body disorders. This observation has two important implications. First, it supports that the cholinergic system in prodromal PD and DLB is impaired and dysfunctional. Second, it suggests that investigations of patients with iRBD may be a key to understand early changes in the cholinergic system related to Lewy body disease.

Another finding of the study was that the affected cortical structures in iRBD are known to receive dense cholinergic projections from the NBM. Furthermore, the cortical tracer uptake was lower in those patients who performed worse on tests of cognitive function. This underlines that early preclinical or prodromal cognitive decline is associated with dysfunction of the cholinergic system in Lewy body disease, and that this dysfunction can be visualized using PET. Furthermore, there is evidence that the cholinergic dysfunction occurs in parallel with nigrostriatal dopaminergic dysfunction, implying that the pathological processes in the NBM and substantia nigra are linked [50, 51].

PET using cholinergic tracers has been used to visualize the peripheral autonomous nervous system. Patients with iRBD show decreased uptake of [^{11}C]donepezil in their colon and small intestine. This signifies a dysfunction of the enteric and parasympathetic nervous system [52]. It may well be that the Lewy pathology was initiated in the peripheral nervous system in those patients with Lewy body dementia that were RBD-positive during their prodromal stage [53]. In iRBD there is pathology in nuclei of the upper brainstem. This means that at the time point of diagnosing iRBD, pathology is already relatively widespread in the brainstem and limbic system. Supposing that pathology in iRBD arose in the peripheral nervous system, and spread to the CNS, it should be theoretically possible to identify cases with pathology confined to the periphery. Pure autonomic failure, another Lewy body disorder, may represent such a population [54].

As such, cholinergic molecular markers are successfully being used to further characterize the prodromal disease stages of RBD-first Lewy body disorders. However, about two-thirds of patients with PD and one-quarter with DLB do not have iRBD in their prodromal stage [55]. The question is then how to identify this group in their prodromal stage? Part of the answer may be MCI-LB—see the next section.

Table 8.1 presents a list of molecular cholinergic human in vivo studies in preclinical and prodromal AD and LBD.

Table 8.1 Human in vivo studies using cholinergic molecular imaging in preclinical and prodromal Alzheimer's disease and Lewy body disease. Studies listed by year of publication from earliest (top) to most recent (buttom). Bold denotes statistical significance. Only studies cited in the text are listed in the table. *AChE* acetylcholinesterase, *AD* Alzheimer's disease, *CN* cognitively normal, *CSF* cerebrospinal fluid, *DLB* dementia with Lewy bodies, *HC* healthy control, *MCI* mild cognitive impairment, *MMSE* mini mental state examination, *iRBD* isolated REM sleep behavior disorder, *SD* standard deviation, *VLMT* verbal learning and memory test

Study	Tracer	Diagnostic group	Results
[38]	[^{11}C] MP4A	MCI ($n = 12$), AD ($n = 13$), HC ($n = 12$) Patients with MCI had subjective memory complaints and showed an impairment greater than 1.5 SD from the mean of healthy controls in at least one memory test	Hippocampus (MCI -17%, AD -27%), frontal cortex (MCI -5%, AD -9%), lateral temporal cortex (MCI -10%, AD -20%), parietal cortex (MCI -8%, AD -13%), thalamus (MCI +11%, AD -2%)
[43]	[^{11}C] MP4A	MCI ($n = 8$), AD ($n = 11$), HC ($n = 21$) MCI fulfilled the Peterson criteria. Four MCI converted to AD during follow-up	Global cortex (MCI -12%, AD *-24%*) MCI who converted to AD had low AChE activity at baseline. Those who remained stable had normal activity
[41]	[^{18}F]FA	MCI ($n = 6$), AD ($n = 17$), HC ($n = 10$) Amnestic MCI	Decreased binding in hippocampus, caudate, frontal, temporal, parietal, and cingulate cortices The MCI cases who converted to AD had low baseline values, those who remained MCI had normal values
[79]	[^{123}I]FA	MCI ($n = 9$), HC ($n = 10$) Amnestic MCI	Reduced uptake in medial temporal lobe of MCI
[40]	[^{18}F]FA	MCI ($n = 8$), AD ($n = 9$), HC ($n = 7$) "Amnestic" MCI ($n = 5$), "multidomain amnestic" MCI ($n = 3$)	In MCI cases who converted to AD: Reduced signal in frontal, parietal, temporal, occipital, posterior cingulate, caudate, right hippocampus, and left anterior cingulate Similar pattern in MCI and AD
[39]	[^{11}C] MP4A	MCI ($n = 10$), AD ($n = 7$), DLB ($n = 4$), HC ($n = 9$) Patients with MCI were described as multidomain amnestic	Prefrontal cortex (MCI *-19%*, AD *-15%*, DLB -13%), superior parietal lobule (MCI *-21%*, AD *-17%*, DLB -6%), inferior parietal lobule (MCI *-21%*, AD *-17%*, DLB *-13%*), temporal lateral cortex (MCI *-23%*, AD *-19%*, DLB *-18%*), occipital lateral cortex (MCI *-23%*, AD *-16%*, DLB *-14%*), hippocampal structures (MCI *-21%*, AD *-19%*, DLB *-22%*), thalamus (MCI *-21%*, AD *-37%*, DLB *-21%*)
[37]	[^{11}C] MP4A	MCI ($n = 17$), HC ($n = 21$) Patients with MCI had memory decline	Total cortex *−10%*. Largest reductions in temporal cortex and limbic regions

Table 8.1 (continued)

Study	Tracer	Diagnostic group	Results
[29]	[^{11}C] MP4A	MCI ($n = 17$), HC ($n = 18$) 16 MCI had signs of neuronal injury and an AD-typical CSF biomarker profile, corresponding to a high likelihood of MCI due to AD. One MCI had signs of neuronal injury but no AD-markers in CSF and classified as intermediate likelihood	Total cortex −13%. Largest reductions in temporal, parietal, and occipital lobes Periventricular white matter lesions negatively correlated with cortical activity of AChE and cognition in both patients and controls. This implies that white matter lesions may disrupt cholinergic projections to the cerebral cortex
[52]	[^{11}C] donepezil	iRBD ($n = 22$), PD ($n = 18$), HC ($n = 16$) iRBD had no parkinsonism or cognitive impairment	Patients with iRBD have decreased binding in the colon and small intestine
[9]	[^{11}C] MP4A	MCI ($n = 14$), HC ($n = 16$) MCI had high probability of AD as they had CSF biomarkers indicative of Alzheimer pathology and signs of neuronal injury. The predominant impairment in all MCI was in the memory domain, five had a purely amnestic MCI subtype, and nine could be classified as multi-domain MCI	Mean cortical AChE activity −11%, most pronounced in lateral temporal, parietal, and occipital lobes, but also including the hippocampi, adjacent medial temporal structures, and frontal areas. The purpose of the study was to investigate the relationship between cholinergic treatment effects and the integrity of the cholinergic system
[72]	[^{18}F] FEOBV	iRBD ($n = 5$), HC ($n = 5$) iRBD group younger and performed better on cognitive measures	Higher uptake in patients with iRBD, particularly brain stem
[80]	[^{11}C] MP4A [^{18}F]FDG	MCI ($n = 19$), HC ($n = 18$) MCI was defined as performance >1.5 standard deviations below the norm in the delayed recall of the VLMT, and > 24 points in the MMSE	Reduced AChE activity in lateral temporal, parietal, and occipital cortices
[74]	[^{18}F] ASEM	MCI ($n = 14$), HC ($n = 17$) MCI at least 1 SD below normal on memory test	Increased binding in cortex including the hippocampus, striatum, thalamus, cerebellum, and basal forebrain
[49]	[^{11}C] donepezil	iRBD ($n = 21$), HC ($n = 10$) iRBD had no parkinsonism or cognitive impairment	Reduced neocortical binding in iRBD
[11]	[^{11}C] donepezil	iRBD ($n = 19$), HC ($n = 27$) iRBD had no parkinsonism or cognitive impairment	Reduced neocortical binding in iRBD. Negative correlation between cortical binding and a marker of inflammation in the basal forebrain
[81]	[^{18}F] FEOBV	MCI ($n = 8$), HC ($n = 10$). Majority of MCI cases were amyloid-negative demonstrated with [^{18}F]florbetaben-PET	MCI cases had reduced cortical uptake of FEOBV. Cholinergic signal correlated with volume of the basal forebrain and hippocampus
[23]	[^{18}F]FA	MCI ($n = 28$), AD ($n = 32$), CN ($n = 42$). Patients with MCI had cognitive impairment in the memory domain	Binding in MCI generally midway between CN and AD in selected subcortical and limbic areas. Preserved hippocampal signal distinguished the MCI group from AD. Alteration may occur early in entorhinal and limbic structures

MCI-LB

MCI plus core features of DLB (MCI-LB) is a prodromal stage of DLB [56]. A recent publication describes the recommendations for identifying prodromal DLB. In short, the prodromal phase may include MCI, delirium-onset, and psychiatric-onset manifestations [56]. So far, no studies using cholinergic in vivo imaging have been published on patients who presented with one of these three phenotypes.

A few recent structural MRI-studies have been published on MCI-LB. A follow-up study investigated gray matter atrophy in

MCI-LB. Comparing patients who remained MCI-LB to those who progressed to DLB, both groups had atrophy in the NBM at baseline [57]. Those who progressed to DLB had more longitudinal atrophy in entorhinal and parahippocampal cortices, temporoparietal association cortices, thalamus, and basal ganglia. Thus, atrophy of the NBM is a feature of prodromal DLB regardless of proximity to dementia and there is gradual atrophy of cortical regions with significant cholinergic innervation. The findings suggest that atrophy of the NBM occurs very early in the pathogenesis of DLB and reaches a plateau when the first cognitive symptoms appear. It seems that the initial phase of MCI-LB is associated with little cortical grey matter atrophy and that the later accelerated cortical grey matter atrophy in MCI-LB is a marker of impending dementia. In the study, RBD was assessed using a questionnaire. Overall, 89% had probable RBD. So far, no studies have focused on RBD-negative MCI-LB, which may represent a separate prodromal phenotype.

In PD without dementia, basal forebrain volume is correlated with cognition and reduced volume predicts future dementia [58–60].

In summary, early patients with MCI-LB show significant atrophy in the NBM [61]. This is followed by atrophy of the entorhinal cortex [57]. Later, on conversion to dementia, there is widespread gray matter atrophy in multiple cortical and subcortical regions, in particular those areas receiving input from the NBM. Both MCI-AD and MCI-LB exhibit atrophy of the NBM, although this is to a lesser degree in MCI-AD [61, 62]. Interestingly, both prodromal groups show evidence of degeneration in the axonal projections from the NBM to the cortex, and the integrity of cholinergic pathways correlate better with clinical features than do atrophy of cholinergic cell bodies [63]. Atrophy of the basal forebrain is closely linked to reduced integrity of its cortical cholinergic projections and cortical cholinergic signal, but it is loss of the projecting axons that is important in the pathological process [64].

Preclinical Changes in Cholinergic Axons

The number of cholinergic neurons in the basal forebrain decreases with age, particularly when transitioning from preclinical to MCI stages of DLB and AD. Morphological abnormalities in the cholinergic axons occur at very early stages of AD. In healthy young brains without AD pathology, the cholinergic axons are thin and homogenous with small uniform varicosities. In middle-aged non-demented persons, axonal abnormalities start to be present. These can include swollen axons, ballooned terminals, less branching, and fewer terminals. The abnormalities increase in non-demented elderly and then decrease in severe ADD, suggesting that the abnormal cholinergic axons atrophy in ADD [65].

The abnormal swellings of the cholinergic axons contain abundant AChE and ChAT. This could explain why some studies find preserved or even locally increased levels of cholinergic markers in prodromal and early disease stages [66, 67]. Also, it suggests that the cholinergic system may be functionally impaired despite preserved or increased levels of cholinergic markers [65]. A post-mortem study found that the increase in cholinergic markers could not be explained by increased number of cholinergic fibers or varicosities [68]. A more likely explanation appears to be an upregulation of proteins and enzymes involved in production and delivery of acetylcholine. This phenomenon has been documented in post-mortem studies [69, 70].

ChAT and VAChT are co-regulated and co-located on the same gene [71]. A recent PET-study found that VAChT may also be upregulated locally in iRBD [72]. The most marked areas of upregulation were found to be in the brainstem which receives most of its cholinergic projections from the PPN/LDT complex on the pontomesencephalic junction. This implies that, in iRBD, the PPN/LDT complex is affected by pathology. This seems reasonable, as iRBD is caused in part by pathology in the nearby subcerulean nucleus. It should be mentioned, however, that the results were based on only five patients with iRBD that were also younger and performed better on cognitive measures compared to their comparison group.

Another study found increased binding of VAChT in the hippocampi of PD patients with normal cognition while PD patients with MCI had normal levels of binding [66]. A possible explanation could be a local upregulation of VAChT due to dysfunctional cholinergic projections from the medial septum and horizontal band to the hippocampus. Local increases in tracer activity have been reported in studies using substrate-tracer for AChE in patients predisposed to PD [73], ligand-tracers for nicotinic receptors in patients with MCI and patients with AD [74, 75], and tracers for muscarinic receptors in patients with PD [76].

Interestingly, axonal swellings may appear prior to accumulation of pathological protein. Reducing axonal transport by genetic modification in mice led to increased levels of axonal swellings and amyloid deposition [77]. Also, reduced expression of VAChT can facilitate Alzheimer pathology in mice [78]. Evidence suggest that similar mechanisms may be at play in humans [65]. Intriguingly, this evidence suggests that cholinergic dysfunction can lead to the accumulation of pathological protein. However, the prevailing understanding is still that it is the accumulation of pathology that causes neuronal dysfunction and degeneration, not the reverse.

To conclude, cholinergic molecular in vivo imaging has made it possible to study early disease stages of dementia and follow progression over time. The studies of neurodegenerative dementias are no longer confined to investigating the cortical cholinergic changes associated with cognitive deficits. Today, we understand that these disorders affect multiple systems that cause a wide range of symptoms and signs, and that changes in the cholinergic system are involved in several of these functions. There is evidence of cholinergic dysfunction in the prodromal stages of ADD and LBD. These changes likely begin during the preclinical stages, but such early patient cases are currently hard to identify. In AD and RBD-negative Lewy body disorders, the earliest changes may occur in cholinergic axons or cell bodies of the basal forebrain. In RBD-positive LBD, the earliest changes most likely occur in cholinergic parasympathetic and intrinsic neurons innervating the internal organs. Overall, this makes cholinergic molecular imaging one of the most interesting, versatile, and promising fields within dementia research.

Acknowledgement To Michel J. Grothe, PhD., Movement Disorders Group, Instituto de Biomedicina de Sevilla (iBiS), for commenting on the manuscript.

References

1. Picciotto MR, Higley MJ, Mineur YS. Acetylcholine as a neuromodulator: cholinergic signaling shapes nervous system function and behavior. Neuron. 2012;76(1):116–29. https://doi.org/10.1016/j.neuron.2012.08.036.
2. Sarter M, Bruno JP. Cognitive functions of cortical acetylcholine: toward a unifying hypothesis. Brain Res Rev. 1997;23(1–2):28–46.
3. Roy R, Niccolini F, Pagano G, Politis M. Cholinergic imaging in dementia spectrum disorders. Eur J Nucl Med Mol Imaging. 2016;43(7):1376–86. https://doi.org/10.1007/s00259-016-3349-x.
4. Bohnen NI, Grothe MJ, Ray NJ, Müller ML, Teipel SJ. Recent advances in cholinergic imaging and cognitive decline—revisiting the cholinergic hypothesis of dementia. Curr Geriatr Rep. 2018;7(1):1–11.
5. Hampel H, Mesulam MM, Cuello AC, Farlow MR, Giacobini E, Grossberg GT, et al. The cholinergic system in the pathophysiology and treatment of Alzheimer's disease. Brain. 2018;141(7):1917–33. https://doi.org/10.1093/brain/awy132.
6. Hampel H, Mesulam MM, Cuello AC, Khachaturian AS, Vergallo A, Farlow MR, et al. Revisiting the cholinergic hypothesis in Alzheimer's disease: emerging evidence from translational and clinical research. J Prev Alzheimers Dis. 2019;6(1):2–15. https://doi.org/10.14283/jpad.2018.43.
7. Pasquini J, Brooks DJ, Pavese N. The cholinergic brain in Parkinson's disease. Mov Disord Clin Pract. 2021;8(7):1012–26. https://doi.org/10.1002/mdc3.13319.
8. Bohnen NI, Yarnall AJ, Weil RS, Moro E, Moehle MS, Borghammer P, et al. Cholinergic system changes in Parkinson's disease: emerging therapeutic approaches. Lancet Neurol. 2022;21:381. https://doi.org/10.1016/s1474-4422(21)00377-x.
9. Richter N, Beckers N, Onur OA, Dietlein M, Tittgemeyer M, Kracht L, et al. Effect of cholinergic treatment depends on cholinergic integrity in early

Alzheimer's disease. Brain. 2018;141(3):903–15. https://doi.org/10.1093/brain/awx356.

10. Kuhl DE, Minoshima S, Fessler JA, Ficaro EP, Wieland DM, Koeppe RA, et al. In vivo mapping of cholinergic terminals in normal aging, Alzheimer's disease, and Parkinson's disease. Ann Neurol. 1996;40(3):399–410.

11. Staer K, Iranzo A, Stokholm MG, Ostergaard K, Serradell M, Otto M, et al. Cortical cholinergic dysfunction correlates with microglial activation in the substantia innominata in REM sleep behavior disorder. Parkinsonism Relat Disord. 2020;81:89–93. https://doi.org/10.1016/j.parkreldis.2020.10.014.

12. Aghourian M, Legault-Denis C, Soucy JP, Rosa-Neto P, Gauthier S, Kostikov A, et al. Quantification of brain cholinergic denervation in Alzheimer's disease using PET imaging with [(18)F]-FEOBV. Mol Psychiatry. 2017;22(11):1531–8. https://doi.org/10.1038/mp.2017.183.

13. Bohnen N, Mueller ML, Kuwabara H, Constantine G, Studenski S. Age-associated leukoaraiosis and cortical cholinergic deafferentation. Neurology. 2009;72(16):1411–6.

14. Kanel P, Bedard MA, Aghourian M, Rosa-Neto P, Soucy JP, Albin RL, et al. Molecular imaging of the cholinergic system in Alzheimer and Lewy body dementias: expanding views. Curr Neurol Neurosci Rep. 2021;21(10):52. https://doi.org/10.1007/s11910-021-01140-z.

15. Berg D, Borghammer P, Fereshtehnejad S-M, Heinzel S, Horsager J, Schaeffer E, et al. Prodromal Parkinson disease subtypes—key to understanding heterogeneity. Nat Rev Neurol. 2021;17(6):349–61.

16. Prado VF, Roy A, Kolisnyk B, Gros R, Prado MA. Regulation of cholinergic activity by the vesicular acetylcholine transporter. Biochem J. 2013;450(2):265–74.

17. Nejad-Davarani S, Koeppe RA, Albin RL, Frey KA, Müller ML, Bohnen NI. Quantification of brain cholinergic denervation in dementia with Lewy bodies using PET imaging with [18 F]-FEOBV. Mol Psychiatry. 2018;1:322.

18. van der Zee S, García DV, Elsinga PH, Willemsen AT, Boersma HH, Gerritsen MJ, et al. [18 F] Fluoroethoxybenzovesamicol in Parkinson's disease patients: quantification of a novel cholinergic positron emission tomography tracer. Mov Disord. 2019;34(6):924–6.

19. Kikuchi T, Okamura T, Zhang MR, Irie T. PET probes for imaging brain acetylcholinesterase. J Labelled Comp Radiopharm. 2013;56(3–4):172–9. https://doi.org/10.1002/jlcr.3002.

20. Nathanson NM. Synthesis, trafficking, and localization of muscarinic acetylcholine receptors. Pharmacol Ther. 2008;119(1):33–43.

21. Dani JA, Bertrand D. Nicotinic acetylcholine receptors and nicotinic cholinergic mechanisms of the central nervous system. Annu Rev Pharmacol Toxicol. 2007;47:699–729.

22. Tiepolt S, Becker G-A, Wilke S, Cecchin D, Rullmann M, Meyer PM, et al. (+)-[18F] Flubatine as a novel α4β2 nicotinic acetylcholine receptor PET ligand—results of the first-in-human brain imaging application in patients with β-amyloid PET-confirmed Alzheimer's disease and healthy controls. Eur J Nucl Med Mol Imaging. 2021;48(3):731–46.

23. Sultzer DL, Lim AC, Gordon HL, Yarns BC, Melrose RJ. Cholinergic receptor binding in unimpaired older adults, mild cognitive impairment, and Alzheimer's disease dementia. Alzheimers Res Ther. 2022;14(1):25. https://doi.org/10.1186/s13195-021-00954-w.

24. Kadir A, Darreh-Shori T, Almkvist O, Wall A, Grut M, Strandberg B, et al. PET imaging of the in vivo brain acetylcholinesterase activity and nicotine binding in galantamine-treated patients with AD. Neurobiol Aging. 2008;29(8):1204–17.

25. Zubieta JK, Koeppe RA, Frey KA, Kilbourn MR, Mangner TJ, Foster NL, et al. Assessment of muscarinic receptor concentrations in aging and Alzheimer disease with [11C] NMPB and PET. Synapse. 2001;39(4):275–87.

26. Liu AKL, Chang RC-C, Pearce RK, Gentleman SM. Nucleus basalis of meynert revisited: anatomy, history and differential involvement in Alzheimer's and Parkinson's disease. Acta Neuropathol. 2015;129(4):527–40.

27. Mesulam MM. Cholinergic circuitry of the human nucleus basalis and its fate in Alzheimer's disease. J Comp Neurol. 2013;521(18):4124–44. https://doi.org/10.1002/cne.23415.

28. Selden NR, Gitelman DR, Salamon-Murayama N, Parrish TB, Mesulam M-M. Trajectories of cholinergic pathways within the cerebral hemispheres of the human brain. Brain J Neurol. 1998;121(12):2249–57.

29. Richter N, Michel A, Onur OA, Kracht L, Dietlein M, Tittgemeyer M, et al. White matter lesions and the cholinergic deficit in aging and mild cognitive impairment. Neurobiol Aging. 2017;53:27–35. https://doi.org/10.1016/j.neurobiolaging.2017.01.012.

30. Iranzo A, Fernández-Arcos A, Tolosa E, Serradell M, Molinuevo JL, Valldeoriola F, et al. Neurodegenerative disorder risk in idiopathic REM sleep behavior disorder: study in 174 patients. PLoS One. 2014;9(2):e89741.

31. Aarsland D, Andersen K, Larsen JP, Lolk A. Prevalence and characteristics of dementia in Parkinson disease: an 8-year prospective study. Arch Neurol. 2003;60(3):387–92.

32. Albert MS, DeKosky ST, Dickson D, Dubois B, Feldman HH, Fox NC, et al. The diagnosis of mild cognitive impairment due to Alzheimer's disease: recommendations from the National Institute on Aging-Alzheimer's Association workgroups on diagnostic guidelines for Alzheimer's disease. Alzheimers Dement. 2011;7(3):270–9. https://doi.org/10.1016/j.jalz.2011.03.008.

33. Mazère J, Lamare F, Allard M, Fernandez P, Mayo W. 123I-Iodobenzovesamicol SPECT imaging of cholin-

ergic systems in dementia with Lewy bodies. J Nucl Med. 2017;58(1):123–8.

34. Shimada H, Hirano S, Shinotoh H, Aotsuka A, Sato K, Tanaka N, et al. Mapping of brain acetylcholinesterase alterations in Lewy body disease by PET. Neurology. 2009;73(4):273–8.

35. Bohnen NI, Kaufer DI, Ivanco LS, Lopresti B, Koeppe RA, Davis JG, et al. Cortical cholinergic function is more severely affected in parkinsonian dementia than in Alzheimer disease: an in vivo positron emission tomographic study. Arch Neurol. 2003;60(12):1745–8.

36. Shimada H, Hirano S, Sinotoh H, Ota T, Tanaka N, Sato K, et al. Dementia with Lewy bodies can be well-differentiated from Alzheimer's disease by measurement of brain acetylcholinesterase activity-a [11C]MP4A PET study. Int J Geriatr Psychiatry. 2015;30(11):1105–13. https://doi.org/10.1002/gps.4338.

37. Haense C, Kalbe E, Herholz K, Hohmann C, Neumaier B, Krais R, et al. Cholinergic system function and cognition in mild cognitive impairment. Neurobiol Aging. 2012;33(5):867–77. https://doi.org/10.1016/j.neurobiolaging.2010.08.015.

38. Rinne JO, Kaasinen V, Järvenpää T, Någren K, Roivainen A, Yu M, et al. Brain acetylcholinesterase activity in mild cognitive impairment and early Alzheimer's disease. J Neurol Neurosurg Psychiatry. 2003;74(1):113–5.

39. Marcone A, Garibotto V, Moresco RM, Florea I, Panzacchi A, Carpinelli A, et al. [11C]-MP4A PET cholinergic measurements in amnestic mild cognitive impairment, probable Alzheimer's disease, and dementia with Lewy bodies: a Bayesian method and voxel-based analysis. J Alzheimers Dis. 2012;31(2):387–99. https://doi.org/10.3233/JAD-2012-111748.

40. Kendziorra K, Wolf H, Meyer PM, Barthel H, Hesse S, Becker GA, et al. Decreased cerebral α4β2* nicotinic acetylcholine receptor availability in patients with mild cognitive impairment and Alzheimer's disease assessed with positron emission tomography. Eur J Nucl Med Mol Imaging. 2011;38(3):515–25.

41. Sabri O, Kendziorra K, Wolf H, Gertz H-J, Brust P. Acetylcholine receptors in dementia and mild cognitive impairment. Eur J Nucl Med Mol Imaging. 2008;35(1):30–45.

42. Vogels O, Broere C, Ter Laak H, Ten Donkelaar H, Nieuwenhuys R, Schulte B. Cell loss and shrinkage in the nucleus basalis Meynert complex in Alzheimer's disease. Neurobiol Aging. 1990;11(1):3–13.

43. Herholz K, Weisenbach S, Kalbe E, Diederich NJ, Heiss W-D. Cerebral acetylcholine esterase activity in mild cognitive impairment. Neuroreport. 2005;16(13):1431–4.

44. Wilson RS, Leurgans SE, Boyle PA, Bennett DA. Cognitive decline in prodromal Alzheimer disease and mild cognitive impairment. Arch Neurol. 2011;68(3):351–6.

45. Grothe M, Heinsen H, Teipel SJ. Atrophy of the cholinergic basal forebrain over the adult age range and in early stages of Alzheimer's disease. Biol Psychiatry. 2012;71(9):805–13. https://doi.org/10.1016/j.biopsych.2011.06.019.

46. Grothe MJ, Ewers M, Krause B, Heinsen H, Teipel SJ, Alzheimer's disease neuroimaging Initiative. Basal forebrain atrophy and cortical amyloid deposition in nondemented elderly subjects. Alzheimers Dement. 2014;10(5 Suppl):S344–53. https://doi.org/10.1016/j.jalz.2013.09.011.

47. Grothe MJ, Heinsen H, Amaro E Jr, Grinberg LT, Teipel SJ. Cognitive correlates of basal forebrain atrophy and associated cortical hypometabolism in mild cognitive impairment. Cereb Cortex. 2016;26(6):2411–26. https://doi.org/10.1093/cercor/bhv062.

48. Schmitz TW, Nathan Spreng R, Alzheimer's Disease Neuroimaging Initiative. Basal forebrain degeneration precedes and predicts the cortical spread of Alzheimer's pathology. Nat Commun. 2016;7:13249. https://doi.org/10.1038/ncomms13249.

49. Gersel Stokholm M, Iranzo A, Ostergaard K, Serradell M, Otto M, Bacher Svendsen K, et al. Cholinergic denervation in patients with idiopathic rapid eye movement sleep behaviour disorder. Eur J Neurol. 2020;27(4):644–52. https://doi.org/10.1111/ene.14127.

50. Stokholm MG, Iranzo A, Østergaard K, Serradell M, Otto M, Svendsen KB, et al. Assessment of neuroinflammation in patients with idiopathic rapid-eye-movement sleep behaviour disorder: a case-control study. Lancet Neurol. 2017;16(10):789–96. https://doi.org/10.1016/s1474-4422(17)30173-4.

51. Braak H, Del Tredici K, Rüb U, De Vos RA, Steur ENJ, Braak E. Staging of brain pathology related to sporadic Parkinson's disease. Neurobiol Aging. 2003;24(2):197–211.

52. Knudsen K, Fedorova TD, Hansen AK, Sommerauer M, Otto M, Svendsen KB, et al. In-vivo staging of pathology in REM sleep behaviour disorder: a multimodality imaging case-control study. Lancet Neurol. 2018;17:618.

53. Horsager J, Andersen KB, Knudsen K, Skjærbæk C, Fedorova TD, Okkels N, et al. Brain-first versus body-first Parkinson's disease: a multimodal imaging case-control study. Brain. 2020;143(10):3077–88.

54. Giannini G, Calandra-Buonaura G, Asioli GM, Cecere A, Barletta G, Mignani F, et al. The natural history of idiopathic autonomic failure: the IAF-BO cohort study. Neurology. 2018;91(13):e1245–e54. https://doi.org/10.1212/WNL.0000000000006243.

55. van de Beek M, van Steenoven I, van der Zande J, Porcelijn I, Barkhof F, Stam C, et al. Characterization of symptoms and determinants of disease burden in dementia with Lewy bodies: DEvELOP design and baseline results. Alzheimers Res Ther. 2021;13(1):1–13.

56. McKeith IG, Ferman TJ, Thomas AJ, Blanc F, Boeve BF, Fujishiro H, et al. Research criteria for the diag-

nosis of prodromal dementia with Lewy bodies. Neurology. 2020;94(17):743–55.

57. Kantarci K, Nedelska Z, Chen Q, Senjem ML, Schwarz CG, Gunter JL, et al. Longitudinal atrophy in prodromal dementia with Lewy bodies points to cholinergic degeneration. Brain Commun. 2022;4:fcac013.

58. Grothe MJ, Labrador-Espinosa MA, Jesus S, Macias-Garcia D, Adarmes-Gomez A, Carrillo F, et al. In vivo cholinergic basal forebrain degeneration and cognition in Parkinson's disease: imaging results from the COPPADIS study. Parkinsonism Relat Disord. 2021;88:68–75. https://doi.org/10.1016/j.parkreldis.2021.05.027.

59. Pereira JB, Hall S, Jalakas M, Grothe MJ, Strandberg O, Stomrud E, et al. Longitudinal degeneration of the basal forebrain predicts subsequent dementia in Parkinson's disease. Neurobiol Dis. 2020;139:104831. https://doi.org/10.1016/j.nbd.2020.104831.

60. Ray NJ, Bradburn S, Murgatroyd C, Toseeb U, Mir P, Kountouriotis GK, et al. In vivo cholinergic basal forebrain atrophy predicts cognitive decline in de novo Parkinson's disease. Brain. 2018;141(1):165–76.

61. Schumacher J, Taylor JP, Hamilton CA, Firbank M, Cromarty RA, Donaghy PC, et al. In vivo nucleus basalis of Meynert degeneration in mild cognitive impairment with Lewy bodies. Neuroimage Clin. 2021;30:102604. https://doi.org/10.1016/j.nicl.2021.102604.

62. Craig CE, Ray NJ, Muller M, Bohnen NI. New developments in cholinergic imaging in Alzheimer and Lewy body disorders. Curr Behav Neurosci Rep. 2020;7(4):278–86. https://doi.org/10.1007/s40473-020-00221-6.

63. Schumacher J, Ray NJ, Hamilton CA, Donaghy PC, Firbank M, Roberts G, et al. Cholinergic white matter pathways in dementia with Lewy bodies and Alzheimer's disease. Brain. 2021;145:1773. https://doi.org/10.1093/brain/awab372.

64. Schmitz TW, Mur M, Aghourian M, Bedard MA, Spreng RN, Alzheimer's disease Neuroimaging Initiative. Longitudinal Alzheimer's degeneration reflects the spatial topography of cholinergic basal forebrain projections. Cell Rep. 2018;24(1):38–46. https://doi.org/10.1016/j.celrep.2018.06.001.

65. Geula C, Nagykery N, Nicholas A, Wu C-K. Cholinergic neuronal and axonal abnormalities are present early in aging and in Alzheimer disease. J Neuropathol Exp Neurol. 2008;67(4):309–18.

66. Legault-Denis C, Aghourian M, Soucy J-P, Rosa-Neto P, Dagher A, Wickens R, et al. Normal cognition in Parkinson's disease may involve hippocampal cholinergic compensation: a PET imaging study with [18F]-FEOBV. Parkinsonism Relat Disord. 2021;91:162. https://doi.org/10.1016/j.parkreldis.2021.09.018.

67. Sanchez-Catasus C, Bohnen NI, D'Cruz N, Muller M. Striatal acetylcholine-dopamine imbalance in Parkinson's disease: in vivo neuroimaging study with dual-tracer PET and dopaminergic PET-informed correlational tractography. J Nucl Med. 2021;62:545. https://doi.org/10.2967/jnumed.121.261939.

68. Ikonomovic MD, Abrahamson EE, Isanski BA, Wuu J, Mufson EJ, DeKosky ST. Superior frontal cortex cholinergic axon density in mild cognitive impairment and early Alzheimer disease. Arch Neurol. 2007;64(9):1312–7.

69. Davis KL, Mohs RC, Marin D, Purohit DP, Perl DP, Lantz M, et al. Cholinergic markers in elderly patients with early signs of Alzheimer disease. JAMA. 1999;281(15):1401–6.

70. DeKosky ST, Ikonomovic MD, Styren SD, Beckett L, Wisniewski S, Bennett DA, et al. Upregulation of choline acetyltransferase activity in hippocampus and frontal cortex of elderly subjects with mild cognitive impairment. Ann Neurol. 2002;51(2):145–55.

71. Woolf NJ. Cholinergic systems in mammalian brain and spinal cord. Prog Neurobiol. 1991;37(6):475–524.

72. Bedard M-A, Aghourian M, Legault-Denis C, Postuma RB, Soucy J-P, Gagnon J-F, et al. Brain cholinergic alterations in idiopathic REM sleep behaviour disorder: a PET imaging study with 18F-FEOBV. Sleep Med. 2019;58:35–41.

73. Liu S-Y, Wile DJ, Fu JF, Valerio J, Shahinfard E, McCormick S, et al. The effect of LRRK2 mutations on the cholinergic system in manifest and premanifest stages of Parkinson's disease: a cross-sectional PET study. Lancet Neurol. 2018;17(4):309–16. https://doi.org/10.1016/s1474-4422(18)30032-2.

74. Coughlin JM, Rubin LH, Du Y, Rowe SP, Crawford JL, Rosenthal HB, et al. High availability of the alpha7-nicotinic acetylcholine receptor in brains of individuals with mild cognitive impairment: a pilot study using (18)F-ASEM PET. J Nucl Med. 2020;61(3):423–6. https://doi.org/10.2967/jnumed.119.230979.

75. Ellis J, Villemagne VL, Nathan PJ, Mulligan RS, Gong SJ, Chan JG, et al. Relationship between nicotinic receptors and cognitive function in early Alzheimer's disease: a 2-[18F] fluoro-A-85380 PET study. Neurobiol Learn Mem. 2008;90(2):404–12.

76. Colloby SJ, Nathan PJ, Bakker G, Lawson RA, Yarnall AJ, Burn DJ, et al. Spatial covariance of cholinergic muscarinic M1/M4 receptors in Parkinson's disease. Mov Disord. 2021;36(8):1879–88. https://doi.org/10.1002/mds.28564.

77. Stokin GB, Lillo C, Falzone TL, Brusch RG, Rockenstein E, Mount SL, et al. Axonopathy and transport deficits early in the pathogenesis of Alzheimer's disease. Science. 2005;307:1282.

78. Kolisnyk B, Al-Onaizi M, Soreq L, Barbash S, Bekenstein U, Haberman N, et al. Cholinergic surveillance over hippocampal RNA metabolism and Alzheimer's-like pathology. Cereb Cortex. 2017;27(7):3553–67. https://doi.org/10.1093/cercor/bhw177.

79. Terrière E, Dempsey MF, Herrmann LL, Tierney KM, Lonie JA, O'Carroll RE, et al. 5-123I-A-85380 binding to the α4β2-nicotinic receptor in mild cognitive impairment. Neurobiol Aging. 2010;31(11):1885–93.

80. Richter N, Nellessen N, Dronse J, Dillen K, Jacobs HIL, Langen KJ, et al. Spatial distributions of cholinergic impairment and neuronal hypometabolism differ in MCI due to AD. Neuroimage Clin. 2019;24:101978. https://doi.org/10.1016/j.nicl.2019.101978.

81. Xia Y, Eeles E, Fripp J, Pinsker D, Thomas P, Latter M, et al. Reduced cortical cholinergic innervation measured using [(18)F]-FEOBV PET imaging correlates with cognitive decline in mild cognitive impairment. Neuroimage Clin. 2022;34:102992. https://doi.org/10.1016/j.nicl.2022.102992.

Neuroinflammation Imaging in Neurodegenerative Diseases

Dima A. Hammoud and Peter Herscovitch

Introduction

Neuroinflammation is a natural response of a competent immune system to any type of CNS insult, and it includes both innate (e.g., monocytes) and adaptive components (lymphocytes). A special characteristic of the CNS is the presence of specialized resident immune cells, the microglia. When faced with a noxious stimulus or injury, microglial cells become activated, increase in size, assume an ameboid shape with shorter processes, and secrete a variety of cytokines and other neurotoxic compounds. An excessive reaction can result in a vicious cycle that eventually results in neuronal injury and death. Microglial activation, however, is only one part of the neuroinflammatory process, with additional contributions from astrocytes, peripherally derived macrophages, and sometimes T-cell lymphocytes (Fig. 9.1).

The potential contribution of neuroinflammation to CNS injury has been extensively studied using molecular imaging with positron emission tomography (PET) in many disease entities, including neurodegenerative diseases (NDDs). Most research using neuroinflammation imaging in NDDs has focused on Alzheimer's disease (AD), with fewer studies evaluating Parkinson's disease (PD) and other movement disorders. The overarching goal of such studies is to understand the role of neuroinflammation in disease pathophysiology and progression. Imaging can also be used to monitor treatment effects and to provide surrogate endpoints in clinical trials of strategies to modify neuroinflammation. While there are many targets that could be used to image neuroinflammation with PET, the most commonly studied target has been the 18-kDa translocator protein (TSPO), an outer mitochondrial membrane receptor that is expressed in many CNS and peripheral immune cells [1]. Basal TSPO expression in the brain parenchyma is low but it is upregulated in inflammatory states. As a result, imaging TSPO has been used to assess the neuroinflammatory process in various diseases including NDDs, and many radioligands have been developed to image TSPO with PET.

However, TSPO as a target to monitor neuroinflammation does have several shortcomings. In the CNS, TSPO is expressed in several cell types. These include resident microglia and monocyte-derived macrophages, astrocytes, and endothelial, choroid plexus and ependymal cells, with low but ubiquitous expression in the parenchyma [2]. Although

D. A. Hammoud (✉)
Radiology and Imaging Sciences, National Institutes of Health/Clinical Center, Bethesda, MD, USA
e-mail: hammoudd@cc.nih.gov

P. Herscovitch
Positron Emission Tomography Department, National Institutes of Health/Clinical Center, Bethesda, MD, USA
e-mail: pherscovitch@cc.nih.gov

D. J. Cross et al. (eds.), *Molecular Imaging of Neurodegenerative Disorders*,
https://doi.org/10.1007/978-3-031-35098-6_9

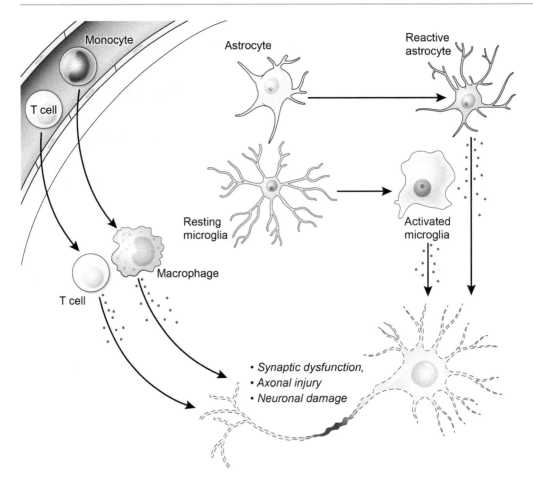

Fig. 9.1 Neuroinflammation and mechanism of neuronal injury: activated microglia, astrocytes, peripherally derived monocytes, and lymphocytes contribute to neuroinflammation. Excess production of cytokines, chemo-kines, and other neurotoxic molecules can result in synaptic loss, axonal degradation, and neuronal cellular damage

generally assumed not to be expressed in neurons, colocalization of TSPO staining with tyrosine hydroxylase has been reported, raising the possibility that dopaminergic neurons also express TSPO [3]. TSPO imaging also cannot distinguish between activated microglia that are harmful (pro-inflammatory M1 phenotype) versus neuroprotective (anti-inflammatory M2), and cannot differentiate microglia from astrocytes, which also participate in the neuroinflammatory process.

The original and most commonly used TSPO PET ligand is [11C]-PK11195, an isoquinolone TSPO antagonist. However, it has several limita-

tions as a PET radiotracer, including low blood–brain barrier permeability and high binding to plasma proteins, limiting tracer entry to brain, and low specific binding to the TSPO target with a poor signal-to-noise ratio in the PET images. As a result, many other ligands have since been and continue to be developed to improve neuroinflammation imaging (Fig. 9.2).

In general, TSPO ligands other than [11C]-PK11195 are referred to as second- or third-generation ligands (Fig. 9.2), with improved affinity and higher specific-to-nonspecific binding. The use of second-generation ligands, however, was immediately hampered because almost

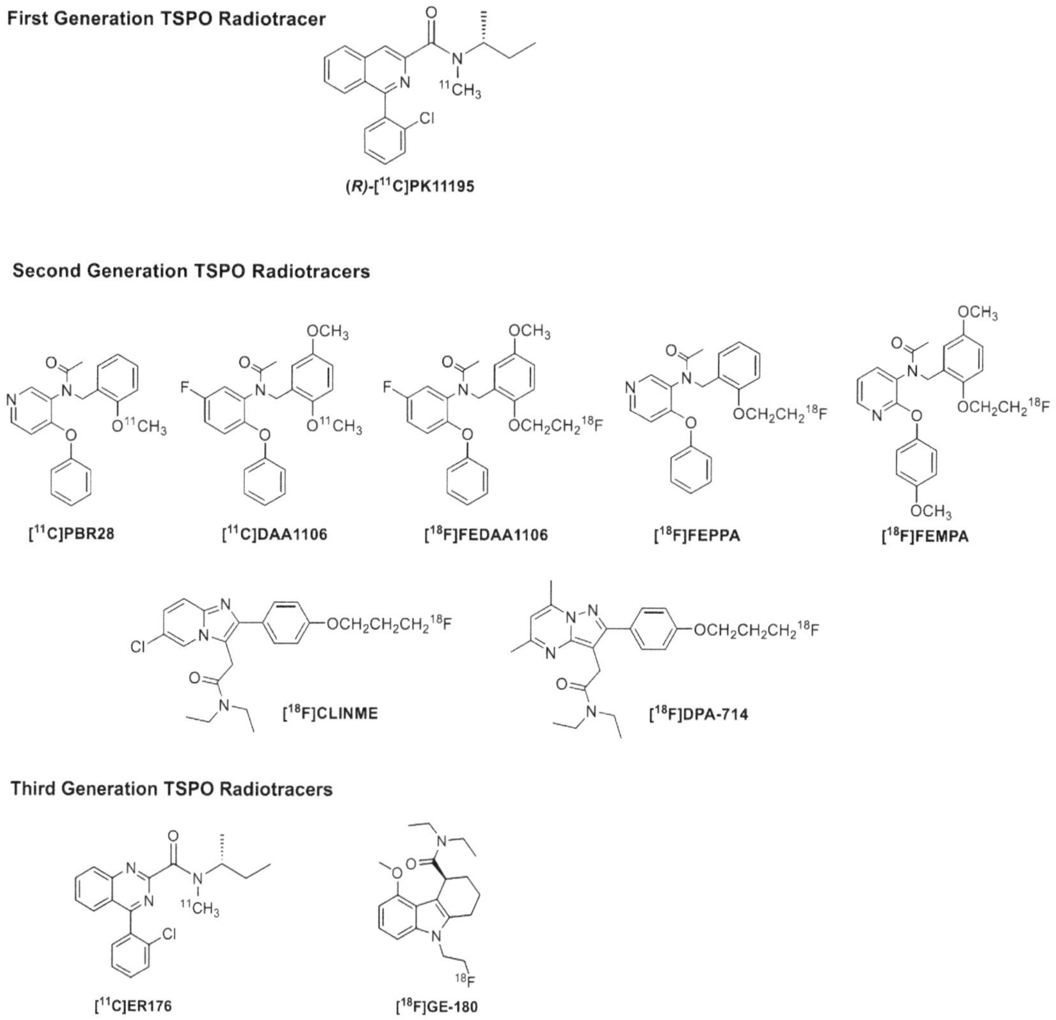

First Generation TSPO Radiotracer

(R)-[¹¹C]PK11195

Second Generation TSPO Radiotracers

[¹¹C]PBR28   [¹¹C]DAA1106   [¹⁸F]FEDAA1106   [¹⁸F]FEPPA   [¹⁸F]FEMPA

[¹⁸F]CLINME   [¹⁸F]DPA-714

Third Generation TSPO Radiotracers

[¹¹C]ER176   [¹⁸F]GE-180

Fig. 9.2 Chemical structures of first-, second-, and third-generation TSPO PET ligands (adapted and reproduced with permission from [65])

10% of subjects showed no specific binding. Upon further evaluation, a polymorphism was discovered in exon 4 of the TSPO gene resulting in a nonconservative amino-acid substitution from alanine to threonine (Ala147Thr). This resulted in three possible binding levels: high-affinity binders (HAB) (C/C; Ala/Ala), medium-affinity binders (MAB) (C/T; Ala/Thr), and low-affinity binders (LAB) (T/T; Thr/Thr) [4, 5]. This necessitates genotyping before imaging and exclusion of almost 10% of the population, as well as the need to increase the sample number to match the binding levels between patients and controls.

Multiple third-generation ligands have subsequently been developed with claims of lower or no sensitivity to polymorphism [6, 7]. However, to our knowledge no ligand has been found that is completely insensitive to polymorphism.

Imaging Neuroinflammation in Alzheimer's Disease

One reason neuroinflammation has been considered a possible factor in the pathophysiology of AD is that the amyloid-β deposition hypothesis seems to be insufficient to explain all aspects of disease pathogenesis. In addition, increased inflammatory markers have been described in AD, and the AD risk genes such as ApoE are known to be associated with innate immune function modulation [8]. Therefore, PET has been widely used to assess the role of neuroinflammation in AD pathogenesis. These PET studies typically include imaging with radiotracers for amyloid and tau to confirm the stage and relation to neuroinflammation of the underlying AD pathophysiological process. Unfortunately, the results of these studies have generally been inconsistent.

Two early studies using [^{11}C]-PK11195 suggested a role for neuroinflammation in AD and mild cognitive impairment (MCI). Cagnin et al. found that while in controls regional binding significantly increased with age in the thalamus, patients with AD showed significantly increased binding in the entorhinal, temporoparietal, and cingulate cortex [9]. Okello et al. showed that amyloid deposition and microglial activation can be detected in about 50% of patients with MCI. However, there was no correlation between regional levels of [^{11}C]-PK11195 and amyloid, suggesting that the two pathologies can co-exist but can also occur independently [10].

Many later studies using second-generation ligands often showed discordant results. Yasuno et al. showed increased [^{11}C]-DAA1106 binding in 10 AD patients [11] and Kreisl et al. found elevated [^{11}C]-PBR28 binding in AD but not in MCI [12]. Two other papers, however, using [^{11}C]-vinpocetine and [^{18}F]-FEDAA1106, showed no difference between AD subjects and age-matched controls [13, 14]. Interestingly, Kreisl et al. found a correlation between neuroinflammation (measured by [^{11}C]-PBR28) and amyloid (imaged with [^{11}C]-PIB), and between neuroinflammation and neurocognitive impairment in AD (although not in MCI patients), contrary to the findings of Okello et al. [10]. Since increased binding of [^{11}C]-PBR28 was seen only in AD, the authors proposed that neuroinflammation occurs after conversion of MCI to AD and worsens with disease progression, thus making its detection possibly useful in marking the conversion from MCI to AD

and in assessing response to experimental treatments.

More recently, many studies using either [^{11}C]-PK11195 or second-generation ligands to assess MCI and AD also demonstrated conflicting results. Some showed no correlation between inflammation, cognition and/or pathologic correlates (amyloid and/or tau burden) [15–17]. However, others showed the opposite, albeit to different degrees or distributions, e.g., in different brain regions or using a global measure of neuroinflammation [18–25].

There are several possible explanations for these discrepant results. The use of different ligands with different imaging characteristics and sensitivities to detect TSPO expression likely is a major factor. This was elegantly demonstrated by Yokokura et al. who used the "gold standard" of receptor blocking experiments to determine the specific binding of two TSPO radiotracers. While [^{11}C]-PK11195 showed small differences between AD and controls in the precuneus, imaging with [^{11}C]-DPA713 demonstrated more impressive increased binding in multiple regions including the anterior and posterior cingulate gyri, thalamus, and precuneus [26] (Fig. 9.3).

Another factor likely underlying the conflicting PET imaging results is the use of different patient populations at different stages of the AD pathophysiological process, often with small sample numbers. A third factor is the use of different image analysis methods to estimate the level of TSPO binding. These include graphical analysis with a measured arterial plasma input function (e.g., [19]), simplified reference tissue methods with various brain regions used to provide information about the delivery of radiotracer to tissue (e.g., [27]), or a semi-quantitative approach using the ratio of local regional radioactivity to radioactivity in the cerebellum which is assumed not to be affected by the disease process (e.g., [28]).

To help reconcile these results, Bradburn et al. performed a meta-analysis of TSPO studies in AD and MCI [29]. The authors concluded that neuroinflammation is increased in AD, with more modest effects in MCI. In the parietal region, the neuroinflammatory effects correlated with Mini-

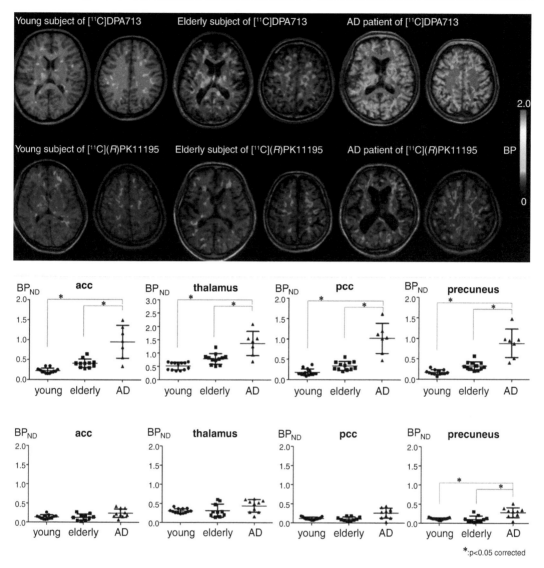

Fig. 9.3 Discrepancy of imaging results between first- and second-generation TSPO PET imaging in AD subjects. While [^{11}C]-PK11195 showed small differences between AD and controls in the precuneus, [^{11}C]-DPA713 demonstrated increased binding in multiple regions, including the anterior and posterior cingulate gyri, thalamus, and precuneus (adapted and reproduced with permission from [26])

Mental State Examination scores in AD. This meta-analysis was published in 2019; the inclusion of more recent studies could provide different results.

Two such studies are noteworthy because they included a large number of subjects who were studied longitudinally [22, 30]. Hamelin et al. used [^{18}F]-DPA714 to evaluate patients who were classified either as prodromal AD (amyloid positive, Clinical Dementia Rating (CDR) score = 0.5)

or demented (amyloid positive, CDR ≥ 1.0 [30]). Follow-up scans in 1–2 years showed two distinctive dynamic patterns of microglial activation: higher initial [^{18}F]-DPA714 binding followed by a slower increase in subjects with slower disease progression, and lower initial [^{18}F]-DPA714 binding followed by a more rapid increase in subjects with accelerated disease progression. This suggested a possible protective role of microglial activation in early stages of AD. This was proposed by Leng and Edison who suggested that an initial microglial response might be protective, thus slowing disease progression (Fig. 9.4). However, subsequent chronic activation eventually causes phenotypic changes in microglia and shifts their behavior toward a pro-inflammatory phenotype, which causes damage to neuronal net-

works and disease progression. On the other hand, AD patients with defective microglial functioning at the onset of disease would undergo a quicker progression and an exaggerated late-stage inflammatory response [31].

Pascoal et al. imaged 130 HAB subjects over the normal aging and AD clinical spectrum, lon-

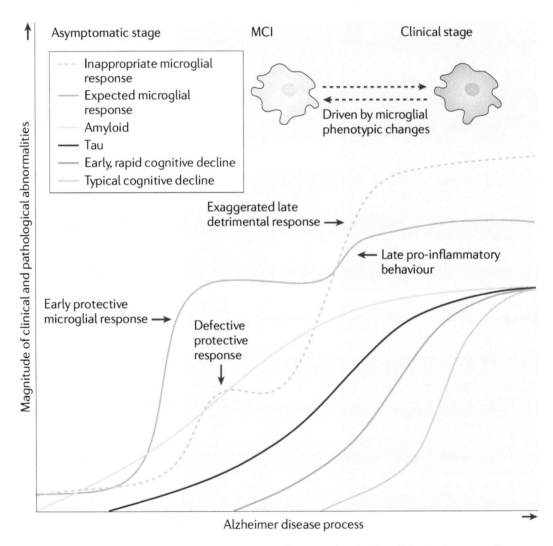

Fig. 9.4 Proposed effect of microglial activation on Alzheimer disease progression [31]. The authors suggest that individual clinical presentation at a given pathological stage in AD might be partly determined by different microglial responses in the early versus late stages of the disease. When microglial activity is deficient, i.e., not protective, at the onset of disease, AD patients might develop cognitive decline at an earlier stage in response to tau and amyloid deposition. This suggests that the initial microglial activation to pathological changes is protective.

However, chronic microglial activation eventually causes phenotypic changes in microglia toward a pro-inflammatory phenotype, with secondary neuronal damage and accelerated symptomatology. In patients with inappropriate early microglial responses, a weak initial protective response results in a quicker transition to worse phenotypes as well as an exaggerated late-stage inflammatory response. MCI: mild cognitive impairment (reproduced with permission from [31])

gitudinally, for TSPO expression and amyloid and tau levels. Neuroinflammation and tau pathology correlated hierarchically with each other following Braak-like stages of neuropathological disease progression. The strongest predictor of cognitive impairment was the co-occurrence of amyloid, tau, and microglial abnormalities. They concluded that amyloid and activated microglia interaction might determine the rate of tau spread across disease stages [22].

In conclusion, neuroinflammation seems to play an important role in the pathophysiology of AD, but a better understanding of this role is needed, especially since many trials of anti-inflammatory drugs did not slow disease progression [32–34]. This is key for future AD clinical trials to suppress pro-inflammatory changes or enhance microglial anti-inflammatory properties, along with anti-amyloid or -tau approaches. Imaging of neuroinflammation in AD should be further refined to serve as a quantitative surrogate endpoint in clinical trials.

Imaging Neuroinflammation in Parkinson's Disease and Other Movement Disorders

Another NDD in which neuroinflammation is suspected to play a role is PD, which is characterized by the degeneration of dopaminergic neurons in the substantia nigra and the pathologic presence of abnormal cytoplasmic inclusions, Lewy bodies, containing alpha-synuclein. PD is classically described as a movement disorder, with bradykinesia, resting tremor, rigidity, and postural instability [35]. More recently, however, it is being thought of as a multi-system disorder, where neuroinflammation and immune dysfunction play a major role, and with non-motor symptoms such as sleep and mood disorders [36] and gastrointestinal dysfunction [37] preceding motor manifestations. Many PD patients also develop dementia in the later stages of the disease.

PET imaging of neuroinflammation in PD patients was first reported by Gerhard et al. who showed increased [11C]-PK11195 binding, although the degree of microglial activation did not correlate with clinical severity or putaminal [18F]-DOPA uptake [38]. A study using a second-generation ligand ([18F]-FEPPA), however, showed no effect of disease or disease x TSPO genotype interaction on ligand binding in any brain region [39]. Interestingly, the same group subsequently showed an interaction between neuroinflammation and amyloid deposition in PD with cognitive decline. They noted that further research is needed to determine whether amyloid deposits cause neuroinflammation and further neurodegeneration, or if increased microglia activation is a protective response [40]. These results likely overlap with prior work showing neuroinflammation in AD.

Using another second-generation ligand, [18F]-DPA714, a third group showed binding that suggested neuroinflammation in the nigrostriatal pathway, more so on the more affected side. However, this did not correlate with symptom severity, dopamine transporter (DAT) binding or disease duration. In the frontal cortex, neuroinflammation did correlate with disease duration [41]. The authors suggested this discrepancy between regions could reflect spreading of pathology in the later stage of the disease [41]. Finally, a study published in 2019 using [11C]-PBR28 in PD patients showed no neuroinflammation despite DAT imaging demonstrating dopaminergic degeneration [42].

A recent meta-analysis of neuroinflammation studies in PD clearly showed the effect of ligand choice on the results. While neuroinflammation was seen in multiple brain regions using [11C]-PK11195, only the midbrain showed significant increases when second-generation ligands were used [43]. Heterogeneity in results was found in many brain regions. This could be due to different ligands, different analysis approaches (e.g., the use of the cerebellum as a reference region), or suboptimal reporting of detailed clinical variables. Of note, the nonspecific binding of [11C]-PK11195 has been reported to be lower in PD patients; this could affect the results of certain analysis methods [44]. Therefore, there is a need for a more uniform approach to performing PET studies and for using large-cohort longitudinal studies to better understand the role of neuroinflammation in PD pathophysiology and progression.

Neuroinflammation imaging has been performed to a lesser extent in other NDDs. In Huntington's disease, for example, several studies identified neuroinflammatory changes, mainly in the globus pallidus and putamen in affected patients [45–47]. In one study, even premanifest HD gene carriers showed increased TSPO expression, although the changes were not significant when compared to controls and affected subjects [46]. In another study, the authors observed further distinct regional and subregional imaging features, which seemed to correspond to phenotypical variability [45]. Imaging studies using first- and second-generation TSPO ligands also identified neuroinflammatory changes in progressive supranuclear palsy patients [23, 48, 49]. In a study by Palleis et al., patients with corticobasal degeneration were also included and showed even more extensive inflammatory changes compared to progressive supranuclear palsy (PSP) subjects. TSPO upregulation, however, was not correlated with measures of disease progression in either PSP or corticobasal degeneration [49]. This contradicts the findings of Malpetti et al., where neuroinflammation (measured with [11C]-PK11195) and tau burden in the brainstem and cerebellum correlated with the subsequent annual rate of PSP disease progression [50]. Additional work is thus needed to better understand the interaction between neuroinflammatory changes and disease progression in different NDDs.

Conclusions

The use of TSPO as an imaging target in NDDs and other CNS diseases remains challenging at multiple levels, and the interpretation of study results should be done with caution. A better understanding of the cellular regulation of TSPO expression and how it changes in relationship to disease progression in NDDs might help determine whether TSPO is an appropriate marker for those diseases, especially AD [51]. Meanwhile, alternative biological targets and radioligands for imaging neuroinflammation are being developed

and may prove superior in the assessment of pro- and anti-inflammatory activity in NDDs [52]. One such radioligand is 11C-BU99008, a novel PET tracer that selectively targets activated astrocytes. A recent study showed higher 11C-BU99008 uptake in eight amyloid positive subjects compared to nine controls in the frontal, temporal, medial temporal, and occipital lobes (regions with high Aβ load) as well as across the whole brain [53], suggesting activated astrocytes in those locations. Other promising targets for imaging neuroinflammation that could be used to evaluate NDDs include cyclooxygenases [54–57], purinergic receptors [58], cannabinoid receptors [59, 60], colony stimulating factor receptor (CSF-1R) [61], inducible nitric oxide synthase (iNOS) [62], and triggering receptor expressed on myeloid cells 1 (TREM1) [63, 64].

References

1. Shah S, Sinharay S, Patel R, Solomon J, Lee JH, Schreiber-Stainthorp W, et al. PET imaging of TSPO expression in immune cells can assess organ-level pathophysiology in high-consequence viral infections. Proc Natl Acad Sci U S A. 2022;119(15):e2110846119.
2. Hammoud DA, Sinharay S, Shah S, Schreiber-Stainthorp W, Maric D, Muthusamy S, et al. Neuroinflammatory changes in relation to cerebrospinal fluid viral load in simian immunodeficiency virus encephalitis. MBio. 2019;10(3):e00970.
3. Gong J, Szego ÉM, Leonov A, Benito E, Becker S, Fischer A, et al. Translocator protein ligand protects against neurodegeneration in the MPTP mouse model of parkinsonism. J Neurosci. 2019;39(19):3752–69.
4. Owen DR, Guo Q, Kalk NJ, Colasanti A, Kalogiannopoulou D, Dimber R, et al. Determination of [(11)C]PBR28 binding potential in vivo: a first human TSPO blocking study. J Cereb Blood Flow Metab. 2014;34(6):989–94.
5. Kreisl WC, Jenko KJ, Hines CS, Lyoo CH, Corona W, Morse CL, et al. A genetic polymorphism for translocator protein 18 kDa affects both in vitro and in vivo radioligand binding in human brain to this putative biomarker of neuroinflammation. J Cereb Blood Flow Metab. 2013;33(1):53–8.
6. Fujita M, Kobayashi M, Ikawa M, Gunn RN, Rabiner EA, Owen DR, et al. Comparison of four (11) C-labeled PET ligands to quantify translocator protein 18 kDa (TSPO) in human brain: (R)-PK11195, PBR28, DPA-713, and ER176-based on recent publications that measured specific-to-non-displaceable ratios. EJNMMI Res. 2017;7(1):84.

7. Lee JH, Simeon FG, Liow JS, Morse CL, Gladding RL, Montero Santamaria JA, et al. In vivo evaluation of six analogs of (11)C-ER176 as candidate (18) F-labeled radioligands for translocator protein 18 kDa (TSPO). J Nucl Med. 2022;63:1252.

8. Zhang HL, Wu J, Zhu J. The immune-modulatory role of apolipoprotein E with emphasis on multiple sclerosis and experimental autoimmune encephalomyelitis. Clin Dev Immunol. 2010;2010:186813, 1.

9. Cagnin A, Brooks DJ, Kennedy AM, Gunn RN, Myers R, Turkheimer FE, et al. In-vivo measurement of activated microglia in dementia. Lancet. 2001;358(9280):461–7.

10. Okello A, Edison P, Archer HA, Turkheimer FE, Kennedy J, Bullock R, et al. Microglial activation and amyloid deposition in mild cognitive impairment: a PET study. Neurology. 2009;72(1):56–62.

11. Yasuno F, Ota M, Kosaka J, Ito H, Higuchi M, Doronbekov TK, et al. Increased binding of peripheral benzodiazepine receptor in Alzheimer's disease measured by positron emission tomography with [11C] DAA1106. Biol Psychiatry. 2008;64(10):835–41.

12. Kreisl WC, Lyoo CH, McGwier M, Snow J, Jenko KJ, Kimura N, et al. In vivo radioligand binding to translocator protein correlates with severity of Alzheimer's disease. Brain. 2013;136(Pt 7):2228–38.

13. Gulyás B, Vas A, Tóth M, Takano A, Varrone A, Cselényi Z, et al. Age and disease related changes in the translocator protein (TSPO) system in the human brain: positron emission tomography measurements with [11C]vinpocetine. NeuroImage. 2011;56(3):1111–21.

14. Varrone A, Mattsson P, Forsberg A, Takano A, Nag S, Gulyás B, et al. In vivo imaging of the 18-kDa translocator protein (TSPO) with [18F]FEDAA1106 and PET does not show increased binding in Alzheimer's disease patients. Eur J Nucl Med Mol Imaging. 2013;40(6):921–31.

15. Knezevic D, Mizrahi R. Molecular imaging of neuroinflammation in Alzheimer's disease and mild cognitive impairment. Prog Neuro-Psychopharmacol Biol Psychiatry. 2018;80(Pt B):123–31.

16. Parbo P, Ismail R, Sommerauer M, Stokholm MG, Hansen AK, Hansen KV, et al. Does inflammation precede tau aggregation in early Alzheimer's disease? A PET study. Neurobiol Dis. 2018;117:211–6.

17. Toppala S, Ekblad LL, Tuisku J, Helin S, Johansson JJ, Laine H, et al. Association of Early β-amyloid accumulation and neuroinflammation measured with [(11)C]PBR28 in elderly individuals without dementia. Neurology. 2021;96(12):e1608–e19.

18. Cisbani G, Koppel A, Knezevic D, Suridjan I, Mizrahi R, Bazinet RP. Peripheral cytokine and fatty acid associations with neuroinflammation in AD and aMCI patients: an exploratory study. Brain Behav Immun. 2020;87:679–88.

19. Dani M, Wood M, Mizoguchi R, Fan Z, Walker Z, Morgan R, et al. Microglial activation correlates in vivo with both tau and amyloid in Alzheimer's disease. Brain. 2018;141(9):2740–54.

20. Klein J, Yan X, Johnson A, Tomljanovic Z, Zou J, Polly K, et al. Olfactory impairment is related to tau pathology and Neuroinflammation in Alzheimer's disease. J Alzheimers Dis. 2021;80(3):1051–65.

21. Malpetti M, Kievit RA, Passamonti L, Jones PS, Tsvetanov KA, Rittman T, et al. Microglial activation and tau burden predict cognitive decline in Alzheimer's disease. Brain. 2020;143(5):1588–602.

22. Pascoal TA, Benedet AL, Ashton NJ, Kang MS, Therriault J, Chamoun M, et al. Microglial activation and tau propagate jointly across braak stages. Nat Med. 2021;27(9):1592–9.

23. Passamonti L, Rodríguez PV, Hong YT, Allinson KSJ, Bevan-Jones WR, Williamson D, et al. [(11)C]PK11195 binding in Alzheimer disease and progressive supranuclear palsy. Neurology. 2018;90(22):e1989–e96.

24. Terada T, Yokokura M, Obi T, Bunai T, Yoshikawa E, Ando I, et al. In vivo direct relation of tau pathology with neuroinflammation in early Alzheimer's disease. J Neurol. 2019;266(9):2186–96.

25. Zou J, Tao S, Johnson A, Tomljanovic Z, Polly K, Klein J, et al. Microglial activation, but not tau pathology, is independently associated with amyloid positivity and memory impairment. Neurobiol Aging. 2020;85:11–21.

26. Yokokura M, Terada T, Bunai T, Nakaizumi K, Takebayashi K, Iwata Y, et al. Depiction of microglial activation in aging and dementia: positron emission tomography with [(11)C]DPA713 versus [(11)C](R)PK11195. J Cereb Blood Flow Metab. 2017;37(3):877–89.

27. Tomasi G, Edison P, Bertoldo A, Roncaroli F, Singh P, Gerhard A, et al. Novel reference region model reveals increased microglial and reduced vascular binding of 11C-(R)-PK11195 in patients with Alzheimer's disease. J Nucl Med. 2008;49(8):1249–56.

28. Lyoo CH, Ikawa M, Liow JS, Zoghbi SS, Morse CL, Pike VW, et al. Cerebellum can serve as a pseudo-reference region in Alzheimer disease to detect neuroinflammation measured with PET radioligand binding to translocator protein. J Nucl Med. 2015;56(5):701–6.

29. Bradburn S, Murgatroyd C, Ray N. Neuroinflammation in mild cognitive impairment and Alzheimer's disease: a meta-analysis. Ageing Res Rev. 2019;50:1–8.

30. Hamelin L, Lagarde J, Dorothée G, Potier MC, Corlier F, Kuhnast B, et al. Distinct dynamic profiles of microglial activation are associated with progression of Alzheimer's disease. Brain. 2018;141(6):1855–70.

31. Leng F, Edison P. Neuroinflammation and microglial activation in Alzheimer disease: where do we go from here? Nat Rev Neurol. 2021;17(3):157–72.

32. Miguel-Álvarez M, Santos-Lozano A, Sanchis-Gomar F, Fiuza-Luces C, Pareja-Galeano H, Garatachea N, et al. Non-steroidal anti-inflammatory drugs as a treatment for Alzheimer's disease: a systematic review and meta-analysis of treatment effect. Drugs Aging. 2015;32(2):139–47.

33. Howard R, Zubko O, Bradley R, Harper E, Pank L, O'Brien J, et al. Minocycline at 2 different dos-

ages vs placebo for patients with mild Alzheimer disease: a randomized clinical trial. JAMA Neurol. 2020;77(2):164–74.

34. Lee J, Howard RS, Schneider LS. The current landscape of prevention trials in dementia. Neurotherapeutics. 2022;19(1):228–47.

35. Tansey MG, Wallings RL, Houser MC, Herrick MK, Keating CE, Joers V. Inflammation and immune dysfunction in Parkinson disease. Nat Rev Immunol. 2022;1-17:657.

36. Lindqvist D, Kaufman E, Brundin L, Hall S, Surova Y, Hansson O. Non-motor symptoms in patients with Parkinson's disease—correlations with inflammatory cytokines in serum. PLoS One. 2012;7(10):e47387.

37. Warnecke T, Schäfer KH, Claus I, Del Tredici K, Jost WH. Gastrointestinal involvement in Parkinson's disease: pathophysiology, diagnosis, and management. NPJ Parkinsons Dis. 2022;8(1):31.

38. Gerhard A, Pavese N, Hotton G, Turkheimer F, Es M, Hammers A, et al. In vivo imaging of microglial activation with [11C](R)-PK11195 PET in idiopathic Parkinson's disease. Neurobiol Dis. 2006;21(2):404–12.

39. Ghadery C, Koshimori Y, Coakeley S, Harris M, Rusjan P, Kim J, et al. Microglial activation in Parkinson's disease using [(18)F]-FEPPA. J Neuroinflammation. 2017;14(1):8.

40. Ghadery C, Koshimori Y, Christopher L, Kim J, Rusjan P, Lang AE, et al. The interaction between neuroinflammation and β-amyloid in cognitive decline in Parkinson's disease. Mol Neurobiol. 2020;57(1):492–501.

41. Lavisse S, Goutal S, Wimberley C, Tonietto M, Bottlaender M, Gervais P, et al. Increased microglial activation in patients with Parkinson disease using [(18)F]-DPA714 TSPO PET imaging. Parkinsonism Relat Disord. 2021;82:29–36.

42. Varnäs K, Cselényi Z, Jucaite A, Halldin C, Svenningsson P, Farde L, et al. PET imaging of [(11)C]PBR28 in Parkinson's disease patients does not indicate increased binding to TSPO despite reduced dopamine transporter binding. Eur J Nucl Med Mol Imaging. 2019;46(2):367–75.

43. Zhang PF, Gao F. Neuroinflammation in Parkinson's disease: a meta-analysis of PET imaging studies. J Neurol. 2022;269(5):2304–14.

44. Laurell GL, Plavén-Sigray P, Jucaite A, Varrone A, Cosgrove KP, Svarer C, et al. Nondisplaceable binding is a potential confounding factor in (11)C-PBR28 translocator protein PET studies. J Nucl Med. 2021;62(3):412–7.

45. Lois C, González I, Izquierdo-García D, Zürcher NR, Wilkens P, Loggia ML, et al. Neuroinflammation in Huntington's disease: new insights with (11)C-PBR28 PET/MRI. ACS Chem Neurosci. 2018;9(11):2563–71.

46. Rocha NP, Charron O, Latham LB, Colpo GD, Zanotti-Fregonara P, Yu M, et al. Microglia activation in basal ganglia is a late event in Huntington disease pathophysiology. Neurol Neuroimmunol Neuroinflamm. 2021;8(3):e984.

47. Politis M, Lahiri N, Niccolini F, Su P, Wu K, Giannetti P, et al. Increased central microglial activation associated with peripheral cytokine levels in premanifest Huntington's disease gene carriers. Neurobiol Dis. 2015;83:115–21.

48. Gerhard A, Trender-Gerhard I, Turkheimer F, Quinn NP, Bhatia KP, Brooks DJ. In vivo imaging of microglial activation with [11C](R)-PK11195 PET in progressive supranuclear palsy. Mov Disord. 2006;21(1):89–93.

49. Palleis C, Sauerbeck J, Beyer L, Harris S, Schmitt J, Morenas-Rodriguez E, et al. In vivo assessment of neuroinflammation in 4-repeat tauopathies. Mov Disord. 2021;36(4):883–94.

50. Malpetti M, Passamonti L, Jones PS, Street D, Rittman T, Fryer TD, et al. Neuroinflammation predicts disease progression in progressive supranuclear palsy. J Neurol Neurosurg Psychiatry. 2021;92(7):769–75.

51. Gouilly D, Saint-Aubert L, Ribeiro MJ, Salabert AS, Tauber C, Péran P, et al. Neuroinflammation PET imaging of the translocator protein (TSPO) in Alzheimer's disease: an update. Eur J Neurosci. 2022;55(5):1322–43.

52. Janssen B, Vugts DJ, Windhorst AD, Mach RH. PET imaging of microglial activation-beyond targeting TSPO. Molecules. 2018;23(3):607.

53. Calsolaro V, Matthews PM, Donat CK, Livingston NR, Femminella GD, Guedes SS, et al. Astrocyte reactivity with late-onset cognitive impairment assessed in vivo using (11)C-BU99008 PET and its relationship with amyloid load. Mol Psychiatry. 2021;26(10):5848–55.

54. Shukuri M, Mawatari A, Takatani S, Tahara T, Inoue M, Arakaki W, et al. Synthesis and preclinical evaluation of (18)F-labeled Ketoprofen methyl esters for Cyclooxygenase-1 imaging in neuroinflammation. J Nucl Med. 2022;63(11):1761.

55. Prabhakaran J, Molotkov A, Mintz A, Mann JJ. Progress in PET imaging of neuroinflammation targeting COX-2 enzyme. Molecules. 2021;26(11):3208.

56. Kumar JSD, Prabhakaran J, Molotkov A, Sattiraju A, Kim J, Doubrovin M, et al. Radiosynthesis and evaluation of [(18)F]FMTP, a COX-2 PET ligand. Pharmacol Rep. 2020;72(5):1433–40.

57. Kim MJ, Lee JH, Juarez Anaya F, Hong J, Miller W, Telu S, et al. First-in-human evaluation of [(11)C]PS13, a novel PET radioligand, to quantify cyclooxygenase-1 in the brain. Eur J Nucl Med Mol Imaging. 2020;47(13):3143–51.

58. Zheng QH. Radioligands targeting purinergic P2X7 receptor. Bioorg Med Chem Lett. 2020;30(12):127169.

59. Ahmad R, Postnov A, Bormans G, Versijpt J, Vandenbulcke M, Van Laere K. Decreased in vivo availability of the cannabinoid type 2 receptor in Alzheimer's disease. Eur J Nucl Med Mol Imaging. 2016;43(12):2219–27.

60. Ahmad R, Koole M, Evens N, Serdons K, Verbruggen A, Bormans G, et al. Whole-body biodistribution and radiation dosimetry of the cannabinoid type 2 receptor

ligand [11C]-NE40 in healthy subjects. Mol Imaging Biol. 2013;15(4):384–90.

61. Horti AG, Naik R, Foss CA, Minn I, Misheneva V, Du Y, et al. PET imaging of microglia by targeting macrophage colony-stimulating factor 1 receptor (CSF1R). Proc Natl Acad Sci U S A. 2019;116(5):1686–91.

62. Herrero P, Laforest R, Shoghi K, Zhou D, Ewald G, Pfeifer J, et al. Feasibility and dosimetry studies for 18F-NOS as a potential PET radiopharmaceutical for inducible nitric oxide synthase in humans. J Nucl Med. 2012;53(6):994–1001.

63. Lucot KL, Stevens MY, Bonham TA, Azevedo EC, Chaney AM, Webber ED, et al. Tracking innate immune activation in a MOUSE model of PARKINSON'S disease using TREM1 and TSPO pet tracers. J Nucl Med. 2022;63:1570.

64. Liu YS, Yan WJ, Tan CC, Li JQ, Xu W, Cao XP, et al. Common variant in TREM1 influencing brain amyloid deposition in mild cognitive impairment and Alzheimer's disease. Neurotox Res. 2020;37(3):661–8.

65. Janssen B, Mach RH. Development of brain PET imaging agents: strategies for imaging neuroinflammation in Alzheimer's disease. Prog Mol Biol Transl Sci. 2019;165:371–99.

Ming-Kai Chen, David Matuskey,
Sjoerd J. Finnema, and Richard E. Carson

Introduction

The recent emergence of positron emission tomography (PET) imaging targeting synapses with synaptic vesicle glycoprotein 2A (SV2A) has opened new avenues for studying neurodegenerative diseases. The general use of this marker in a wide range of diseases makes it par-

M.-K. Chen (✉)
Department of Radiology and Biomedical Imaging,
Yale University School of Medicine,
New Haven, CT, USA
e-mail: ming-kai.chen@yale.edu

D. Matuskey
Department of Radiology and Biomedical Imaging,
Yale University School of Medicine,
New Haven, CT, USA

Department of Psychiatry, Yale University School of Medicine, New Haven, CT, USA

Department of Neurology, Yale University School of Medicine, New Haven, CT, USA
e-mail: david.matuskey@yale.edu

S. J. Finnema
Neuroscience Discovery Research, Translational Imaging, AbbVie, North Chicago, IL, USA
e-mail: sjoerd.finnema@abbvie.com

R. E. Carson
Department of Radiology and Biomedical Imaging,
Yale University School of Medicine,
New Haven, CT, USA

Department of Biomedical Engineering, Yale University, New Haven, CT, USA
e-mail: richard.carson@yale.edu

ticularly suitable for human research, including disease diagnosis and differentiation and therapeutic monitoring. In many cases, pairing SV2A-PET with a second PET radioligand with a disease-specific focus has provided unique multimodal information on brain pathophysiology. Here, we review SV2A glycoproteins, SV2A-PET tracers, and the potential application of SV2A-PET in various neurodegenerative diseases, including Alzheimer's disease (AD), frontotemporal dementia (FTD), Parkinson's disease (PD), dementia with Lewy bodies (DLB), progressive supranuclear palsy (PSP), corticobasal degeneration (CBD), and Huntington's disease (HD).

SV2A PET as a Measure of Synaptic Density

Synaptic vesicle glycoprotein 2 (SV2) is a glycoprotein located on secretory vesicles in neurons and endocrine cells. SV2 is essential for synaptic function and is involved in vesicle trafficking and exocytosis, although research on its exact function continues (see reviews [1, 2]). SV2 has three distinctly distributed isoforms in the brain. SV2A is ubiquitously expressed in almost all synapses, while SV2B is more restricted, and SV2C is only observed in a few rat brain regions [1, 2]. Among glutamatergic and GABAergic neurons, SV2A is thought to be located in both classes, while SV2B might be more restricted to the former and SV2C to the latter [2]. Therefore, SV2A is a promising biomarker of synaptic density with little variation in copy number per vesicle [3].

SV2A has been shown to be a therapeutic target of the antiepileptic drug levetiracetam [4]. Consequently, the first attempt to develop a SV2A-PET radioligand was ^{11}C-levetiracetam [5]. Later, higher affinity SV2A-selective ligands were synthesized and evaluated [6]. Three of the SV2A ligands were radiolabeled as ^{11}C-UCB-A [7], ^{18}F-UCB-H [8], and ^{11}C-UCB-J [9], and all were evaluated in nonhuman primates. Of these, ^{11}C-UCB-J has the most suitable pharmacokinetics with rapid and high brain uptake, reversible binding kinetics, and relatively low nonspecific binding in white matter [9]. However, the short half-life of carbon-11 (20.4 min) limits the production of ^{11}C-UCB-J to PET centers with cyclotrons. Based on the initial success of ^{11}C-UCB-J, fluorine-18 (half-life ~110 min) labeled SV2A radioligands with slightly modified chemical structure have attracted more interest for potential broader applicability in multicenter studies. Initial work focused on ^{18}F-UCB-J, which provided similar pharmacokinetic results to ^{11}C-UCB-J [10], however, the radiosynthetic process was not suitable for routine production. Subsequent focus was on the mono- and difluorinated UCB-J analogs, ^{18}F-SynVesT-1 (^{18}F-SDM-8, ^{18}F-MNI-1126) [11, 12] and ^{18}F-SynVesT-2 (^{18}F-SDM-2) [13]. In humans, ^{18}F-SynVesT-1 displayed outstanding characteristics with very high brain uptake, fast and reversible kinetics, excellent test-retest reproducibility, and binding specificity to SV2A [14, 15]. Compared to ^{11}C-UCB-J, ^{18}F-SynVesT-1 displayed higher binding potential (BP_{ND}) due to lower nonspecific binding. Recent human PET scans with ^{18}F-SynVesT-2 showed slightly lower BP_{ND}, but with faster kinetics. The availability of these fluorine-18 labeled SV2A-PET radioligands provides great opportunities for multicenter clinical studies in various neurodegenerative diseases.

To examine whether SV2A-PET provides an index of synaptic density, a correlation study between in vivo SV2A-PET and in vitro bioassays was conducted [16]. A baboon underwent a ^{11}C-UCB-J scan, followed by postmortem brain tissue studies. ^{11}C-UCB-J distribution volume (V_T) measured by PET correlated well with the regional SV2A density measured by homogenate binding assay and Western blot [16]. Importantly, there was also good correlation between SV2A and the "gold standard" synaptic density marker synaptophysin in Western blot and confocal microscopy experiments, i.e., SV2A can be used as a surrogate for synaptophysin to quantify synapse density [16]. Further studies in postmortem human tissue are ongoing to further validate SV2A as a biomarker of synaptic density.

Pharmacokinetic modeling studies of SV2A-PET in humans revealed that the best models to quantify V_T values are the one-tissue compartment model (1TC) for ^{11}C-UCB-J [17], ^{18}F-SynVesT-1 [15], and ^{18}F-SynVesT-2, and Logan graphical analysis for ^{18}F-UCB-H [18]. Excellent test-retest reproducibility and low noise V_T images can be obtained with the 1TC model for ^{11}C-UCB-J [17] and ^{18}F-SynVesT-1 [14, 15]. Please see the references and Chap. 12 by Carson and colleagues for more details of modeling methodology. Here, we focus on the potential clinical application of SV2A-PET as a biomarker of synapse density in various neurodegenerative diseases as reported below (summarized in Table 10.1).

Table 10.1 Literature with SV2A PET in human studies of neurodegenerative disorders, listed in chronological order per disorder

Populations	Subjects	Tracer(s)	Outcome measure	Major finding	Reference
AD and CN	10 AD/ MCI	^{11}C-UCB-J	BP_{ND}	41% lower binding in the hippocampus of AD	[27]
AD and CN	24 AD/ MCI	^{18}F-UCB-H	V_T	Lower binding in the hippocampus (31%), cortical (11–18%) and thalamus (16%) of AD	[28]
AD and CN	34 AD/ MCI	^{11}C-UCB-J	DVR_{Cb}	Extensive cortical and subcortical reductions of DVR_{Cb} in AD	[29]
AD and CN	45 AD / MCI	^{11}C-UCB-J	DVR_{Cb}	Positive association between global synaptic density and global cognition as well as performance	[31]
AD and CN	38 AD/ MCI	^{11}C-UCB-J ^{11}C-PiB	DVR_{Cb}	Inverse association between global amyloid deposition and hippocampal SV2A binding in participants with aMCI, but not mild dementia	[32]
AD and CN	10 AD/ MCI	^{11}C-UCB-J ^{18}F-flortaucipir	DVR_{Cb}	Entorhinal cortical tau inversely associated with hippocampal synaptic density	[35]
AD and CN	14 AD/ MCI	^{11}C-UCB-J ^{18}F-FDG	DVR_{Cb}	Similar reduction of ^{11}C-UCB-J and FDG in medial temporal lobe of AD, but smaller reduction of ^{11}C-UCB-J in neocortex than FDG	[36]
AD and CN	12 AD	^{18}F-UCB-H	V_T	33% decrease in right hippocampus in AD (trend level)	[40]
Presymptomatic C9orf72 mutation carriers and CN	3 carriers	^{11}C-UCB-J	BP_{ND}	Decrease in thalamus in carriers	[39]
bvFTD and CN	1 bvFTD	^{11}C-UCB-J	BP_{ND}	Lower binding in frontotemporal and subcortical regions	[39]
bvFTD and CN	12 bvFTD	^{18}F-UCB-H	V_T	41% decrease in right parahippocampus in bvFTD (trend level)	[40]
PD and CN	12 PD	^{11}C-UCB-J	BP_{ND}	Up to 45% lower binding in PD, largest in SN (45%) with multiple cortical areas included	[45]
PD (early drug-naive) and CN	12 PD	^{11}C-UCB-J	V_T	Lower binding in PD ranged from 15% (CAU) to 8% in multiple areas, SN was 7%	[46]
PD and CN	30 PD	^{11}C-UCB-J	BP_{ND}	Lower binding in PD from 15%, largest in SN	[47]
PD and CN	21 PD	^{11}C-UCB-J	SUVR-1	Lower binding in PD in SN	[51]
DLB/PDD and CN	13 DLB/ PDD	^{11}C-UCB-J	SUVR-1	Lower binding in DLB/ PDD in multiple areas	[51]
PSP and CN	14 PSP	^{11}C-UCB-J	BP_{ND}	Up to 50% lower binding in cortical and subcortical areas	[55]
CBD and CN	15 CBD	^{11}C-UCB-J	BP_{ND}	Up to 50% lower binding in cortical and subcortical areas	[55]
HD (premanifest and early stage) and CN	18 HD	^{11}C-UCB-J	BP_{ND}	Lower binding in PUT (−19%), CAU (−16%) in premanifest; PUT (−33%), CAU (−31%), whole gray matter (−12%) in early stage	[59]

AD Alzheimer's disease, *bvFTD* behavioral-variant FTD, *CBD* corticobasal degeneration, *CN* cognitively normal, *DLB* Lewy body dementia, *FTD* frontotemporal dementia, *HD* Huntington's disease, *MCI* mild cognitive impairment, *PD* Parkinson's disease, *PDD* PD-dementia, *PSP* progressive supranuclear palsy, BP_{ND} binding potential, DVR_{Cb} distribution volume ratio (cerebellum reference), *SUV* standardized uptake value, *SUVR* SUV ratio, V_T volume of distribution, *CAU* caudate, *PUT* putamen, *SN* substantia nigra

Alzheimer's Disease

Dementia is abnormal cognitive decline that is greater than expected as compared to age matched controls, often causing disability and eventually affecting the ability to independently perform daily living activities. Dementia can be attributed to many causes, the most common is Alzheimer's disease (AD), accounting for more than 50–60% of dementia, while 15–25% of cases are due to frontotemporal dementia (FTD) and 15–25% of cases due to dementia with Lewy bodies (DLB), respectively [19]. According to the Alzheimer's Association, an estimated 6.2 million Americans aged 65 and older are living with AD in 2021 [20]. This number could grow to 13.8 million by 2060 barring the development of medical breakthroughs to prevent, slow, or cure AD [20].

From a diagnostic perspective, AD is viewed as a continuum from preclinical AD to mild cognitive impairment (MCI), and to AD dementia. The clinical dementia stage of AD has a distinct pathology of plaques composed of β-amyloid (Aβ), neurofibrillary tangles, and loss of synaptic density [21]. Synapses are crucial for cognitive function, and synaptic density loss is a robust and consistent pathology in AD [22]. Synaptic density impairment including loss of synapses and presynaptic proteins is observed in the early stages of clinical AD [23]. Therefore, the ability to assess synaptic density in vivo is extremely valuable in AD research, as well as to monitor the efficacy of potential therapies.

PET imaging is used extensively in AD research to measure glucose metabolism (i.e., ^{18}F-FDG), β-amyloid plaques, and neurofibrillary tangles in the framework of amyloid-tau-neurodegeneration (AT(N)) [24]. ^{18}F-FDG PET is widely used clinically to differentiate AD from FTD, and to track disease progression by measuring neuronal activity. However, ^{18}F-FDG is metabolized by both neurons and glial cells (astrocytes, microglia, and oligodendrocytes) and is not a direct biomarker of synaptic density. ^{18}F-FDG uptake is also affected by stimulation, medication, and blood glucose levels [25]. SV2A-PET has shown itself to be a stable measure not affecting by blood flow [17, 26], thus it can provide a direct indicator of synaptic density in AD.

In the first SV2A-PET AD study with ^{11}C-UCB-J, 10 AD (all Aβ+) and 11 cognitively normal (CN) subjects were compared [27]. Reduced hippocampal ^{11}C-UCB-J binding was hypothesized based on early degeneration of entorhinal cortical cell projections to the hippocampus via the perforant pathway and hippocampal SV2A reduction observed in a postmortem study [23]. BP_{ND} using centrum semiovale (CS) as the reference region was lower by 41% in the hippocampus of AD compared to CN, which was greater than the volume loss (22%) measured by MRI [27]. When combining AD and CN groups, statistically significant correlations were found between hippocampus BP_{ND} and cognitive tests including an episodic memory score and a clinical dementia rating [27]. Bastin and colleagues reported the evaluation of ^{18}F-UCB-H in 24 patients with MCI or AD (all Aβ+) and 19 CN [28] and found that V_T was lower in the hippocampus (31%), cortical regions (11–18%), and thalamus (16%). The difference in the hippocampal binding was directly related to patients' cognitive decline and unawareness of memory problems.

In a subsequent ^{11}C-UCB-J study in a larger cohort of early AD ($n = 34$) and CN ($n = 19$), broader cortical and subcortical reductions in SV2A binding were seen, which were more widespread than reductions in gray matter volume [29]. Here, the outcome measure was distribution volume ratio with cerebellum as an alternative reference region, which provided a more reliable signal than the small CS reference region. These findings better reflect the pathological findings of reduced cortical synaptic density in AD postmortem studies [30]. Recently, Mecca and colleagues also showed a significant positive association between global synaptic density and global cognition as well as performance on five individual cognitive domains (verbal memory, language, executive function, processing speed, and visuospatial ability) among 45 participants with early AD [31]. These results further support the use of synaptic imaging as a potential surrogate biomarker outcome for therapeutic trials that is well-correlated with clinical measures [31].

The relationships between SV2A-PET for synaptic density with amyloid [32], tau [33–35], and FDG [36] have also been investigated in AD. We measured ^{11}C-UCB-J distribution volume ratio and ^{11}C-PiB for Aβ deposition and observed a significant inverse association between global Aβ deposition and hippocampal SV2A binding in participants with MCI, but not in mild dementia [32]. A "paradoxical" positive association between hippocampal Aβ and SV2A binding was found [32], suggesting that fibrillar Aβ is still accumulating in the early stages of the disease before plateauing at later stages [32].

A study of 10 MCI and 10 CN subjects found an inverse association between tau deposition (^{18}F-MK-6240) and ^{11}C-UCB-J within the medial temporal lobe [33]. There was decreased ^{11}C-UCB-J binding mainly in substructures of the medial temporal lobe (48%–51%) and increased ^{18}F-MK6240 binding (42%–44%) in the same region, spreading to association cortices [33]. Decreased performance on cognitive tests was associated with both increased tau and decreased SV2A binding in the hippocampus,

although in a multivariate analysis only tau binding was significantly related to cognitive performance [33]. Likewise, in a small cohort study of 7 AD, higher regional ^{18}F-flortaucipir uptake and lower ^{11}C-UCB-J uptake across the subjects were reported [34]. Higher ^{18}F-flortaucipir and lower ^{11}C-UCB-J uptake were also associated with altered synaptic function by magnetoencephalography spectral measures [34]. A third correlation study between ^{11}C-UCB-J and ^{18}F-flortaucipir in 10 AD and 10 CN participants showed that entorhinal cortical (ERC) tau was inversely correlated with hippocampal synaptic density ($r = -0.59$, $P = 0.009$) [35]. After correction for partial volume effects, the association of ERC tau with hippocampal synaptic density was stronger in the overall sample ($r = -0.61$, $P = 0.007$) and in the AD group where the effect size was large, but not statistically significant ($r = -0.58$, $P = 0.06$) [35]. This inverse association of ERC tau and hippocampal synaptic density may reflect synaptic failure due to tau pathology in ERC neurons projecting to the hippocampus [35].

A study comparing ^{11}C-UCB-J and ^{18}F-FDG in 14 AD and 11 CN participants found that these measures showed similar reductions in the medial temporal lobe of AD [36]. However, the magnitude of reduction of ^{11}C-UCB-J in the neocortex was smaller than that of ^{18}F-FDG. The highest inter-tracer correlations were found in the medial temporal cortex (see representative images in Fig. 10.1). Interestingly, the patterns of ^{11}C-UCB-J delivery/perfusion (e.g., K_1) and ^{18}F-FDG uptake (e.g., Patlak K_i) are very similar. Thus, synaptic loss and perfusion/metabolism measures that can be obtained from a single dynamic ^{11}C-UCB-J scan provide complementary information on AD pathophysiology [36].

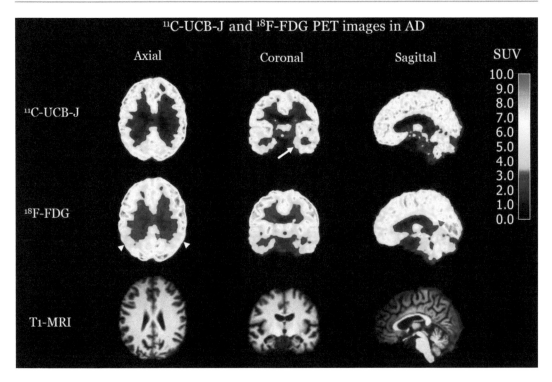

Fig. 10.1 Representative ^{11}C-UCB-J and ^{18}F-FDG PET (SUV) and MRI images in AD. Evident reduction of ^{11}C-UCB-J binding in the hippocampus of AD was noted (arrow denotes the left hippocampus). Evident hypome-tabolism was also noted in temporal and parietal cortices of AD (white arrowhead denotes the parietal cortices) as well as posterior cingulate (red arrow heads)

Frontotemporal Dementia

FTD is also commonly misdiagnosed as AD or other neuropsychiatric disorders because it has two major patterns involving gradual or progressive changes in behavioral or language impairments. The affected population is generally younger than AD (35 to 75 years old), and 20%–40% of patients have a positive family history of FTD [37]. Previous studies have provided evidence for synaptic dysfunction and loss in FTD [38]. Malpetti and colleagues assessed in vivo synaptic density in three presymptomatic C9orf72 mutation carriers, one symptomatic patient with a behavioral variant (bvFTD) and 19 healthy controls [39]. In the presymptomatic group, they reported a marked decrease in thalamic ^{11}C-UCB-J binding, and a slight decrease in the cortex. The patient with bvFTD demonstrated extensive synaptic loss in frontotemporal regions. Salmon et al. assessed ^{18}F-UCB-H PET in 12 patients with probable bvFTD compared to 12 CN and 12 AD and reported decreased binding in the right anterior parahippocampal gyrus in bvFTD [40]. In that study, anosognosia was correlated with synaptic density in the caudate nucleus and the anteromedial prefrontal cortex. Ongoing studies in bvFTD are being conducted to further characterize this disorder.

Parkinson's Disease

Parkinson's disease (PD) is a long-term degenerative disorder that has prominent motor and nonmotor symptoms [41]. The most obvious early motor symptoms of PD are tremor, rigidity, and bradykinesia, while nonmotor symptoms can consist of cognitive, emotional, and autonomic changes. PD symptoms have primarily been related to a nigrostriatal dopaminergic deficit [41], and assessment of this pathway with dopamine transporter single photon emission CT (DaT-SPECT) has been approved by the US Food and Drug Administration and the European Medicines Agency to support the differential diagnosis between parkinsonism versus essential tremor. More recent research in PD has demonstrated the involvement of several neurotransmitter systems beyond dopamine, however, giving an importance to using new tools and biomarkers to investigate this condition [42, 43]. Growing evidence has drawn attention to the significance of exploring synaptic changes in this context [44].

Matuskey et al. conducted the first in vivo investigation of SV2A/synaptic density in 12 subjects with mild bilateral PD and 12 matched CN using ^{11}C-UCB-J. Lower BP_{ND} was found in PD, with between-group differences in subcortical regions including the substantia nigra (SN) (−45%), red nucleus (−31%), and locus coeruleus (−17%). Interestingly, lower synaptic density was also observed in cortical areas including the posterior cingulate cortex (−15%), parahippocampal gyrus (−12%), orbitofrontal cortex (−11%), and ventromedial prefrontal cortex (−11%) [45].

In a related multi-tracer PET study, Wilson and colleagues compared SV2A (^{11}C-UCB-J), mitochondrial complex 1 (^{18}F-BCPP-EF), and sigma 1 receptor (^{11}C-SA-4503) in 12 drug-naive early PD patients and 16 CN [46]. The PD group had significantly lower ^{11}C-UCB-J V_T in the striatum, thalamus, brainstem, dorsal raphe, and cortical regions. Differences in this cohort were less pronounced in the SN (−7%). Interestingly, no significant changes were detected in ^{18}F-BCPP-EF V_T for mitochondrial complex 1 and ^{11}C-SA-4503 V_T for sigma receptor in the same regions between groups [46]. This study also investigated the correlation between clinical symptoms and V_T values, revealing an inverse correlation between synaptic density in the brainstem and clinical rating scores. Furthermore, eight PD patients underwent longitudinal ^{11}C-UCB-J PET scan at a 1-year interval and no significant changes were detected [46].

In a third study, Delva and colleagues compared ^{11}C-UCB-J measures among 30 PD and 20 CN [47] and reported significantly lower BP_{ND} in the SN (−15%) of PD. They also reported non-significantly lower BP_{ND} in dorsal striatum (−7%), caudate (−6%), and putamen (−6%) in the PD group. No correlation between BP_{ND} values and clinical symptoms was found.

These investigations with ^{11}C-UCB-J PET have shown its ability to assess differences in PD and have the potential to increase the understanding of the pathophysiology and potentially improve the diagnosis of PD. Further studies with larger samples are currently underway to achieve these goals.

Dementia with Lewy Body and Parkinson's Disease Dementia (PDD)

As PD progresses, a considerable portion of patients with PD develop cognitive impairments and dementia [48]. DLB is closely related to PD with four major characteristics: parkinsonism, visual hallucinations, cognitive fluctuations, and REM-sleep behavior disorder [49]. The differential diagnosis between DLB and other types of dementia such as AD is usually difficult because of overlapping symptoms. FDG PET can be very useful for the initial clinical diagnosis due to distinct regional hypometabolic patterns among various types of dementia [19]. DaT-SPECT has also been used clinically for detecting the dopaminergic deficit of DLB. However, the diagnosis and treatment for DLB remains challenging and new imaging biomarkers are needed to develop better understanding of the pathophysiology.

Nicastro et al. reported decreased ^{11}C-UCB-J binding in parietal and occipital regions of two patients with DLB [50], which is similar to the regional hypometabolism of FDG PET in DLB observed clinically [19]. Andersen and colleagues conducted ^{11}C-UCB-J PET to compare synaptic density in 21 non-demented PD (nPD) subjects, 13 patients with PD-dementia or DLB (DLB/PDD), and 15 age matched CN using standardized uptake ratio (SUVR)-1 binding as the outcome with cerebellar white matter as a reference region [51]. The nPD group showed lower values compared to CN only in the SN. The brain changes in DLB/PDD group were more extensive, with significantly lower SUVR-1 values in the SN, occipital cortices, parietal cortices, primary sensorimotor cortex, middle frontal gyrus, and orbitofrontal cortex [51].

Progressive Supranuclear Palsy and Corticobasal Degeneration

PSP and CBD are both neurodegenerative primary tauopathies and have similarities in clinical symptoms (e.g., motor, behavioral, and cognitive abnormalities) [52], but are considered different disorders as different tau strains and brain regions are affected [53]. Previous work has suggested that oligomeric tau leads to synaptic loss [54], which may play an essential role in PSP and CBD. Recently, Holland et al. found widespread (up to 50%) cortical and subcortical reduction of ^{11}C-UCB-J binding in both PSP (n = 14) and CBD (n = 15) compared to controls [55], consistent with postmortem data [54]. They also reported a negative correlation between global ^{11}C-UCB-J binding and the PSP and CBD rating scales and a positive correlation with the revised Addenbrooke's Cognitive Examination [55].

Huntington's Disease

HD is an autosomal dominant disease caused by an expanded CAG triplet in the Huntington chromosome. Clinical characterizations of HD are progressive movement disorders (including chorea), cognitive deficits (culminating in dementia), and psychiatric symptoms (e.g., depression) [56]. The pathogenesis of HD is not clear, but studies have found synaptic and neuronal dysfunction and cell death in the cortex and striatum in HD [57]. Lower SV2A levels (~25%) were observed in cortical area in HD gene carriers compared to controls by ^{3}H-UCB-J autoradiography and SV2A immunofluorescence in human brain tissue [58]. Recently, a cross-sectional human PET study found significant loss of SV2A in multiple regions including the putamen (−28%), caudate (−25%), and whole GM (−9%) in the HD group (n = 11) compared to CN (n = 15). In the same study, reduced FDG uptake in the HD group compared to CN was restricted to the caudate and putamen and not found in the pallidum, cerebral cortex, or cerebellum [59]. The discrepancy between regional SV2A loss and hypometabolism could be due to miscoupling of synaptic density and neuronal activity in GABAergic predominant regions or due to increased FDG uptake from microglial activation [59]. In the premanifest HD mutation carriers group (n = 7), both ^{11}C-UCB-J and FDG PET showed significant reductions in putamen and caudate only [59]. Striatal ^{11}C-UCB-J binding was positively correlated with clinical measures in motor and cognitive domains [59]. The study suggests the loss of presynaptic terminal integrity in early HD, which begins in the striatum in the early manifest phase, and correlates with motor impairment [59]. Furthermore, the study also suggests that ^{11}C-UCB-J PET is more sensitive than ^{18}F-FDG PET for the detection of extrastriatal changes in early HD [59].

Limitations

Despite the success of SV2A-PET as a potential biomarker for synaptic density in a wide variety of neurodegenerative diseases, several important questions have been raised (see a recent comprehensive review by Rossi et al. [60]). First, the biological function and the expressional properties of SV2A in synaptic vesicles have not been fully elucidated. The exact interaction between SV2A and the recently developed tracers including ^{11}C-UCB-J can be further clarified. Whether these tracers are able to bind to all the synaptic vesicles in the synaptic terminal or only a subset of them could lead to different interpretations of PET results. However, given the high specific binding signal of ^{11}C-UCB-J, it is likely that the tracers bind to most SV2A sites. Furthermore, SV2A expression seems to have stronger association with the GABAergic than the glutamatergic transmission in some brain regions, despite its ubiquitous presence throughout the brain [61]. The sensitivity and specificity for SV2A-PET to detect synaptic density loss will surely differ among various neurodegenerative diseases, partly depending on the relative involvement of inhibitory or excitatory neurons. Furthermore, SV2A expression seems to be modified in a more complicated pattern, including dynamic changes, especially in epilepsy (see review [60]). A very fundamental question remains to be further examined "What really is detected with SV2A-PET?" It is important to develop more detailed understanding of the biological changes underlying a reduction in SV2A-PET signal. Further validation studies between in vivo PET and post-mortem in vitro studies are ongoing to address some of these questions.

Summary

In conclusion, PET imaging of SV2A provides a direct measure of synaptic vesicles and is considered as a proxy for synaptic density. High-quality PET radioligands labeled with carbon-11 and fluorine-18 have been developed and validated for use in human studies. The potential versatility of synaptic imaging has facilitated the widespread use of these tools. Here, we focused on SV2A-PET studies in neurodegenerative disorders (Table 10.1). Overall, these PET studies show that SV2A loss is specific to disease-associated brain regions and is consistent with loss of synaptic density. While loss of synaptic density may not be specific to neurodegeneration, regional patterns of synaptic loss may provide valuable insights for distinguishing various types of dementia.

The utility of SV2A as a general marker of synapse density is promising but requires formal validation by comparing in vivo SV2A PET signals with postmortem assessments of SV2A and synaptic levels in human brain tissue. Further studies using fluorine-18 labeled radioligands in larger patient cohorts are also required to identify potential clinical applications of SV2A-PET imaging, including early detection of synaptic

density loss, differential diagnosis of different types of dementia, and monitoring of disease progression. SV2A-PET can also be used as an outcome measure for disease-modifying therapy trials, especially those targeting synaptic preservation and restoration. SV2A-PET holds great promise as a novel in vivo biomarker for dementia and neurodegeneration.

References

1. Mendoza-Torreblanca JG, Vanoye-Carlo A, Phillips-Farfan BV, Carmona-Aparicio L, Gomez-Lira G. Synaptic vesicle protein 2A: basic facts and role in synaptic function. Eur J Neurosci. 2013;38(11):3529–39.
2. Bartholome O, Van den Ackerveken P, Sanchez Gil J, de la Brassinne BO, Leprince P, Franzen R, et al. Puzzling out synaptic vesicle 2 family members functions. Front Mol Neurosci. 2017;10:148.
3. Mutch SA, Kensel-Hammes P, Gadd JC, Fujimoto BS, Allen RW, Schiro PG, et al. Protein quantification at the single vesicle level reveals that a subset of synaptic vesicle proteins are trafficked with high precision. J Neurosci. 2011;31(4):1461–70.
4. Lynch BA, Lambeng N, Nocka K, Kensel-Hammes P, Bajjalieh SM, Matagne A, et al. The synaptic vesicle protein SV2A is the binding site for the antiepileptic drug levetiracetam. Proc Natl Acad Sci U S A. 2004;101(26):9861–6.
5. Cai H, Mangner TJ, Muzik O, Wang M-W, Chugani DC, Chugani HT. Radiosynthesis of 11C-levetiracetam: a potential marker for PET imaging of SV2A expression. ACS Med Chem Lett. 2014;5(10):1152–5.
6. Mercier J, Archen L, Bollu V, Carré S, Evrard Y, Jnoff E, et al. Discovery of heterocyclic nonacetamide synaptic vesicle protein 2A (SV2A) ligands with single-digit nanomolar potency: opening avenues towards the first SV2A positron emission tomography (PET) ligands. ChemMedChem. 2014;9(4):693–8.
7. Estrada S, Lubberink M, Thibblin A, Sprycha M, Buchanan T, Mestdagh N, et al. [11C]UCB-A, a novel PET tracer for synaptic vesicle protein 2 A. Nucl Med Biol. 2016;43(6):325–32.
8. Warnock GI, Aerts J, Bahri MA, Bretin F, Lemaire C, Giacomelli F, et al. Evaluation of 18F-UCB-H as a novel PET tracer for synaptic vesicle protein 2A in the brain. J Nucl Med. 2014;55(8):1336–41.
9. Nabulsi NB, Mercier J, Holden D, Carre S, Najafzadeh S, Vandergeten MC, et al. Synthesis and preclinical evaluation of ^{11}C-UCB-J as a PET tracer for imaging the synaptic vesicle glycoprotein 2A in the brain. J Nucl Med. 2016;57(5):777–84.
10. Li S, Cai Z, Zhang W, Holden D, Lin SF, Finnema SJ, et al. Synthesis and in vivo evaluation of [^{18}F] UCB-J for PET imaging of synaptic vesicle glyco-

protein 2A (SV2A). Eur J Nucl Med Mol Imaging. 2019;46(9):1952–65.

11. Li S, Cai Z, Wu X, Holden D, Pracitto R, Kapinos M, et al. Synthesis and in vivo evaluation of a novel PET radiotracer for imaging of synaptic vesicle glycoprotein 2A (SV2A) in nonhuman primates. ACS Chem Neurosci. 2019;10(3):1544–54.

12. Constantinescu CC, Tresse C, Zheng M, Gouasmat A, Carroll VM, Mistico L, et al. Development and in vivo preclinical imaging of Fluorine-18-labeled synaptic vesicle protein 2A (SV2A) PET tracers. Mol Imaging Biol. 2019;21(3):509–18.

13. Cai Z, Li S, Zhang W, Pracitto R, Wu X, Baum E, et al. Synthesis and preclinical evaluation of an (18) F-labeled synaptic vesicle glycoprotein 2A PET imaging probe: [(18)F]SynVesT-2. ACS Chem Neurosci. 2020;11:592.

14. Li S, Naganawa M, Pracitto R, Najafzadeh S, Holden D, Henry S, et al. Assessment of test-retest reproducibility of [(18)F]SynVesT-1, a novel radiotracer for PET imaging of synaptic vesicle glycoprotein 2A. Eur J Nucl Med Mol Imaging. 2021;48(5):1327–38.

15. Naganawa M, Li S, Nabulsi N, Henry S, Zheng MQ, Pracitto R, et al. First-in-human evaluation of (18)F-SynVesT-1, a radioligand for PET imaging of synaptic vesicle glycoprotein 2A. J Nucl Med. 2021;62(4):561–7.

16. Finnema SJ, Nabulsi NB, Eid T, Detyniecki K, Lin SF, Chen MK, et al. Imaging synaptic density in the living human brain. Sci Transl Med. 2016;8(348):348ra96.

17. Finnema SJ, Nabulsi NB, Mercier J, Lin SF, Chen MK, Matuskey D, et al. Kinetic evaluation and test-retest reproducibility of [(11)C]UCB-J, a novel radioligand for positron emission tomography imaging of synaptic vesicle glycoprotein 2A in humans. J Cereb Blood Flow Metab. 2018;38(11):2041–52.

18. Bahri MA, Plenevaux A, Aerts J, Bastin C, Becker G, Mercier J, et al. Measuring brain synaptic vesicle protein 2A with positron emission tomography and [(18)F]UCB-H. Alzheimers Dement (N Y). 2017;3(4):481–6.

19. Brown RK, Bohnen NI, Wong KK, Minoshima S, Frey KA. Brain PET in suspected dementia: patterns of altered FDG metabolism. Radiographics. 2014;34(3):684–701.

20. Alzheimer's Association. 2021 Alzheimer's disease facts and figures. Alzheimers Dement. 2021;17(3):327–406.

21. Overk CR, Masliah E. Pathogenesis of synaptic degeneration in Alzheimer's disease and Lewy body disease. Biochem Pharmacol. 2014;88(4):508–16.

22. Selkoe DJ. Alzheimer's disease is a synaptic failure. Science. 2002;298(5594):789–91.

23. Robinson JL, Molina-Porcel L, Corrada MM, Raible K, Lee EB, Lee VM, et al. Perforant path synaptic loss correlates with cognitive impairment and Alzheimer's disease in the oldest-old. Brain. 2014;137(Pt 9):2578–87.

24. Jack CR Jr, Bennett DA, Blennow K, Carrillo MC, Dunn B, Haeberlein SB, et al. NIA-AA research framework: toward a biological definition of Alzheimer's disease. Alzheimers Dement. 2018;14(4):535–62.

25. Ishibashi K, Onishi A, Fujiwara Y, Ishiwata K, Ishii K. Relationship between Alzheimer disease-like pattern of 18F-FDG and fasting plasma glucose levels in cognitively normal volunteers. J Nucl Med. 2015;56(2):229–33.

26. Smart K, Liu H, Matuskey D, Chen MK, Torres K, Nabulsi N, et al. Binding of the synaptic vesicle radiotracer [(11)C]UCB-J is unchanged during functional brain activation using a visual stimulation task. J Cereb Blood Flow Metab. 2021;41(5):1067–79.

27. Chen MK, Mecca AP, Naganawa M, Finnema SJ, Toyonaga T, Lin SF, et al. Assessing synaptic density in Alzheimer disease with synaptic vesicle glycoprotein 2A positron emission tomographic imaging. JAMA Neurol. 2018;75(10):1215–24.

28. Bastin C, Bahri MA, Meyer F, Manard M, Delhaye E, Plenevaux A, et al. In vivo imaging of synaptic loss in Alzheimer's disease with [18F]UCB-H positron emission tomography. Eur J Nucl Med Mol Imaging. 2020;47(2):390–402.

29. Mecca AP, Chen MK, O'Dell RS, Naganawa M, Toyonaga T, Godek TA, et al. In vivo measurement of widespread synaptic loss in Alzheimer's disease with SV2A PET. Alzheimers Dement. 2020;16(7):974–82.

30. de Wilde MC, Overk CR, Sijben JW, Masliah E. Meta-analysis of synaptic pathology in Alzheimer's disease reveals selective molecular vesicular machinery vulnerability. Alzheimers Dement. 2016;12(6):633–44.

31. Mecca AP, O'Dell RS, Sharp ES, Banks ER, Bartlett HH, Zhao W, et al. Synaptic density and cognitive performance in Alzheimer's disease: a PET imaging study with [(11) C]UCB-J. Alzheimers Dement. 2022;18:2527.

32. O'Dell RS, Mecca AP, Chen MK, Naganawa M, Toyonaga T, Lu Y, et al. Association of Aβ deposition and regional synaptic density in early Alzheimer's disease: a PET imaging study with [(11)C]UCB-J. Alzheimers Res Ther. 2021;13(1):11.

33. Vanhaute H, Ceccarini J, Michiels L, Koole M, Sunaert S, Lemmens R, et al. In vivo synaptic density loss is related to tau deposition in amnestic mild cognitive impairment. Neurology. 2020;95:e545.

34. Coomans EM, Schoonhoven DN, Tuncel H, Verfaillie SCJ, Wolters EE, Boellaard R, et al. In vivo tau pathology is associated with synaptic loss and altered synaptic function. Alzheimers Res Ther. 2021;13(1):35.

35. Mecca AP, Chen M-K, O'Dell RS, Naganawa M, Toyonaga T, Godek TA, et al. Association of entorhinal cortical tau deposition and hippocampal synaptic density in older individuals with normal cognition and early Alzheimer's disease. Neurobiol Aging. 2021;111:44.

36. Chen MK, Mecca AP, Naganawa M, Gallezot JD, Toyonaga T, Mondal J, et al. Comparison of [(11)C] UCB-J and [(18)F]FDG PET in Alzheimer's disease: a tracer kinetic modeling study. J Cereb Blood Flow Metab. 2021;41:271678X211004312.

37. McKhann GM, Albert MS, Grossman M, Miller B, Dickson D, Trojanowski JQ. Clinical and pathological diagnosis of frontotemporal dementia: report of the work group on frontotemporal dementia and Pick's disease. Arch Neurol. 2001;58(11):1803–9.
38. Marttinen M, Kurkinen KM, Soininen H, Haapasalo A, Hiltunen M. Synaptic dysfunction and septin protein family members in neurodegenerative diseases. Mol Neurodegener. 2015;10:16.
39. Malpetti M, Holland N, Jones PS, Ye R, Cope TE, Fryer TD, et al. Synaptic density in carriers of C9orf72 mutations: a [(11) C]UCB-J PET study. Ann Clin Transl Neurol. 2021;8(7):1515–23.
40. Salmon E, Bahri MA, Plenevaux A, Becker G, Seret A, Delhaye E, et al. In vivo exploration of synaptic projections in frontotemporal dementia. Sci Rep. 2021;11(1):16092.
41. Goetz CG. The history of Parkinson's disease: early clinical descriptions and neurological therapies. Cold Spring Harb Perspect Med. 2011;1(1):a008862.
42. Picconi B, Piccoli G, Calabresi P. Synaptic dysfunction in Parkinson's disease. Adv Exp Med Biol. 2012;970:553–72.
43. Jellinger KA. Neuropathology of sporadic Parkinson's disease: evaluation and changes of concepts. Mov Disord. 2012;27(1):8–30.
44. Villalba RM, Smith Y. Differential striatal spine pathology in Parkinson's disease and cocaine addiction: a key role of dopamine? Neuroscience. 2013;251:2–20.
45. Matuskey D, Tinaz S, Wilcox KC, Naganawa M, Toyonaga T, Dias M, et al. Synaptic changes in Parkinson disease assessed with in vivo imaging. Ann Neurol. 2020;87(3):329–38.
46. Wilson H, Pagano G, de Natale ER, Mansur A, Caminiti SP, Polychronis S, et al. Mitochondrial complex 1, sigma 1, and synaptic vesicle 2A in early drug-naive Parkinson's disease. Mov Disord. 2020;35(8):1416–27.
47. Delva A, Van Weehaeghe D, Koole M, Van Laere K, Vandenberghe W. Loss of presynaptic terminal integrity in the substantia Nigra in early Parkinson's disease. Mov Disord. 2020;35(11):1977–86.
48. Aarsland D, Kurz MW. The epidemiology of dementia associated with Parkinson's disease. Brain Pathol. 2010;20(3):633–9.
49. McKeith IG, Boeve BF, Dickson DW, Halliday G, Taylor JP, Weintraub D, et al. Diagnosis and management of dementia with Lewy bodies: fourth consensus report of the DLB consortium. Neurology. 2017;89(1):88–100.
50. Nicastro N, Holland N, Savulich G, Carter SF, Mak E, Hong YT, et al. (11)C-UCB-J synaptic PET and multimodal imaging in dementia with Lewy bodies. Eur J Hybrid Imaging. 2020;4(1):25.
51. Andersen KB, Hansen AK, Damholdt MF, Horsager J, Skjaerbaek C, Gottrup H, et al. Reduced synaptic density in patients with lewy body dementia: an [(11) C]UCB-J PET imaging study. Mov Disord. 2021;36(9):2057–65.
52. Burrell JR, Hodges JR, Rowe JB. Cognition in corticobasal syndrome and progressive supranuclear palsy: a review. Mov Disord. 2014;29(5):684–93.
53. Sanders DW, Kaufman SK, DeVos SL, Sharma AM, Mirbaha H, Li A, et al. Distinct tau prion strains propagate in cells and mice and define different tauopathies. Neuron. 2014;82(6):1271–88.
54. Bigio EH, Vono MB, Satumtira S, Adamson J, Sontag E, Hynan LS, et al. Cortical synapse loss in progressive supranuclear palsy. J Neuropathol Exp Neurol. 2001;60(5):403–10.
55. Holland N, Jones PS, Savulich G, Wiggins JK, Hong YT, Fryer TD, et al. Synaptic loss in primary tauopathies revealed by [(11) C]UCB-J positron emission tomography. Mov Disord. 2020;35(10):1834–42.
56. Nithianantharajah J, Hannan AJ. Dysregulation of synaptic proteins, dendritic spine abnormalities and pathological plasticity of synapses as experience-dependent mediators of cognitive and psychiatric symptoms in Huntington's disease. Neuroscience. 2013;251:66–74.
57. Fourie C, Kim E, Waldvogel H, Wong JM, McGregor A, Faull RL, et al. Differential changes in postsynaptic density proteins in postmortem Huntington's disease and Parkinson's disease human brains. J Neurodegener Dis. 2014;2014:938530, 1.
58. Bertoglio D, Verhaeghe J, Wyffels L, Miranda A, Stroobants S, Mrzljak L, et al. Synaptic vesicle glycoprotein 2A is affected in the CNS of Huntington's disease mice and post-mortem human HD brain. J Nucl Med. 2021;
59. Delva A, Michiels L, Koole M, Van Laere K, Vandenberghe W. Synaptic damage and its clinical correlates in people with early Huntington disease: a PET study. Neurology. 2021;98:e83.
60. Rossi R, Arjmand S, Bærentzen SL, Gjedde A, Landau AM. Synaptic vesicle glycoprotein 2A: features and functions. Front Neurosci. 2022;16:864514.
61. Bajjalieh SM, Frantz GD, Weimann JM, McConnell SK, Scheller RH. Differential expression of synaptic vesicle protein 2 (SV2) isoforms. J Neurosci. 1994;14(9):5223–35.

MR Imaging of Neurodegeneration

11

1

2

Tammie L. S. Benzinger and Saurabh Jindal

Key Points

- Recent innovations in MR imaging allow not only to rule out organic dementia but also to differentiate various dementia subtypes and quantify the atrophic changes.
- The use of advanced imaging biomarkers such as volumetric, functional, and diffusion MRI provides early detection of neurodegeneration impacting disease management.

Introduction

The prevalence of neurodegenerative diseases is increasing with the increase in the aging population. Alzheimer's disease (AD) is the most common neurodegenerative disorder estimated to globally impact 67 million individuals by the year 2030, respectively [1]. Neuroimaging serves as a noninvasive tool to investigate the structural and functional aspects of the brain. Magnetic resonance imaging (MRI) is the first line modal-

T. L. S. Benzinger (✉)
Neuroradiology Section, Department of Radiology, Mallinckrodt Institute of Radiology, Washington University in St. Louis, Saint Louis, MO, USA
e-mail: benzingert@wustl.edu

S. Jindal
Neuroimaging Laboratories-Research Center, Mallinckrodt Institute of Radiology, Washington University in St. Louis, Saint Louis, MO, USA
e-mail: jindals@wustl.edu

ity in the workup of patients with slowly progressive dementia [2]. It allows for qualitative and quantitative detection of changes. It also aids in the tracking of disease progression. In this chapter, we will discuss the application of structural and functional MRI techniques in various dementia subtypes.

Structural Imaging

Protocol Considerations

A standardized imaging protocol optimized to detect dementia-related changes is essential. A magnetic field strength of ≥ 1.5 Tesla (T) is required to appreciate subtle volume changes. A good quality structural MRI requires a high signal-to-noise ratio (SNR). Three-dimensional (3D) T1-weighted imaging (WI) with 256 mm field of view and $\leq 1.2 \times 1.2 \times 1.2$ mm resolution offers high spatial resolution and is best for morphometric images [3]. Magnetization prepared rapid acquisition echo (MPRAGE) (Siemens), spoiled gradient recalled sequence (SPGR) (General Electronic), and 3D turbo field echo (Philips) are the most commonly used sequences. The rest of the protocol can be tailored based on the setting whether clinical or research. In clinical practice, two-dimensional (2D) fluid-attenuated inversion recovery (FLAIR) and 2D gradient recall echo/susceptibility weighted

1

© The Author(s), under exclusive license to Springer Nature Switzerland AG 2023
D. J. Cross et al. (eds.), *Molecular Imaging of Neurodegenerative Disorders*,
https://doi.org/10.1007/978-3-031-35098-6_11

imaging (GRE/SWI) are generally obtained. A 2D T2-WI, diffusion weighted imaging (DWI), post-contrast imaging, and magnetic resonance angiography are optional depending on the suspected etiology and availability of time [3]. Suggested guidelines for image acquisition of these sequences is available from the American College of Radiology [4]. For research purposes, 1 mm thick sagittal 3D FLAIR, 3 mm thick 3D GRE/SWI, resting-state functional MRI (rsfMRI) with a repetition time (TR) of 2000 ms, and diffusion tensor imaging (DTI) having ≥30 directions may be acquired with optional arterial spin labeling (ASL) images [3]. The Alzheimer's Disease Neuroimaging Initiative (ADNI) has published guidelines for performance of MRI for dementias and is a useful resource [5]. Protocol for serial longitudinal scans should be consistent for accurate follow-up. In particular, if assessing for serial microbleeds or siderosis, consistent field strength and choice of GRE or SWI sequence is critical for accurate assessment of change, which is important in the setting of antibody based anti-amyloid immunotherapies which can have complications of amyloid related imaging abnormality (ARIA) [6].

Role of Structural Imaging in Neurodegeneration

It serves as a vital tool to rule out surgically amenable focal lesions such as tumors, hematoma, and vascular malformations. It also helps to differentiate AD from non-AD dementia by identifying patterns of gray-white matter atrophy which are best appreciated on 3D-T1WI. FLAIR is helpful in identifying white matter (WM) changes seen as chronic small vessel ischemia in vascular dementia (VD). Degree of vascular damage can be assessed on T2* GRE/SWI images where bleeds are seen as dark blooming foci. DWI and post-gadolinium images are crucial in the diagnostic workup of suspected rapidly progressive dementia with an infectious or inflammatory etiology. DWI is also helpful in excluding acute infarction in the setting of VD and hippocampal lesions in transient global

amnesia [7]. ARIA in antibody treated AD individuals are seen as parenchymal edema or sulcal effusion on FLAIR and microbleeds or superficial siderosis on T2* GRE/SWI [6]. A stepwise approach can help narrow down the likely etiology of dementia (Fig. 11.1).

Degree of Atrophy

Visual assessment scales can be used to grade atrophy.

1. Global cortical atrophy scale (Pasquier scale): It is a 4-step scale that evaluates sulcal and ventricular dilation in various regions of the brain on T1 or FLAIR images. Graded as 0—normal/no ventricular enlargement, 1—opening of sulci/mild enlargement, 2—gyral atrophy/moderate enlargement, 3—"knife blade" gyral atrophy/severe enlargement [8].
2. ii. Medial temporal lobe atrophy scale (Scheltens' Scale): Based on width of choroid fissure & temporal horn, and height of hippocampal formation, atrophy can be assessed on a scale of 0–4 with very good sensitivity in senile-onset AD [9].

Loco-Regional Pattern of Atrophy

Loco-regional pattern analysis can help determine the type of dementia in some cases (Table 11.1) [7].

These visual assessments for volume loss require expert training and are limited by inter-rater variability. Recent trends involve the use of more sensitive automated quantitative techniques that allow cross-sectional and longitudinal analyses of the volumetric data from which patterns of atrophy and its progression in dementia can be evaluated. The commonly used volumetric software tools work either by cortical thickness-based or tissue-based segmentation. NeuroQuant (https://www.cortechs.ai/products/neuroquant/, USA) [10], Neuroreader (https://brainreader.net/, Denmark) [11], and Siemens Brain Morphometry (https://www.siemens-healthineers.com/, Germany) are approved by the United States Food and Drug Administration. Freesurfer (https://surfer.nmr.mgh.harvard.edu/, USA) [12], Voxel-Based Morphometry (https://neuro-jena.

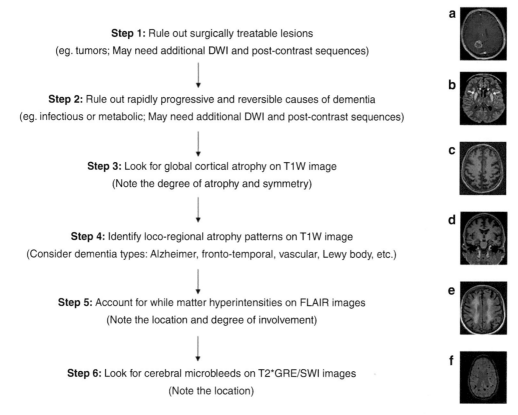

Step 1: Rule out surgically treatable lesions
(eg. tumors; May need additional DWI and post-contrast sequences)

Step 2: Rule out rapidly progressive and reversible causes of dementia
(eg. infectious or metabolic; May need additional DWI and post-contrast sequences)

Step 3: Look for global cortical atrophy on T1W image
(Note the degree of atrophy and symmetry)

Step 4: Identify loco-regional atrophy patterns on T1W image
(Consider dementia types: Alzheimer, fronto-temporal, vascular, Lewy body, etc.)

Step 5: Account for while matter hyperintensities on FLAIR images
(Note the location and degree of involvement)

Step 6: Look for cerebral microbleeds on T2*GRE/SWI images
(Note the location)

Fig. 11.1 Flowchart showing a stepwise approach to the diagnosis of dementia by imaging (DWI-diffusion weighted imaging, T1WI- T1 weighted imaging, FLAIR-fluid-attenuated inversion recovery, GRE- gradient recall echo, SWI- susceptibility weighted imaging). Data taken from [7]. (**a**) Coronal post-contrast image showing peripherally enhancing right temporal lobe tumor, (**b**) Axial DWI image showing restricted diffusion in bilateral corti- ces in Creutzfeldt-Jakob disease, (**c**) Axial T1W image showing bilateral parietal lobe atrophy, (**d**) Coronal T1W image showing bilateral temporal lobe atrophy, (**e**) Axial FLAIR image showing periventricular and deep white matter hyperintensities, (**f**) Axial T2*GRE image showing blooming foci in left temporal region representing microhemorrhages

Table 11.1 Loco-regional atrophy patterns and possible dementia subtypes. Data taken and modified from [7]

Location/pattern of atrophy	Possible dementia subtype
Hippocampus and/or medial temporal lobe	Usually AD (Fig. 11.2a), FTLD (Fig. 11.3c)
Posterior cingulate sulci and precuneus	Pre-senile AD (Fig. 11.2b, c)
Parietal lobes	Posterior cortical atrophy, usually AD (Fig. 11.2b, c)
Occipital lobes	Posterior cortical atrophy, mostly AD, dementia with Lewy bodies
Frontal and/or temporal lobes	FTLD (Fig. 11.3a, b) (right predominant-behavioral variant, left predominant- semantic variant)
Ventriculomegaly with disproportionate changes in subarachnoid spaces	Normal pressure hydrocephalus
Midbrain	Posterior supranuclear palsy
Pons with cerebellum	Multiple system atrophy
Cerebellum	Creutzfeldt-Jakob disease

AD Alzheimer's disease, *FTLD* frontotemporal lobar degeneration

github.io/software.html#vbm, Germany) [13] and FSL (https://fsl.fmrib.ox.ac.uk/fsl/fslwiki/, UK) [14] are used widely in research setting. The FreeSurfer quantified volumes can be plotted on individual longitudinal participant graphs comparing the results to a normative database [15] (Fig. 11.2d–f and 11.3d–h).

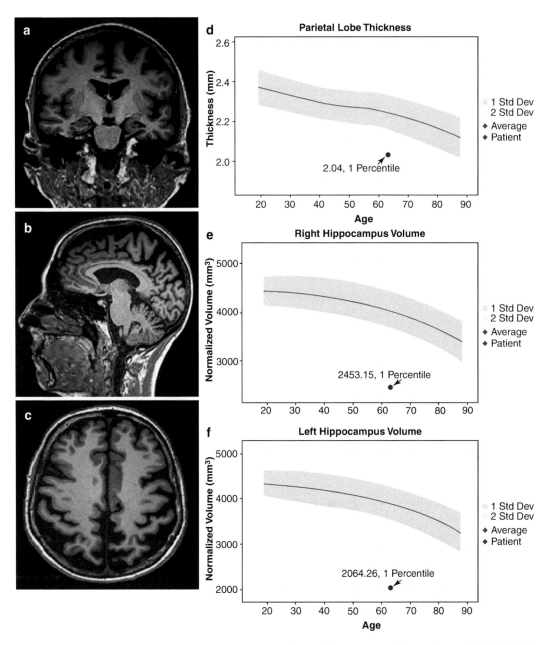

Fig. 11.2 MRI of 63-year-old white female with Alzheimer's dementia. (**a**) Coronal T1-WI showing bilateral hippocampal and temporal lobe atrophy (L > R) with Sylvian fissure widening. (**b**, **c**) Sagittal and axial sections of T1WI, respectively, showing gyral atrophy in parietal lobes including the precuneus with regional sulcal widening. Atrophy appears fairly symmetrical in either hemi-sphere with antero-posterior gradient. (**d–f**) Individual longitudinal participant (ILP) graphs showing FreeSurfer quantified volumes for parietal lobes and hippocampi at first percentile (< 2SD) compared to a normal database. (Image courtesy: Dr. Farzaneh Rahmani, Department of Radiology, Washington University in St. Louis)

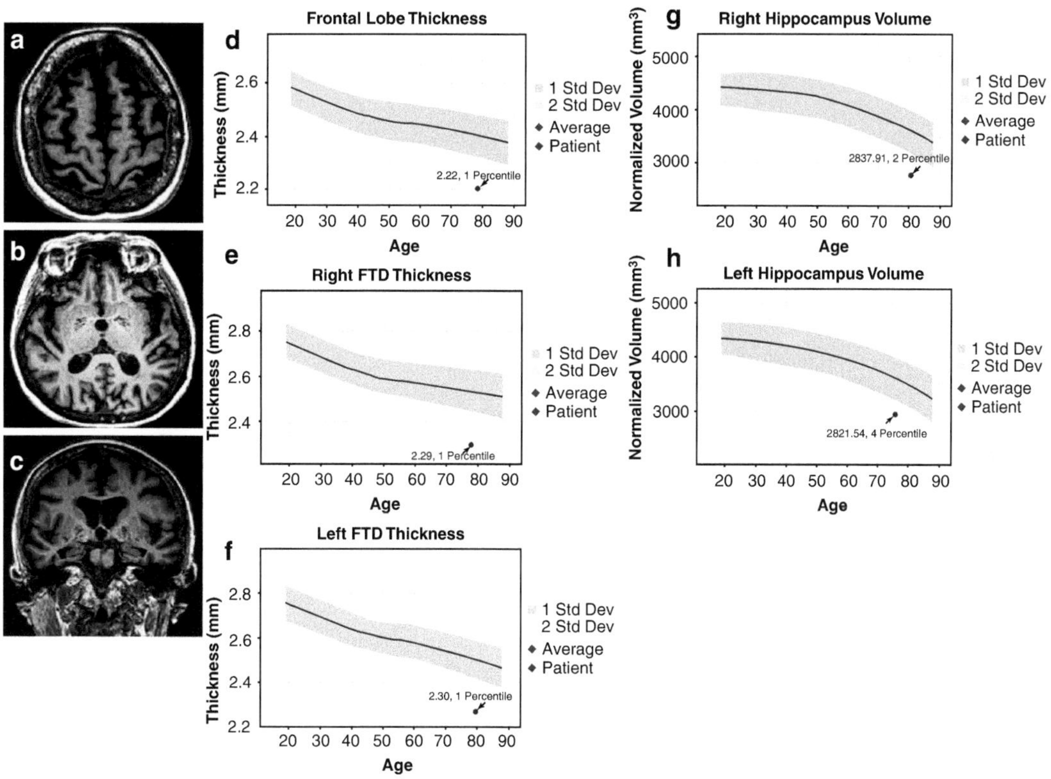

Fig. 11.3 MRI of 78-year-old white female with Frontotemporal lobar degeneration. (**a, b**) Axial sections of T1WI images showing gyral atrophy in bilateral frontal and temporal lobes, respectively, with regional sulcal widening. Atrophy appears slightly asymmetrical (L > R) in either hemisphere with an antero-posterior gradient. (**c**) Coronal T1-WI showing bilateral hippocampal and temporal lobe atrophy with Sylvian fissure widening. (**d–f**) Individual longitudinal participants (ILP) graphs showing FreeSurfer quantified volumes for frontal lobes and combined frontotemporal lobes at first percentile (< 2SD) when compared to a normal database. (**g, h**) ILP graphs showing FreeSurfer quantified volumes for right and left hippocampus at second and fourth percentile, respectively, when compared to a normal database. (Image courtesy: Dr. Farzaneh Rahmani, Department of Radiology, Washington University in St. Louis)

White Matter Hyperintensities (WMH)

WMH should be assessed for their location and degree of involvement. They can be periventricular, subcortical, and/or deep in location. Fazekas scoring is used to grade these changes in the periventricular and deep WM (Table 11.2) [16].

Cerebral microbleeds and Siderosis

Brain hemorrhages, most commonly consisting of cerebral microbleeds and/or superficial siderosis, are found in about 20% and 60% of patients with AD and VD, respectively, while seen only in 10% of the aging population [7]. They are also important component of ARIA in the setting of anti-amyloid immunotherapy [6]. Microbleeds are defined as 2–10 mm round hypointensities on T2*GRE/SWI images. They are better appreciated on SWI due to greater susceptibility and higher resolution. Lobar microhemorrhages are frequently seen with cerebral amyloid angiopathy, whereas central (basal ganglia, thalamus, and brainstem) microhemorrhages are more common with hypertensive encephalopathy. Superficial siderosis represents hemosiderin deposition along the leptomeninges, seen on MRI as hypointense signal with blooming on T2*GRE/SWI images.

Table 11.2 Fazekas scoring system. Data taken from [16]

Score	Periventricular WMH	Deep WMH	Inference
0	Absent	Absent	Normal
1	Caps	Punctate foci	Normal before 65 years
2	Smooth halo	Early confluence	Abnormal before 70 years
3	Irregular and extending to deep white matter	Large confluent areas	Always abnormal with poor cognitive outcomes

WMH white matter hyperintensities

Diffusion MRI Techniques

Diffusion MRI is an advanced imaging tool based on the property of diffusion of water molecules within the tissue at micron level. It assesses the integrity of axonal WM tracts along with their density and myelination characteristics. Imaging relies on fast diffusion encoding sequences such as echo-planar imaging (EPI). DTI and diffusion kurtosis imaging (DKI) are the commonly used diffusion techniques to assess the pathophysiology of neurodegenerative diseases [17].

Diffusion Tensor Imaging

DTI provides a quantitative evaluation of anisotropic diffusion of water molecules in the WM of brain using four metrics: fractional anisotropy (FA), mean diffusivity (MD), axial diffusivity, and radial diffusivity (RD). An increase in MD is seen in AD individuals due to disruption of cellular membrane impeding diffusion of water molecules. An abnormally decreased fractional anisotropy is also seen in AD due to loss of tract integrity [17]. DTI is also used in the diagnosis of Parkinson disease, amyotrophic lateral sclerosis, and traumatic brain injury (Table 11.3).

Limitations: (1) DTI is unable to detect GM changes as there is no information on the non-Gaussian diffusion of water molecules. (2) Presence of CSF and single compartment approximation results in a partial volume effect at the gray-white matter junction.

Table 11.3 Summary of the diffusion MRI findings in AD and PD. Data taken from [17–21]

Diffusion technique		AD	PD
DTI	MD	↑	↑
	FA	↓	↓
	Affected regions	Cingulate gyrus, precuneus, temporal lobe	Substantia nigra, frontal lobe, temporal lobe
	Special note	Volumetric MRI is superior for medial temporal lobe atrophy in early AD	DTI is not considered as diagnostic in early PD
DKI	MK	↓	↓
	AK	↓	–
	RK	↓	–
	Affected regions	White matter in the genu of corpus callosum, cingulum, temporal, frontal, and occipital regions	Substantia nigra, red nuclei, and anterior cingulum
	Special note	Changes in MK and AK have shown correlation with MMSE scores in occipital lobes	Together with QSM has a diagnostic accuracy of ~80–100%

AD Alzheimer disease, *PD* Parkinson disease, *DTI* diffusion tensor imaging, *MD* mean diffusivity, *FA* fractional anisotropy, *DKI* diffusion kurtosis imaging, *MK* mean kurtosis, *AK* axial kurtosis, *RK* radial kurtosis, *MMSE* mini-mental status examination, *QSM* quantity susceptibility mapping

Diffusion Kurtosis Imaging

DKI is useful in assessing GM by measuring the non-gaussian distribution of water molecules at the voxel level. A higher value of diffusion kurtosis corresponds with the deviation of water molecules from the Gaussian distribution, suggesting a more restricted environment. The opposite of this happens in neuronal loss. DKI describes the brain metrics using mean kurtosis (MK), axial kurtosis (AK), and radial kurtosis (RK). It has a role in the diagnosis of AD and PD (Table 11.3). It has been shown that DKI metrics are less affected by WMH and are more sensitive than DTI metrics in AD [17].

Resting-State Functional MRI

Principle and Acquisition

Hemodynamic changes are induced by regional neuronal activity due to neurovascular coupling. These changes result in dilution of the deoxygenated hemoglobin which acts as an endogenous contrast resulting in T2* prolongation and an increase in T2* MRI signals. This signal change is known as blood oxygen level dependent (BOLD) effect. Individuals with dementia are likely to have difficulty performing demanding cognitive tasks as a part of task-based fMRI. rsfMRI overcomes this limitation by acquiring continuous BOLD contrast images at rest. Acquisition of rsfMRI requires EPI with a TR of 2–3 s for 150–300 EPI volumes taken over 5–10 min of scan time [22]. The principle of rsfMRI by Biswal [23] and the default mode network (DMN) by Raichle [24] provided strong research evidence for use of rsfMRI in the evaluation of dementia in clinical setting.

Data Analysis

The rsfMRI data can be analyzed through various software packages such as statistical parametric mapping (http://www.fil.ion.ucl.ac.uk/spm/doc/) and FSL (http://fsl.fmrib.ox.ac.uk/fsl/fslwiki/). Functional connectivity between two remote brain regions is reflected by interregional correlation between low frequency (0.08–0.1 Hz) fluctuations. Correlation can be tested by paired region of interest (ROI), seed-to-voxel functional connectivity analysis or independent component analysis (ICA) [22, 23]. Seed-to-voxel analysis is a model-based method and easily comprehensible. ICA is a model-free analysis that generates resting-state network (RSN) maps with their individual temporal signal variations. ICA can be used to filter the physiological noise from pulsations in CSF [22]. RSN analysis can be done at an individual or group level each having their own advantages and disadvantages [25].

Role in Dementia Diagnosis

Individuals with AD have shown decreased resting-state functional connectivity compared to controls using seed-based ROI analysis (Fig. 11.4). Seed-based analysis of rsfMRI in 510 AD cases performed by Brier et al. showed abnormal RSN connectivity [26]. Reduced functional connectivity has been shown between in posterior cingulate cortex and hippocampus using seed-based analysis and ICA in AD [27, 28]. Classification performance based on combined seed- and ICA-based analysis was 97% in AD vs. controls advocating the usefulness of rsfMRI in AD diagnosis [29]. Easy technique and low burden on patients and radiologists permit the use of rsfMRI in clinical practice [22].

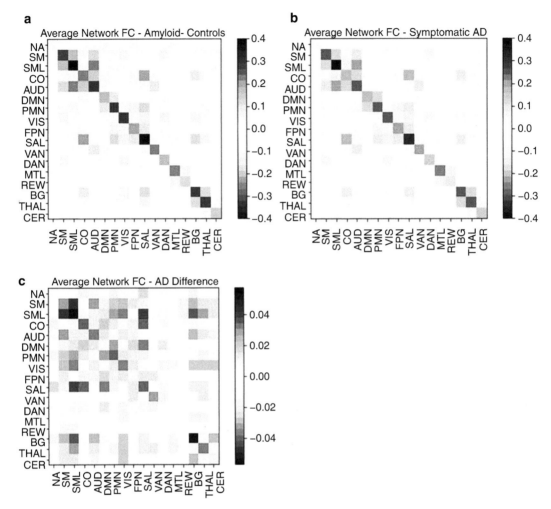

Fig. 11.4 AD-related differences in resting-state functional connectivity (RSFC). (**a**) Average RSFC within (along diagonal) and between networks (off diagonal) in amyloid-negative controls. (**b**) Average RSFC within and between networks in symptomatic AD participants. (**c**) Difference in RSFC between AD participants and controls. **Key.** For A and B, warm and cool colors indicate stronger positive and negative correlations, respectively. For C, cool colors indicate networks reduced connectivity in AD. *NA* unassigned regions, *SM* somatomotor network, *SML* lateral somatomotor network, *CO* cingulo-opercular network, *AUD* auditory network, *DMN* default mode network, *PMN* parietal memory network, *VIS* visual network, *FPN* fronto-parietal network, *SAL* salience network, *VAN* ventral attention network, *DAN* dorsal attention network, *MTL* medial temporal lobe network, *RE* reward network, *BG* basal ganglia network, *THAL* thalamus network, *CER* cerebellum network. ROIs and networks defined from Seitzman et al. [30]. (Image courtesy: Dr. Peter R. Millar, Department of Neurology, Washington University in St. Louis)

Magnetic Resonance Spectroscopy (MRS)

Principle and Acquisition

MRS is a noninvasive imaging tool to detect various metabolites and their concentrations in tissues based on the phenomenon of chemical shift imaging. Local magnetic field differences can produce a chemical shift due to changes in the resonance frequencies of the target nuclei (e.g., 1H). Results are plotted on a graph with chemical shift in ppm on x-axis and signal amplitude on y-axis. The area under the peak is proportional to the metabolite concentration. 1.5 T and 3 T scanners are able to show choline, creatine (Cr), glutamine, myoinositol (mIns), and N-acetyle aspartate (NAA). Height of the peak changes with echo time (TE) which varies from 18 to 288 ms. Short TE has higher signal intensity and detects mIns. However, there is baseline distortion and peak superimposition at shorter TE leading to metabolite quantification errors. Volume localization in single-volume MRS can be obtained by stimulated echo acquisition mode and point-resolved spectroscopy [22].

Role of MR Spectroscopy in Dementia Diagnosis

A correlation between reduced NAA and senile plaques was shown by Klunk and colleagues [31]. Decrease in NAA or NAA/Cr by ~10–15% was seen in hippocampus, posterior cingulate, and precuneus in AD. These reductions are also seen in frontal lobe in frontotemporal lobar degeneration (FTLD), and occipital lobes in dementia with Lewy body [22]. Miller et al. demonstrated elevated mIns in addition to decreased NAA in the demented brain [32]. MRS alone is 64–94.1% sensitive and 72.7–92.3% specific in differentiating AD from healthy controls, while in conjunction with volumetric MRI sensitivity and specificity increases to 97% and 94%, respectively [33].

Caution is advised when interpreting metabolite derangements as age-related increase in Cr and decrease in NAA can be confounding factors. Metabolite changes on MRS can be observed before structural changes aiding in clinical diagnosis of dementia. In comparison to positron emission tomography, MRS can be done at the time of MRI examination making it fast and cost-effective. Concerns with acquisition parameters, quantitative assessment, and unavailability of standard values limit its clinical utility [22].

Arterial Spin Labeling MR Perfusion

Principle and Acquisition

Noninvasive MR perfusion imaging technique that uses inverted spins of arterial blood as an endogenous contrast. A perfusion-related signal is extracted by subtracting control images with normal spins from these labeled arterial blood images. 30–50 sets of these two sets of images have to be acquired over 4–5 min to increase SNR. 3 T MRI theoretically doubles the SNR compared to 1.5 T MRI although it increases the recovery time of inverted spins (1.6 s at 3 T vs. 1.4 s at 1.5 T). Acquisition of labeled images to quantify relative cerebral blood flow (rCBF) is delayed by 1.5–2 s for 3 T scanners to account for the arterial transit time (ATT). Patient motion and field inhomogeneity due to sinuses or implants could also interfere with rCBF [22].

Types

Pulsed ASL is easier to implement but has low SNR and higher sensitivity to ATT prolongation. Continuous ASL has a better signal in rCBF measurement due to longer labeling duration but also has a higher specific absorption rate. Pulsed-continuous ASL with short labeling pulses overcomes the disadvantage of higher absorption [22].

Role of ASL in Dementia Diagnosis

Although rCBF changes in dementia have been evaluated with single-photon emission computerized tomography (SPECT), ASL has higher spatial resolution and can be co-registered to a high-resolution 3D anatomical image overcoming partial volume effects in cortical GM voxels. Perfusion abnormalities seen with ASL in parietal lobes of AD individuals are consistent with changes seen on nuclear imaging studies [34, 35]. Efficacy of ASL in differentiating AD vs healthy subjects supports its clinical feasibility as a screening tool [36]. ASL is also useful in differentiating AD from FTLD by showing distinct areas of hypoperfusion [37].

Treatable and Reversible Dementias

Acute and treatable dementias have an atypical presentation. Prompt identification is critical for appropriate and effective treatment.

Infections

Sporadic Creutzfeldt-Jakob disease shows the areas of restricted diffusion on DWI images in thalamus (pulvinar sign), caudate, putamen, and cortex in the early stage of the disease with corresponding hyperintensities on T2/FLAIR images. Generalized brain atrophy with cortical thinning is evident in late stages. It should be differentiated from corticobasal degeneration which can present with myoclonus but shows caudate lobe and asymmetric premotor atrophy. **HIV-associated neurocognitive dysfunction/disorders** present with generalized brain atrophy, and T2/FLAIR subcortical and periventricular WMH without mass effect or enhancement. DTI reveals MD and FA abnormalities in the subcortical WM. **Progressive multifocal Leukoencephalopathy** is seen in immunocompromised patients (HIV or transplant recipients) as asymmetric multifocal T1 and T2 hyperintensities in the subcortical and periventricular WM along with U-fiber involvement. **Neuro-syphilis** is characterized by subcortical lesions in the temporal apex and insular gyri with meningeal enhancement, granulomas, and vasculitis-related basal ganglia infarctions [22].

Neoplasm

Lesions such as lymphomatosis cerebri and intravascular B-cell lymphomatosis can present with cognitive symptoms. Lymphomatosis cerebri appears as non-enhancing diffuse leukoencephalopathy on MRI. Intravascular B-cell lymphomatosis shows multifocal infarction-like findings inconsistent with regions of arterial supply and pontine hyperintensities that need differentiation from osmotic demyelination [22].

Chronic Subdural Hematoma (SDH)

AD mimicker and a known cause of reversible dementia especially, in elderly individuals. A meta-analysis of case-control studies showed traumatic brain injury as a risk factor for AD. It may exacerbate pre-existing dementia. Evacuation of the bleed has been shown to

improve cognition and mental status in these patients [38].

Metabolic

Wernicke Encephalopathy occurs secondary to thiamine deficiency appearing as symmetrically enhancing T2/FLAIR hyperintensities in the thalamus, hypothalamus, and periaqueductal regions. **Hypoglycemic Encephalopathy** shows the areas of restricted diffusion in the corpus callosum, corona radiate, or internal capsule on DWI. Cortical and basal ganglia involvement denotes poor prognosis [22].

Post-Icteric Encephalopathy

It appears as T2/FLAIR hyperintensities and swelling of the cerebellum, hippocampus, amygdala, thalamus, and cortex with restricted diffusion on DWI Imaging plays an important role in differentiating it from encephalitis and metabolic encephalopathy thus prevent its progression to epilepsy [22].

Recent Advances in Imaging of Neurodegeneration

7T MRI

Ultrahigh-resolution MRI with ability to detect hippocampus atrophy at subfield level in mild cognitive impairment. Increased sensitiveness to susceptibility changes allows detection of microbleeds and iron-dense amyloid plaques invisible on routine imaging [39]. It can differentiate AD from controls with a specificity of 94.4% taking ≥ 5 microinfarcts as a cutoff [40].

Quantitative Susceptibility Mapping (QSM)

Iron is present in Aβ plaques and neurofibrillary tangles. QSM is based on multi-echo 3D GRE images and can help quantify iron overload associated with AD, PD, and VD. A systemic review by Ravanfar and colleagues reported increased susceptibility changes or iron deposition in amygdala and dorsal striatum of AD subjects and in substantia nigra of PD individuals [41].

Neuroinflammation Imaging (NII) Using Diffusion

NII is an in vivo MR diffusion-based imaging technique developed to clinically image and quantify WM inflammation and damage in AD. Increased NII-derived cellular diffusivity was seen in both preclinical and early symptomatic phases of AD while decreased FA and increased RD indicating WM damage was only appreciated in symptomatic AD [42].

Quantitative Gradient Recalled Echo (qGRE) MRI

Identifies dark matter as a new imaging biomarker of neurodegeneration that precedes tissue atrophy in early AD. Kothapalli et al. used qGRE R2t* to identify hippocampal subfields with very low neuronal content (dark matter) and relatively preserved neurons (viable tissue). Compared to morphometric MRI, more significant differentiation was found between dark matter and viable tissue volume measurements between mild AD and controls [43].

Magnetization Transfer Imaging

It is based on the exchange of magnetization between macromolecules bound protons and free protons. By using off-resonance pulses and improving the image contrast it helps to provide information at the microstructural level. Colonna et al. found decreased magnetization transfer ratios in cortical, subcortical, and WM regions in AD individuals [44].

Summary

Brain MRI is an important tool for differential diagnosis and monitoring of neurodegenerative disorders and monitoring of therapy-related adverse events. Awareness of the applications of advanced structural and functional imaging biomarkers is essential for optimization of dementia imaging protocols.

Further Reading

For further overview and detailed explanations of imaging in various dementia subtypes and advanced MRI techniques refer to textbooks [7] and [22].

Acknowledgements Dr. Farzaneh Rahmani, M.D., Department of Radiology, Washington University in St. Louis.

Dr. Peter R. Millar, Ph.D., Department of Neurology, Washington University in St. Louis.

Grants NIH/NIA P50AG005681 NIH/NIA P01AG026276. NIH/NIA P01AG003991.

References

1. Prince M, Bryce R, Albanese E, Wimo A, Ribeiro W, Ferri CP. The global prevalence of dementia: a systematic review and meta analysis. Alzheimers Dement. 2013;9(1):63–75.e2. https://doi.org/10.1016/j.jalz.2012.11.007.
2. McKhann GM, Knopman DS, Chertkow H, et al. The diagnosis of dementia due to Alzheimer's disease: recommendations from the National Institute on Aging-Alzheimer's Association workgroups on diagnostic guidelines for Alzheimer's disease. Alzheimers Dement. 2011;7(3):263–9. https://doi.org/10.1016/j.jalz.2011.03.005.
3. Park M, Moon WJ. Structural MR imaging in the diagnosis of Alzheimer's disease and other neurodegenerative dementia: current imaging approach and future perspectives. Korean J Radiol. 2016;17(6):827–45. https://doi.org/10.3348/kjr.2016.17.6.827.
4. Accreditation Support [Internet]. MRI exam-specific parameters: head and neck module. 2022. https://accreditationsupport.acr.org/support/solutions/articles/11000061019-mri-exam-specific-parameters-

head-and-neck-module-revised-4-6-2022-. Accessed 4 June 2022.

5. Jack CR Jr, Bernstein MA, Fox NC, et al. The Alzheimer's disease neuroimaging initiative (ADNI): MRI methods. J Magn Reson Imaging. 2008;27(4):685–91. https://doi.org/10.1002/jmri.21049.

6. Sperling RA, Jack CR Jr, Black SE, et al. Amyloid-related imaging abnormalities in amyloid-modifying therapeutic trials: recommendations from the Alzheimer's Association research roundtable workgroup. Alzheimers Dement. 2011;7(4):367–85. https://doi.org/10.1016/j.jalz.2011.05.2351.

7. Barkhof F, Fox NC, Bastos-Leite AJ, Scheltens P. Neuroimaging in dementia. Berlin: Springer; 2011.

8. Pasquier F, Leys D, Weerts JG, Mounier-Vehier F, Barkhof F, Scheltens P. Inter- and intraobserver reproducibility of cerebral atrophy assessment on MRI scans with hemispheric infarcts. Eur Neurol. 1996;36(5):268–72. https://doi.org/10.1159/000117270.

9. Scheltens P, Launer LJ, Barkhof F, Weinstein HC, van Gool WA. Visual assessment of medial temporal lobe atrophy on magnetic resonance imaging: interobserver reliability. J Neurol. 1995;242(9):557–60. https://doi.org/10.1007/BF00868807.

10. Brewer JB. Fully-automated volumetric MRI with normative ranges: translation to clinical practice. Behav Neurol. 2009;21(1):21–8. https://doi.org/10.3233/BEN-2009-0226.

11. Ahdidan J, Raji CA, DeYoe EA, et al. Quantitative neuroimaging software for clinical assessment of hippocampal volumes on MR imaging. J Alzheimers Dis. 2016;49(3):723–32. https://doi.org/10.3233/JAD-150559.

12. Dale AM, Fischl B, Sereno MI. Cortical surface-based analysis. I segmentation and surface reconstruction. Neuroimage. 1999;9(2):179–94. https://doi.org/10.1006/nimg.1998.0395.

13. Ashburner J, Friston KJ. Voxel-based morphometry—the methods. NeuroImage. 2000;11(6 Pt 1):805–21. https://doi.org/10.1006/nimg.2000.0582.

14. Jenkinson M, Beckmann C, Behrens TEJ, Woolrich MW, Smith SM. FSL. NeuroImage. 2012;62(2):782–90. https://doi.org/10.1016/j.neuroimage.2011.09.015.

15. Koenig LN, Day GS, Salter A, et al. Select atrophied regions in Alzheimer disease (SARA): an improved volumetric model for identifying Alzheimer disease dementia. Neuroimage Clin. 2020;26:102248. https://doi.org/10.1016/j.nicl.2020.102248.

16. Fazekas F, Chawluk JB, Alavi A, Hurtig HI, Zimmerman RA. MR signal abnormalities at 1.5 T in Alzheimer's dementia and normal aging. AJR Am J Roentgenol. 1987;149(2):351–6. https://doi.org/10.2214/ajr.149.2.351.

17. Kamagata K, Andica C, Kato A, et al. Diffusion magnetic resonance imaging-based biomarkers for neurodegenerative diseases. Int J Mol Sci. 2021;22(10):5216. Published 2021 May 14. https://doi.org/10.3390/ijms22105216.

18. Teipel SJ, Wegrzyn M, Meindl T, et al. Anatomical MRI and DTI in the diagnosis of Alzheimer's disease: a European multicenter study. J Alzheimers Dis. 2012;31(Suppl 3):S33–47. https://doi.org/10.3233/JAD-2012-112118.

19. Atkinson-Clement C, Pinto S, Eusebio A, Coulon O. Diffusion tensor imaging in Parkinson's disease: review and meta-analysis. Neuroimage Clin. 2017;16:98–110. https://doi.org/10.1016/j.nicl.2017.07.011. Published 2017 Jul 15.

20. Yuan L, Sun M, Chen Y, et al. Non-Gaussian diffusion alterations on diffusion kurtosis imaging in patients with early Alzheimer's disease. Neurosci Lett. 2016;616:11–8. https://doi.org/10.1016/j.neulet.2016.01.021.

21. Ito K, Ohtsuka C, Yoshioka K, et al. Differential diagnosis of parkinsonism by a combined use of diffusion kurtosis imaging and quantitative susceptibility mapping. Neuroradiology. 2017;59(8):759–69. https://doi.org/10.1007/s00234-017-1870-7.

22. Matsuda H, Asada T, Tokumaru AM, editors. Neuroimaging diagnosis for Alzheimer's disease and other dementias. Springer: Tokyo; 2017.

23. Biswal B, Yetkin FZ, Haughton VM, Hyde JS. Functional connectivity in the motor cortex of resting human brain using echo-planar MRI. Magn Reson Med. 1995;34(4):537–41. https://doi.org/10.1002/mrm.1910340409.

24. Raichle ME, MacLeod AM, Snyder AZ, Powers WJ, Gusnard DA, Shulman GL. A default mode of brain function. Proc Natl Acad Sci U S A. 2001;98(2):676–82. https://doi.org/10.1073/pnas.98.2.676.

25. Cole DM, Smith SM, Beckmann CF. Advances and pitfalls in the analysis and interpretation of resting-state FMRI data. Front Syst Neurosci. 2010;4:8. https://doi.org/10.3389/fnsys.2010.00008. Published 2010 Apr 6.

26. Brier MR, Thomas JB, Snyder AZ, et al. Loss of intranetwork and internetwork resting state functional connections with Alzheimer's disease progression. J Neurosci. 2012;32(26):8890–9. https://doi.org/10.1523/JNEUROSCI.5698-11.2012.

27. Zarei M, Beckmann CF, Binnewijzend MA, et al. Functional segmentation of the hippocampus in the healthy human brain and in Alzheimer's disease. NeuroImage. 2013;66:28–35. https://doi.org/10.1016/j.neuroimage.2012.10.071. [published correction appears in Neuroimage. 2013 Dec;83:1109].

28. Greicius MD, Srivastava G, Reiss AL, Menon V. Default-mode network activity distinguishes Alzheimer's disease from healthy aging: evidence from functional MRI. Proc Natl Acad Sci U S A. 2004;101(13):4637–42. https://doi.org/10.1073/pnas.0308627101.

29. Koch W, Teipel S, Mueller S, Benninghoff J, Wagner M, Bokde ALW, Hampel H, Coates U, Reiser M, Meindl T. Diagnostic power of default mode network

resting state fMRI in the detection of Alzheimer's disease. Neurobiol Aging. 2012;33(3):466–78. https://doi.org/10.1016/j.neurobiolaging.2010.04.013.

30. Seitzman BA, Gratton C, Marek S, et al. A set of functionally-defined brain regions with improved representation of the subcortex and cerebellum. NeuroImage. 2020;206:116290. https://doi.org/10.1016/j.neuroimage.2019.116290.

31. Klunk WE, Panchalingam K, Moossy J, McClure RJ, Pettegrew JW. N-acetyl-L-aspartate and other amino acid metabolites in Alzheimer's disease brain: a preliminary proton nuclear magnetic resonance study. Neurology. 1992;42(8):1578–85. https://doi.org/10.1212/wnl.42.8.1578.

32. Miller BL, Moats RA, Shonk T, Ernst T, Woolley S, Ross BD. Alzheimer disease: depiction of increased cerebral myo-inositol with proton MR spectroscopy. Radiology. 1993;187(2):433–7. https://doi.org/10.1148/radiology.187.2.8475286.

33. Westman E, Wahlund LO, Foy C, et al. Combining MRI and MRS to distinguish between Alzheimer's disease and healthy controls. J Alzheimers Dis. 2010;22(1):171–81. https://doi.org/10.3233/JAD-2010-100168.

34. Binnewijzend MA, Kuijer JP, Benedictus MR, et al. Cerebral blood flow measured with 3D pseudocontinuous arterial spin-labeling MR imaging in Alzheimer disease and mild cognitive impairment: a marker for disease severity. Radiology. 2013;267(1):221–30. https://doi.org/10.1148/radiol.12120928.

35. Musiek ES, Chen Y, Korczykowski M, et al. Direct comparison of fluorodeoxyglucose positron emission tomography and arterial spin labeling magnetic resonance imaging in Alzheimer's disease. Alzheimers Dement. 2012;8(1):51–9. https://doi.org/10.1016/j.jalz.2011.06.003.

36. Mak HK, Qian W, Ng KS, et al. Combination of MRI hippocampal volumetry and arterial spin labeling MR perfusion at 3-tesla improves the efficacy in discriminating Alzheimer's disease from cognitively normal

elderly adults. J Alzheimers Dis. 2014;41(3):749–58. https://doi.org/10.3233/JAD-131868.

37. Hu WT, Wang Z, Lee VM, Trojanowski JQ, Detre JA, Grossman M. Distinct cerebral perfusion patterns in FTLD and AD. Neurology. 2010;75(10):881–8. https://doi.org/10.1212/WNL.0b013e3181f11e35.

38. Sahyouni R, Goshtasbi K, Mahmoodi A, Tran DK, Chen JW. Chronic subdural hematoma: a perspective on subdural membranes and dementia. World Neurosurg. 2017;108:954–8. https://doi.org/10.1016/j.wneu.2017.09.063.

39. McKiernan EF, O'Brien JT. 7T MRI for neurodegenerative dementias in vivo: a systematic review of the literature. J Neurol Neurosurg Psychiatry. 2017;88(7):564–74. https://doi.org/10.1136/jnnp-2016-315022.

40. van Rooden S, Goos JD, van Opstal AM, et al. Increased number of microinfarcts in Alzheimer disease at 7-T MR imaging. Radiology. 2014;270(1):205–11. https://doi.org/10.1148/radiol.13130743.

41. Ravanfar P, Loi SM, Syeda WT, et al. Systematic review: quantitative susceptibility mapping (QSM) of brain iron profile in neurodegenerative diseases. Front Neurosci. 2021;15:618435. https://doi.org/10.3389/fnins.2021.618435. Published 2021 Feb 18.

42. Wang Q, Wang Y, Liu J, et al. Quantification of white matter cellularity and damage in preclinical and early symptomatic Alzheimer's disease. Neuroimage Clin. 2019;22:101767. https://doi.org/10.1016/j.nicl.2019.101767.

43. Kothapalli SVVN, Benzinger TL, Aschenbrenner AJ, et al. Quantitative gradient Echo MRI identifies dark matter as a new imaging biomarker of neurodegeneration that precedes tissue atrophy in early Alzheimer's disease. J Alzheimers Dis. 2022;85(2):905–24. https://doi.org/10.3233/JAD-210503.

44. Colonna I, Koini M, Pirpamer L, et al. Microstructural tissue changes in Alzheimer disease brains: insights from magnetization transfer imaging. AJNR Am J Neuroradiol. 2021;42(4):688–93. https://doi.org/10.3174/ajnr.A6975.

PET Quantification and Kinetic Analysis

12

Richard E. Carson ⓘ, Mika Naganawa,
and Jean-Dominique Gallezot

Introduction

PET provides vast opportunities to interrogate normal and pathophysiological brain functions with appropriately designed radiotracers. After injection of each radiotracer, the PET scanner measures radioactivity concentrations throughout the brain. To produce physiological measures, quantification procedures for PET data begin with full pharmacokinetic modeling of dynamic data. The results from such analyses are quantitative measures tailored to provide meaningful data for a specific research or clinical question. Based on these approaches, often simplified analyses are developed, to yield comparable measures with simpler methodology, e.g., shorter scans or less invasive procedures.

PET kinetic analysis methods typically have a small number (e.g., 1–2) of parameters that are achievable outcome measures. These parameters (1) are equal or proportional to the underlying physiological variable; and (2) can be determined with sufficient precision. Depending on the study, different outcome measures may be determined. For example, PET studies can use tracers with either reversible or irreversible kinetics.

Irreversible tracers are completely or mostly trapped in tissue, at least for the duration of the study. Reversible radiotracers show substantial clearance within the time frame of the scan. Different outcome measures are produced for reversible and irreversible tracers. Irreversible tracers are often used for metabolic or enzymatic processes (e.g., glucose metabolism using [18F] FDG), while receptor studies more commonly employ reversible tracers.

In this chapter, we use the term "receptor" or "target" when the radiotracer binds selectively to a protein of interest, which could be a receptor, transporter, enzyme, or other protein, and the goal is to assess a value proportional to concentration of the protein. For such compounds, the research community adopted nomenclature for the quantitative outcome measures derived from kinetic analyses [1]. Here we will focus on tracers with reversible characteristics, since, it has generally been found that quantification strategies have had more successful applications with this class of compounds. Often, irreversible tracers have uptake that is limited by tracer delivery and blood flow [2].

Tracers and Models

PET quantification of ligand-receptor binding is derived from in vitro pharmacology methods, based on the receptor density (B_{max}, nM) and the

R. E. Carson (✉) · M. Naganawa · J.-D. Gallezot
Department of Radiology and Biomedical Imaging,
Yale PET Center, Yale University,
New Haven, CT, USA
e-mail: richard.carson@yale.edu;
mika.naganawa@yale.edu;
jean-dominique.gallezot@yale.edu

equilibrium dissociation constant (K_D, nM), the concentration of ligand producing 50% target occupancy. The equilibrium relationship of free ligand concentration (C_F) to specifically bound ligand concentration (C_S) follows the Michaelis–Menten equation:

$$C_S = \frac{B_{max}C_F}{K_D + C_F} \quad (12.1)$$

Most PET studies administer tracer levels of radioligand, so the concentration of bound radioligand is negligible ($C_S < <B_{max}$), with typically <5% occupancy of the target, thus avoiding pharmacological effects. Such molecules are termed *radiotracers*. Under tracer conditions, $C_F \ll K_D$, and Eq. (12.1) simplifies to:

$$\frac{C_S}{C_F} = \frac{B_{max}}{K_D} \quad (12.2)$$

This specifically bound-to-free ratio is the y-intercept on a Scatchard plot. At tracer doses, only unoccupied or *available* receptors will be detectable, i.e., receptors occupied by endogenous neurotransmitters or drugs are not measured. In this case, B_{max} is replaced by B_{avail} in the above equations.

One important measure used to assess receptor binding is the volume of distribution (V_T, mL/cm^3), the concentration ratio, *at equilibrium*, of radiotracer in tissue to that in the arterial plasma. The units of V_T reflect the fact that radioactivity concentrations measured in blood (from samples) and tissue (from PET data) are different. It is called a volume since it reflects the volume of plasma that contains the same radioactivity as 1 cm^3 of tissue. V_T reflects the radiotracer that is specifically bound to the receptor, as well as free or nonspecifically bound tracer. Since competing agents do not displace the latter two components, they are termed "nondisplaceable." Mathematically,

$$V_T = V_{ND} + V_S \quad (12.3)$$

where subscripts T, ND, and S, refer to total, nondisplaceable, and specific, respectively. Most PET studies use bolus injection of a radiotracer, so modeling is used to estimate the equilibrium

ratio by estimating V_T from the kinetic parameters from a model fit to the dynamic data.

The other commonly used outcome measure is the binding potential, *BP*, the equilibrium ratio of the concentration of specifically bound radiotracer to that in a reference fluid (or region). There are three versions of *BP*, using different references: free plasma radiotracer (BP_F), total plasma (BP_P), or the tissue nondisplaceable component (BP_{ND}). The most used term is BP_{ND} (V_S/V_{ND}), which can be estimated using reference region techniques (see below). Ideal reference (REF) regions have no specific binding ($V_S = 0$), so V_T in this region is equal to V_{ND} in the target region-of-interest (ROI). All binding potentials can be calculated from V_T, e.g.,

$$BP_{ND} = \frac{V_{T,ROI} - V_{T,REF}}{V_{T,REF}} = \frac{V_S}{V_{ND}} \quad (12.4)$$

All forms of the binding potential are linearly proportional to the available target concentration (B_{avail}). V_T provides am indirect index of specific binding; it is linearly related to the specific binding component (V_S), but since it includes nonspecific uptake, it is less sensitive to detecting differences in specific binding. The V_T outcome measurement typically requires arterial blood sampling and is generally used when no reference region is available.

PET Data Acquisition

Image Data Acquisition

PET studies begin with the intravenous administration of the radiotracer that contains a positron-emitting isotope. The radiotracer circulates throughout the body and is deposited in all organs. Ultimately, each radioactive atom decays and the detected event allows for reconstruction of the spatial distribution of the radiotracer. Typically, events are grouped into distinct time frames (typically 0.5–10 min), and the number of events follows a Poisson distribution. Shorter time frames provide improved temporal resolution, albeit with higher variance.

Image Reconstruction

The raw count data are converted to the 3D distribution of radioactivity using reconstruction algorithms to produce images with pixel or voxel values. Modern systems use statistical algorithms that account for the Poisson nature of the count data [3]. The images are calibrated in absolute units (Becquerels/cm^3, Bq/cm^3). Dynamic acquisition produces a 4D dataset of concentration images versus time, amenable to tracer kinetic modeling.

PET images have finite resolution, i.e., they are a blurred version of the true underlying distribution of radioactivity. At the boundary between gray and white matter, the radiotracer concentration can abruptly change. However, this abrupt change is blurred in a PET dataset. This is known as the partial volume effect (PVE) and causes underestimation of concentration in high-activity areas and overestimation of low-activity areas. There are many partial volume correction (PVC) methods [4] and typically, PVC methods will increase signal in gray matter regions, often with an increase in noise. There is statistical noise in all PET data depending on the number of radioactive counts in each image frame. With higher counts, the coefficient of variation of PET data (standard deviation/mean) decreases.

PET Image Processing

Brain regions of interest (ROI) are identified, typically using automated template methods [5] based on an anatomical MRI image from the same subject. First, a PET image is rigidly registered to the anatomical MRI image, which is normalized to a template image that has predefined ROIs such as the AAL template [5]. These combined registrations are then used to project the ROI onto the PET images or to transform the PET data into a normalized space for voxelwise comparisons.

Input Functions

Some PET applications require measurement of the arterial input function, the concentration of radiotracer in arterial plasma over the period of the scan. This forms the input function for analysis of brain data since all brain radiotracer is derived from blood. Interpretation of brain signal alone is often misleading without consideration of changes in radiotracer availability in the blood. Since PET radiotracers that are administered intravenously usually exhibit rapid kinetics, arterial plasma is used instead of venous, since there can be large differences between arterial and venous concentrations, especially at early times postinjection.

Radiotracers can be metabolized in the body, so it is important to measure the time course of the parent (unmetabolized) compound. It is generally assumed that polar radiolabeled metabolites do not enter the brain. Arterial blood samples are acquired, and the radioactivity concentration in plasma (Bq/mL) is assayed. Second, the fraction of radioactivity due to parent radiotracer (parent fraction) must be determined, generally using chromatography techniques [6]. The parent fraction is usually measured for a subset of 6–10 discrete blood samples and the fraction curve over time is then fit to a mathematical function. The final arterial plasma input function (C_p) is the product of the measured total plasma radioactivity concentration and the parent fraction function.

Image-derived input function (IDIF) methods have been proposed to obviate the need for arterial blood sampling. IDIFs use the radioactivity in the blood vessels in the PET images to estimate the input function. IDIF methods only estimate the radioactivity in the whole blood, thus, blood sampling may be required for metabolite correction. Many IDIF methods have been proposed for brain studies, but this is challenging depending on what arterial blood vessels are in the field of view. For example, the carotid arteries have an average diameter of ~4–6 mm, thus the PVE causes errors. Total body PET systems can avoid this error if the aorta is in the field of view [7].

Kinetic Analysis

Tracer kinetic modeling has been used for many years to measure the uptake, retention, and metabolism of radiotracers [8]. These approaches depend on the *tracer* assumption, i.e., that the mass concentration of the radiotracer is small, so it does not alter the saturation of any enzyme or the occupancy of any receptor or transporter (e.g., mass concentration $<< K_D$). This leads to linear differential equations with constant coefficients, and compartment modeling approaches are used. PET measures the activity in the brain directly. To analyze such data, we need information about the radiotracer's plasma concentration, i.e., the input function. With the input function and the time-activity curve (TAC) for each region or each voxel, compartment models are derived which can best fit the dynamic data.

For a review of commonly used compartment models in PET, see [9]. Other simplified methods have been used to extract a subset of model parameters, without definition of a specific model configuration [10, 11]. Other important developments were methods that inferred the input function, by use of the TAC in a reference region [12–14], thus avoiding arterial samples. These reference approaches have been most widely used in the brain if there are brain regions completely or nearly devoid of the target receptor.

Compartment Modeling

The solution of compartmental models can always be written as $C_T(t) = C_P(t) \otimes h(t)$ where $\otimes$ is the convolution operator and $h(t)$ is the tissue impulse response function, i.e., a sum of n exponentials, where n is the number of tissue compartments in the model. To choose the best way to quantify a new radiotracer, various compartment models are tested and compared, to determine the simplest model that accurately fits the TACs.

In some cases, the data can be well described by a one-tissue compartment model (1TC, Fig. 12.1a). The 1TC differential equation is:

$$\frac{dC_T(t)}{dt} = K_1 C_P(t) - k_2 C_T(t) \quad (12.5)$$

Transfer of radiotracer from plasma (C_P) to the tissue is described by the rate constant K_1 (mL/min/cm³) while efflux is described by k_2 (min⁻¹). The volume of distribution is an equilibrium measures, derived by setting the derivative to 0:

$$V_T = \frac{C_T}{C_P} = \frac{K_1}{k_2} \quad (12.6)$$

For both 1TC and 2TC (see below) models, K_1 describes the rate of tracer transfer from the arterial plasma to the tissue, and consequently depends on both blood flow (F) and the extraction fraction of radiotracer from the capillary into the tissue (E), such that $K_1 = F \times E$.

A second common model is the two-tissue compartment model (2TC, Fig. 12.1b). The first compartment contains the free plus nonspecific uptake of radiotracer in the tissue (nondisplaceable; C_{ND}) and the second compartment contains specific uptake (i.e., binding to the target) in the tissue (C_S). The additional rate constants describe

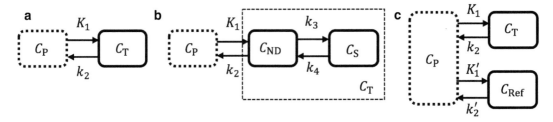

Fig. 12.1 PET compartment models. (**a**) The one-tissue compartment (1TC) model with two rate constants (K_1 and k_2), describing exchanges between the tissue (C_T) and the plasma input (C_P). (**b**) The two-tissue compartment (2TC) model with four rate constants (K_1, k_2, k_3, and k_4) describing exchanges between the free plus nonspecific pool in the tissue, i.e., the nondisplaceable pool (C_{ND}) and

C_P, and binding of the radiotracer in a specific compartment (C_S); the tissue concentration C_T is the sum of C_{ND} and C_S. (**c**) The simplified reference tissue model (SRTM), with three constants ($R_1 = K_1 / K_1'$, k_2, and k_2'), which assumes that both the target and reference tissue can be described by the 1TC model

specific binding association, k_3 (min^{-1}), and dissociation, k_4 (min^{-1}). The total activity in tissue $C_T = C_{ND} + C_S$. The differential equations for this model are

$$\frac{dC_{ND}(t)}{dt} = K_1 C_P(t) - [k_2 + k_3] C_{ND}(t) + k_4 C_S(t)$$

$$(12.7)$$

$$\frac{dC_S(t)}{dt} = k_3 C_{ND}(t) - k_4 C_S(t) \qquad (12.8)$$

The nondisplaceable, specific, and total volumes of distribution are:

$$V_{ND} = \frac{C_{ND}}{C_P} = \frac{K_1}{k_2}$$

$$V_S = \frac{C_S}{C_P} = \frac{K_1 k_3}{k_2 k_4} \qquad (12.9)$$

$$V_T = \frac{C_T}{C_P} = \frac{K_1}{k_2}\left(1 + \frac{k_3}{k_4}\right)$$

Ideally, the binding potential $BP_{ND} = V_S/V_{ND}$ could be computed from k_3/k_4. However, unconstrained fits to PET data rarely separate specific and nondisplaceable components accurately, so such results require validation. Thus, BP_{ND} is best computed with a reference region, as in Eq. (12.4).

Parameter Estimation

To estimate the model parameters [15], an optimization algorithm is used to minimize the sum of the squared differences between the observed radiotracer concentration (C_i) at time frame i (t_i) and the modeled radiotracer concentration ($C(t_i,k)$) based on the parameters (k). If there is substantial inter-frame variation in image noise (e.g., due to different frame durations or isotope decay), a weighted sum of squares is more appropriate, with lower weight for the higher-noise frames. $C(t_i,k)$ may also include a correction for the radioactivity concentration measured in the blood, modeled as the product of the local blood volume (V_B) and the whole blood concentration(C_B(t)). V_B can be fixed to an a priori value, generally 0.05 in gray matter, or esti-

mated from model fitting. After finding the parameter set that produces the minimum sum of squares, the uncertainty of the parameter estimates, i.e., the standard error (SE), can be obtained and can be compared to each parameter estimate to assess if it is reliably estimated.

The kinetic constants K_1, k_2, k_3, k_4 are known as microparameters, which may not always be reliably estimated (i.e., with small %SE). However, the macroparameter V_T is generally estimated reliably. Thus, the most common outcome measures from compartment modeling are V_T and K_1.

Choosing which model best describes the data is an important part of the characterization of a radiotracer. The "best" model is the simplest one that accurately describes the data, and provides parameter estimates with reasonable standard errors. Model selection is often based on the F-test or the Akaike Information Criterion (AIC) [15]. In many cases, the 1TC model produces a slight lack of fit compared to 2TC, but V_T values between the two models are in close agreement [16].

Reference Region Methods

The modeling methods described above depend on accurate input function measurement from arterial blood sampling and metabolite determination. Instead, reference region approaches were developed to estimate BP_{ND} by using a region devoid of specific radiotracer binding as a proxy of nondisplaceable kinetics. Ideally, the assumption of negligible specific binding in a reference region should be validated with blocking studies, which should show no change in the reference region V_T between baseline and blocking scans. Also, V_{ND} in all brain regions is assumed to be uniform, an assumption that can also be evaluated with blocking studies.

The simplified reference tissue model (SRTM, Fig. 12.1c) [13] which has three parameters is widely used. It assumes that the 1TC model is appropriate for *both* target and reference regions, in which case the solution to the 1TC differential equation is

$$C_T(t) = R_1 C_{REF}(t) + R_1 \{k_2' - k_2\} C_{REF}(t) \otimes \exp(-k_2 t)$$

(12.10)

where $C_{REF}(t)$ is the concentration of radiotracer in the reference region, K_1' and k_2' are the reference region influx and efflux rate constants, respectively, k_2 is the efflux constant in the target tissue, and $R_1 = K_1 / K_1'$. The SRTM model is fit to the observed PET data and BP_{ND} can be calculated from the three parameters (R_1, k_2, k_2') as follows:

$$BP_{ND} = \frac{V_T}{V_{ND}} - 1 = \frac{K_1 / k_2}{K_1' / k_2'} - 1 = \frac{R_1 k_2'}{k_2} - 1$$

(12.11)

The term V_T/V_{ND} is also known as the distribution volume ratio, or *DVR*, which equals $BP_{ND} + 1$. SRTM can be estimated efficiently with a basis function approach at the voxel level [17]. Noise can be reduced in SRTM by determining one global value of k_2' using the SRTM2 approach [18], however, this approach depends more strongly on the 1TC assumption than SRTM.

Linearizations

The above methods require the definition of an a priori model for the radiotracer. To provide rapid model-free estimation, linearized approaches have been developed to produce stable estimates with computational efficiency. Linearized methods were first developed for tracers that bind irreversibly. Mathematical rearrangement of the plasma and tissue TACs produces a straight line, with the slope being the net uptake rate parameter (K_i); this is called the Patlak plot [19]. These approaches were generalized for reversible radiotracers to yield the Logan plot [11]:

$$\left(\frac{\int_0^t C_T(\tau) d\tau}{C_T(t)} \right) = V_T \left(\frac{\int_0^t C_P(\tau) d\tau}{C_T(t)} \right) + b, t > t^*$$

(12.12)

Plotting the two terms in parentheses against each other produces a linear graph, with slope equal to V_T and intercept b. This relationship becomes linear after some time t^*, which is determined empirically. The Logan plot can be used for any reversible radiotracer, without specifying the number and arrangement of the compartments. However, this method can produce biased V_T estimates when there is noise in the tissue TAC [20]. Other linearized methods have been derived to reduce noise-induced bias, such as Multilinear Analysis 1 (MA1) [10] and Likelihood Estimation in Graphical Analysis (LEGA) [21]. MA1 fits the tissue TAC directly:

$$C_T(t) = -\frac{V_T}{b} \int_0^t C_P(\tau) d\tau + \frac{1}{b} \int_0^t C_T(\tau) d\tau, t > t^*$$

(12.13)

Typically, graphical V_T estimates are on the 1TC assumption since they use only a portion of the TAC data. These estimates are typically less variable than 2TC estimates, since only two parameters are estimated.

Linearized reference region approaches have also been developed for BP_{ND} (or DVR). The equation for the Logan reference region approach [14] is as follows:

$$\frac{\int_0^t C_T(\tau) d\tau}{C_T(t)} = \frac{V_T}{V_{ND}} \left\{ \frac{\int_0^t C_{REF}(\tau) d\tau}{C_T(t)} + \frac{C_{REF}(t)}{k_2' C_T(t)} \right\} + b, t > t^*$$

(12.14)

The slope is $DVR (1 + BP_{ND})$. The parameter k_2' can be fixed a priori if it is well characterized. Alternatively, if the $C_{REF}(t)/C_T(t)$ term becomes constant quickly, then this term can be lumped with the intercept (b) and fixing the k_2' parameter is unnecessary, although t^* tends to

be later in those cases. Like the plasma version, the Logan reference approach also underestimates BP_{ND} in situations of high noise. To avoid this bias, the multilinear reference tissue model (MRTM [12]), analogous to MA1 was developed:

$$C_{T}(t) = -\frac{BP_{ND}}{b}\left\{\int_{0}^{t}C_{REF}(\tau)d\tau + \frac{1}{k_{2}^{'}}C_{REF}(t)\right\} + \frac{1}{b}\int_{0}^{t}C_{T}(\tau)d\tau, t > t^{*}$$

$$(12.15)$$

As with SRTM and SRTM2, a single $k_{2}^{'}$ value can be estimated, and then parameter estimation is performed again with a 2-parameter fit, a method known as MRTM2 [12].

Constant Infusion

For some tracers, a simple approach to estimate V_T is equilibrium analysis, where the radiotracer is continuously infused until constant decay-corrected concentrations (i.e., equilibrium) are obtained in plasma and all target tissues. In practice, a bolus plus infusion is used to reach equilibrium more quickly [22]. If the radiotracer's kinetic parameters are known from bolus injection studies, then the optimal bolus fraction can be determined by simulation to establish equilibrium quickly in all regions. Once true equilibrium is established, V_T is calculated as C_T/C_P. If venous and arterial blood are in equilibrium, arterial samples can be avoided [23]. For reference region analysis, BP_{ND} is $C_T/C_{REF}-1$.

This paradigm is only practical for some radiotracers, i.e., those with sufficiently rapid kinetics and a suitably long isotope half-life, Additionally, if there are interindividual differences in radiotracer kinetics, then the quality of equilibrium will vary, introducing bias and variability; corrections for lack of equilibrium have been developed [24].

Model Simplification

Simplified quantification methods are advantageous in studies with large cohorts or with participants where it is challenging to undergo a long PET scan or invasive arterial blood sampling. The standard uptake value (SUV), which is the regional activity concentration during a short scan normalized by dose per body weight, is used as an alternative to compartment modeling because: (1) it is easy to compute; (2) the scan duration is typically 10–30 min, and (3) the SUV method does not require arterial blood sampling. Alternatively, a ratio of activity in one region to a reference region (SUVR) may be used as a surrogate for DVR (or SUVR-1 can act a s surrogate for BP_{ND}). For example, as shown in Fig. 12.2, a large human cohort study with ^{11}C-UCB-J showed that imaging 60–90 min postinjection provided the best match between SUVR-1 (centrum semiovale reference) and the gold standard BP_{ND} calculated from 1TC modeling [25].

Parametric Imaging

Images of model parameters can be produced by extracting a TAC from each voxel, processing it using the modeling method of choice to produce one or more parameter estimates, and constructing images consisting of these parameter estimates. An example is shown in Fig. 12.3 for human brain images from ^{11}C-PHNO [26] which binds to the dopamine D_2 and D_3 receptors, located primarily in the basal ganglia and the substantia nigra. Using the dynamic images (sample time frames shown in Fig. 12.3a–c), parametric images were created with SRTM2 [18], using cerebellum as reference: BP_{ND} (Fig. 12.3d) and R_1 (Fig. 12.3e) images. R_1 images show the conventional pattern of high delivery (flow) in gray matter regions, and lower flow in white matter. BP_{ND} images shows the specific binding pattern.

Many of the previously described methods are directly applicable and easily implemented on a voxel-by-voxel basis. For linear model equations, such as Logan plots (Eqs. 12.12 and 12.14), MA1 (Eq. 12.13), and MRTM (Eq. 12.15), the parameters can be estimated directly using ordinary or weighted least squares [15]. For models with one nonlinear parameter, such as 1TC and SRTM, rapid voxel-by-voxel calculations are possible, and are generally implemented as a basis function method [27].

When computing parametric images, some form of noise reduction is often needed. Noise reduction can be done in the temporal and/or spatial domains. Spatially, Gaussian smoothing is

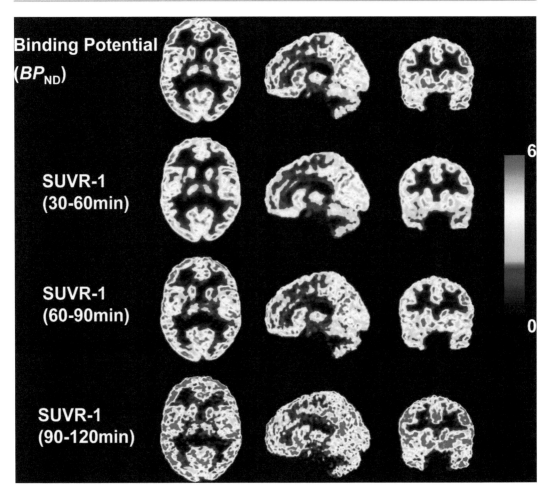

Fig. 12.2 Representative 1TC BP_{ND} parametric images for a ^{11}C-UCB-J PET scan with the corresponding SUVR-1 images for 30–60, 60–90, and 90–120 min time windows

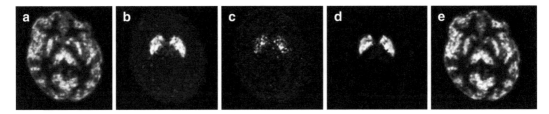

Fig. 12.3 Parametric images from a ^{11}C-PHNO study calculated with SRTM2. (**a–c**) Dynamic tracer concentration images at 0–10 min (**a**), 40–60 min (**b**), and 90–120 min (**c**) postinjection. (**d**) BP_{ND} images on a scale of 0–3. (**e**) R_1 images on a scale of 0–2. Radiotracer deliv-ery is seen to be uniform in gray matter regions in the R_1 images. Specific binding to dopamine D_2 and D_3 receptors in the striatum is evident in the BP_{ND} images. Tracer concentration images at any time point contain various mixtures of the information in the BP_{ND} and R_1 images

the simplest method to reduce noise, but at the cost of poorer resolution. Many algorithms have been applied including other linear or nonlinear filters or constraints based on registered MR images. More recently, deep learning methods have been widely applied for image denoising [28]. In the temporal domain, a simple approach to reduce noise is to limit the range of the basis functions used in models such as 1TC and SRTM, i.e., raise the lower limit on the range of the k_2 values which reduces outlier V_T values [26]. There are also a large number of combined spatiotemporal smoothing methods, including principal component analysis, clustering algorithms, and the HYPR method that uses a set of lower-noise composite images to reduce noise without sacrificing resolution [29].

Usually, parametric images are computed by first reconstructing a series of image frames, and then applying kinetic modeling to each voxel TAC; this is called the indirect method. Alternatively, modeling can be incorporated directly within the reconstruction algorithm; this is called the direct method which has statistical advantages. Direct reconstruction algorithms produce parametric images with lower variability at equivalent dose [30].

Example of Model Development and Validation

Optimization and validation of modeling methods is an important step. Here, we use the SV2A tracer ^{11}C-UCB-J as an example [31]. Cross validation of in vivo values with in vitro measures is highly desirable. To validate ^{11}C-UCB-J as a marker of synaptic density, a baboon PET scan was performed, after which the animal was sacrificed, and the brain dissected. Tissues were sampled from 12 regions and analyzed by Western blotting and SV2A homogenate binding assays. The regional SV2A Western blot measurements correlated well with in vivo V_T values and also with in vitro regional synaptophysin measurements. In vitro B_{max} values from homogenate binding also correlated well with V_T and with the SV2A Western blot data. These data indicated that PET can accurately quantify SV2A density in vivo.

Modeling studies of ^{11}C-UCB-J in humans revealed that the 1TC model was optimal to quantify V_T values, and excellent test-retest reproducibility and low noise V_T images can be obtained [16]. Activation studies in humans showed that V_T was unaffected by visual stimula-

tion, while K_1, the tracer influx constant related to blood flow, increased in the visual cortex [32].

For quantification of specific binding, a reference tissue is required, and the centrum semiovale (CS) was proposed based on in vitro biochemical data [31], showing negligible specific binding. However, there was a small displacement of ^{11}C-UCB-J in CS with competing drugs levetiracetam and brivaracetam [31], consistent with autoradiography data, and CS V_T overestimates the gray matter (GM) nondisplaceable distribution volume (V_{ND}) [33]. Nevertheless, CS V_T is significantly correlated with V_{ND}, suggesting that it remains a useful, albeit imperfect, reference region [33] for disorders without white matter pathology. Alternative outcome measures are V_T or V_T normalized by plasma protein binding (f_P).

For reference tissue modeling, since 1TC is the optimal model, SRTM and SRTM2 were suitable. However, estimating k_2', the efflux rate from the CS, is challenging due to high noise in this small region. SRTM2 with a population average k_2' has been found to be useful to generate BP_{ND} images, however, this approach requires validation in each population.

Receptor Dynamics

Endogenous Neurotransmitters

As described above, PET imaging is sensitive to *available* receptor sites, i.e., those not occupied by endogenous or exogenous compounds. Thus, PET can provide measures of neurotransmission in the living brain. Quantification is based on the classical occupancy model [34], based on extensive evidence that increases in extracellular dopamine directly compete with radiotracers binding at D_2/D_3 receptors.

The protocol to measure changes in neurotransmitter levels is like that of drug occupancy studies (see below), except that low amounts of "occupancy" by neurotransmitters are expected. Most commonly, a baseline scan is acquired, the stimulus or drug is administered leading to increases (or decreases) in neurotransmitter concentrations, and a second scan is acquired. BP_{ND} is estimated for the baseline and post-activation scan, and the percent change in BP_{ND} is determined. Such a two-scan approach can be performed in 1 day with a ^{11}C-labeled radiotracer with two radiosyntheses. An alternative approach is to assess both baseline and post-stimulus BP_{ND} with a single scan using a constant infusion [35]. This approach is best suited for longer lived ^{18}F-labeled radiotracers.

More sophisticated approaches attempt to directly model the effect of time-varying receptor availability on the PET signal [36]. This type of analysis is best accomplished with radiotracers with rapid kinetics, where the PET signal more closely follows the neurotransmitter dynamics, such as ^{11}C-raclopride.

Drug-Induced Occupancy

PET imaging is important in CNS drug development for validation of target engagement and determination of target occupancy [37], i.e., to relate a drug's dose or blood concentration to target occupancy. PET has been widely used in early-stage studies to quantify this relationship, e.g., in kappa opioid receptors [38]. Using this information, further clinical trials can be halted if the desired level of receptor occupancy cannot be achieved at the maximal tolerable drug dose.

Receptor occupancy (r, range: 0–1) can be measured quantitatively if the drug and the radiotracer bind to the same site. This is typically performed with two scans in each subject, one at baseline (base) and one at a suitable time after drug administration (post). Assuming no change in nondisplaceable binding induced by the drug, Eq. (12.3) becomes

$$V_{T,post} = V_{ND} + (1-r)V_S \quad (12.16)$$

With a reference region, BP_{ND} (Eq. 12.4) in the post-drug scan is

$$BP_{ND,post} = \frac{V_{ND} + (1-r)V_{S,ROI} - V_{T,REF}}{V_{T,REF}} \quad (12.17)$$

and r can be determined independently for each ROI

$$r = \frac{BP_{ND,base} - BP_{ND,post}}{BP_{ND,base}} \quad (12.18)$$

Without a reference region devoid of receptors, r can be determined using V_T values from multiple regions with the "occupancy plot," if r and nondisplaceable binding (V_{ND}) are uniform across brain regions [39]. The occupancy equation is

$$V_{T,base} - V_{T,post} = r\left(V_{T,base} - V_{ND}\boldsymbol{u}\right) \quad (12.19)$$

Here, $V_{T,base}$ and $V_{T,post}$ are vectors of the regional V_T values at baseline and post-drug administration, respectively, and $\boldsymbol{u}$ is a vector of ones. Plotting $V_{T,base} - V_{T,post}$ (y-axis) against $V_{T,base}$ (x-axis) produces a linear relationship with a slope of r and x-intercept of V_{ND}. Like other PET linearizations, this approach is not statistically optimal, and alternative methods have been developed [37].

Ultimately, r values are related to drug dose (D) or drug plasma concentration (C) to estimate the ID_{50} or IC_{50}, respectively, i.e., the dose or concentration that produces 50% occupancy of the target. This estimation can be performed as a 1-parameter fit (assuming 100% maximal occupancy) or a 2-parameter fit, which also estimates the maximal occupancy (r_{max}) [40]:

$$r = \frac{C}{C + IC_{50}}$$

$$r = \frac{r_{max}C}{C + IC_{50}} \quad (12.20)$$

This analysis is typically done by combining data from multiple subjects, often using multiple post-drug scans at different plasma drug levels.

Summary

With modern PET scanners and tracer kinetic modeling methods, quantitative measurements of physiological parameters can be made throughout the brain with high accuracy and precision. Development and optimization of appropriate kinetic models for each radiotracer is an important step for the proper application of these molecules for the study of the healthy brain and for studies of neuropsychiatric disorders. Properly validated models also provide a firm basis for simplifications of acquisition and analysis strategies to improve patient comfort and facilitate multi-center trials.

References

1. Innis RB, Cunningham VJ, Delforge J, Fujita M, Gjedde A, Gunn RN, et al. Consensus nomenclature for in vivo imaging of reversibly binding radioligands. J Cereb Blood Flow Metab. 2007;27(9):1533–9.
2. Koeppe RA, Frey KA, Snyder SE, Meyer P, Kilbourn MR, Kuhl DE. Kinetic modeling of N-[11C] methylpiperidin-4-yl propionate: alternatives for analysis of an irreversible positron emission tomography trace for measurement of acetylcholinesterase activity in human brain. J Cereb Blood Flow Metab. 1999;19(10):1150–63.
3. Lange K, Carson R. EM reconstruction algorithms for emission and transmission tomography. J Comput Assist Tomogr. 1984;8(2):306–16.
4. Erlandsson K, Buvat I, Pretorius PH, Thomas BA, Hutton BF. A review of partial volume correction techniques for emission tomography and their applications in neurology, cardiology and oncology. Phys Med Biol. 2012;57(21):R119–59.
5. Tzourio-Mazoyer N, Landeau B, Papathanassiou D, Crivello F, Etard O, Delcroix N, et al. Automated anatomical labeling of activations in SPM using a macroscopic anatomical parcellation of the MNI MRI single-subject brain. NeuroImage. 2002;15(1):273–89.
6. Hilton J, Yokoi F, Dannals RF, Ravert HT, Szabo Z, Wong DF. Column-switching HPLC for the analysis of plasma in PET imaging studies. Nucl Med Biol. 2000;27(6):627–30.
7. Badawi RD, Shi H, Hu P, Chen S, Xu T, Price PM, et al. First human imaging studies with the EXPLORER total-body PET scanner. J Nucl Med. 2019;60(3):299–303.
8. Cobelli C, Foster D, Toffolo G. Tracer kinetics in biomedical research: from data to model. New York, NY: Plenum Publishing; 2001.
9. Gunn RN, Gunn SR, Cunningham VJ. Positron emission tomography compartmental models. J Cereb Blood Flow Metab. 2001;21(6):635–52.
10. Ichise M, Toyama H, Innis RB, Carson RE. Strategies to improve neuroreceptor parameter estimation by linear regression analysis. J Cereb Blood Flow Metab. 2002;22(10):1271–81.
11. Logan J, Fowler JS, Volkow ND, Wolf AP, Dewey SL, Schlyer DJ, et al. Graphical analysis of reversible radioligand binding from time-activity measurements applied to [N-11C-methyl]-(−)-cocaine PET studies in human subjects. J Cereb Blood Flow Metab. 1990;10(5):740–7.
12. Ichise M, Liow JS, Lu JQ, Takano A, Model K, Toyama H, et al. Linearized reference tissue parametric imaging methods: application to [11C]DASB
13. Lammertsma AA, Hume SP. Simplified reference tissue model for PET receptor studies. NeuroImage. 1996;4(3 Pt 1):153–8.
14. Logan J, Fowler JS, Volkow ND, Wang GJ, Ding YS, Alexoff DL. Distribution volume ratios without blood sampling from graphical analysis of PET data. J Cereb Blood Flow Metab. 1996;16(5):834–40.
15. Carson RE. Tracer kinetic modeling. In: Valk PE, Bailey DL, Townsend DW, Maisey MN, editors. Positron emission tomography: basic science and clinical practice. London: Springer; 2003. p. 147–79.
16. Finnema SJ, Nabulsi NB, Mercier J, Lin SF, Chen MK, Matuskey D, et al. Kinetic evaluation and test-retest reproducibility of [(11)C]UCB-J, a novel radioligand for positron emission tomography imaging of synaptic vesicle glycoprotein 2A in humans. J Cereb Blood Flow Metab. 2018;38(11):2041–52.
17. Gunn RN, Lammertsma AA, Hume SP, Cunningham VJ. Parametric imaging of ligand-receptor binding in PET using a simplified reference region Model. NeuroImage. 1997;6(4):279–87.
18. Wu Y, Carson RE. Noise reduction in the simplified reference tissue model for neuroreceptor functional imaging. J Cereb Blood Flow Metab. 2002;22(12):1440–52.
19. Patlak CS, Blasberg RG, Fenstermacher JD. Graphical evaluation of blood-to-brain transfer constants from multiple-time uptake data. J Cereb Blood Flow Metab. 1983;3(1):1–7.
20. Slifstein M, Laruelle M. Effects of statistical noise on graphic analysis of PET neuroreceptor studies. J Nucl Med. 2000;41(12):2083–8.
21. Ogden RT. Estimation of kinetic parameters in graphical analysis of PET imaging data. Stat Med. 2003;22(22):3557–68.
22. Carson RE. PET physiological measurements using constant infusion. Nucl Med Biol. 2000;27(7):657–60.
23. Park E, Sullivan JM, Planeta B, Gallezot JD, Lim K, Lin SF, et al. Test-retest reproducibility of the metabotropic glutamate receptor 5 ligand [(18)F]FPEB with bolus plus constant infusion in humans. Eur J Nucl Med Mol Imaging. 2015;42(10):1530–41.
24. Hillmer AT, Carson RE. Quantification of PET infusion studies without true equilibrium: a tissue clearance correction. J Cereb Blood Flow Metab. 2020;40(4):860–74.
25. Naganawa M, Gallezot JD, Finnema SJ, Matuskey D, Mecca A, Nabulsi NB, et al. Simplified quantification of (11)C-UCB-J PET evaluated in a large human cohort. J Nucl Med. 2021;62(3):418–21.
26. Gallezot JD, Zheng MQ, Lim K, Lin SF, Labaree D, Matuskey D, et al. Parametric imaging and test-retest variability of 11C-(+)-PHNO binding to D2/D3 dopamine receptors in humans on the high-resolution research Tomograph PET scanner. J Nucl Med. 2014;55:960.

27. Gunn RN, Lammertsma AA, Hume SP, Cunningham VJ. Parametric imaging of ligand-receptor binding in PET using a simplified reference region model. NeuroImage. 1997;6(4):279–87.

28. Gong K, Guan J, Liu CC, Qi J. PET image Denoising using a deep neural network through fine tuning. IEEE Trans Radiat Plasma Med Sci. 2019;3(2):153–61.

29. Christian BT, Vandehey NT, Floberg JM, Mistretta CA. Dynamic PET denoising with HYPR processing. J Nucl Med. 2010;51(7):1147–54.

30. Germino M, Gallezot JD, Yan J, Carson RE. Direct reconstruction of parametric images for brain PET with event-by-event motion correction: evaluation in two tracers across count levels. Phys Med Biol. 2017;62(13):5344–64.

31. Finnema SJ, Nabulsi NB, Eid T, Detyniecki K, Lin SF, Chen MK, et al. Imaging synaptic density in the living human brain. Sci Transl Med. 2016;8(348):348ra96.

32. Smart K, Liu H, Matuskey D, Chen MK, Torres K, Nabulsi N, et al. Binding of the synaptic vesicle radiotracer [(11)C]UCB-J is unchanged during functional brain activation using a visual stimulation task. J Cereb Blood Flow Metab. 2021;41(5):1067–79.

33. Rossano S, Toyonaga T, Finnema SJ, Naganawa M, Lu Y, Nabulsi N, et al. Assessment of a white matter reference region for (11)C-UCB-J PET quantification. J Cereb Blood Flow Metab. 2020;40(9):1890–901.

34. Laruelle M. Imaging synaptic neurotransmission with in vivo binding competition techniques & colon; a critical review. J Cereb Blood Flow Metab. 2000;20(3):423–51.

35. Carson RE, Breier A, de Bartolomeis A, Saunders RC, Su TP, Schmall B, et al. Quantification of amphetamine-induced changes in [11C]raclopride binding with continuous infusion. J Cereb Blood Flow Metab. 1997;17(4):437–47.

36. Morris ED, Yoder KK, Wang C, Normandin MD, Zheng QH, Mock B, et al. ntPET: a new application of PET imaging for characterizing the kinetics of endogenous neurotransmitter release. Mol Imaging. 2005;4(4):473–89.

37. Naganawa M, Gallezot JD, Rossano S, Carson RE. Quantitative PET imaging in drug development: estimation of target occupancy. Bull Math Biol. 2017;81:3508.

38. Naganawa M, Dickinson GL, Zheng MQ, Henry S, Vandenhende F, Witcher J, et al. Receptor occupancy of the kappa-opioid antagonist LY2456302 measured with positron emission tomography and the novel radiotracer 11C-LY2795050. J Pharmacol Exp Ther. 2016;356(2):260–6.

39. Cunningham VJ, Rabiner EA, Slifstein M, Laruelle M, Gunn RN. Measuring drug occupancy in the absence of a reference region: the Lassen plot re-visited. J Cereb Blood Flow Metab. 2010;30(1):46–50.

40. Finnema SJ, Rossano S, Naganawa M, Henry S, Gao H, Pracitto R, et al. A single-center, open-label positron emission tomography study to evaluate brivaracetam and levetiracetam synaptic vesicle glycoprotein 2A binding in healthy volunteers. Epilepsia. 2019;60(5):958–67.

Semi-Quantitative Analysis: Software-Based Imaging Interpretation: NEUROSTAT/SPM

13

Kazunari Ishii

Key Points

The usefulness of semi-quantitative methods in the interpretation of molecular images is described. Semi-quantitative values are useful for interpreting metabolic and perfusion imaging in degenerative brain diseases, and voxel-based statistical analysis of images with SPM or 3D-SSP is used in clinical practice as an aid to diagnostic interpretation. In amyloid imaging, the measurement of the standardized uptake value ratio (SUVR) is also useful.

Introduction

In the field of degenerative diseases, absolute values of metabolic and blood flow parameters are not as necessary as in the field of cerebrovascular diseases.

For neurodegenerative disease, the interpretation of molecular imaging such as that acquired with fluorodeoxyglucose (FDG)-PET is based on visual inspection.

Three-dimensional stereotactic surface projections (3D-SSP), which form the basis of the NEUROSTAT program and statistical parametric mapping (SPM), have become indispensable tools for the analysis of brain imaging obtained from modalities such a PET, SPECT, and fMRI. These 3D-SSP methods are used to convert individual brains into a standard coordinate system (stereotaxic brain coordinates) through anatomical standardization, after which statistical analysis can be performed on each voxel.

In statistical analysis methods for images such as those in SPM and 3D-SSP, individual brains of different sizes and shapes are deformed and aligned to a standard brain (in stereotaxic brain coordinates). This procedure is called "anatomical standardization," and after this process, statistical analysis is performed on each voxel for analytical or diagnostic purposes.

The conventional analytical method of setting a region of interest (ROI) for the analysis has the following problems: (a) the size and range of the ROI may not be standardized and may not be consistent across observers, (b) it is very difficult to set ROIs in the same region for each target brain, (c) ROI settings vary across observers, (d) ROI settings may be arbitrary, (e) the whole brain may not be analyzed, only the region covered by the ROI. Therefore, some areas may be overlooked. In comparison, statistical image analysis methods such as SPM and 3D-SSP permit voxel-by-voxel analysis of the whole brain of each subject, thereby providing an objective method that can overcome the above problems.

K. Ishii (✉)
Department of Radiology, Kindai University Faculty
of Medicine, Osakasayama, Japan
e-mail: ishii@med.kindai.ac.jp

© The Author(s), under exclusive license to Springer Nature Switzerland AG 2023
D. J. Cross et al. (eds.), *Molecular Imaging of Neurodegenerative Disorders*,
https://doi.org/10.1007/978-3-031-35098-6_13

SPM (Statistical Parametric Mapping)

SPM was first developed by Friston et al. as software for the analysis of brain activation studies using PET [1]. SPM has since undergone many improvements and SPM12 (Fig. 13.1) is currently available for free download from https: //www.fil.ion.ucl.ac.uk/spm/. SPM was originally developed as a tool for analyzing brain activation tests in normal subjects but has also been applied to group comparisons between normal and diseased subjects. SPM is now an indispensable tool for the analysis of functional MRI (fMRI), and also allows voxel-based morphometry to be performed on 3D T1 MRI brain imaging [2].

The process for SPM analysis is as follows.

Realignment and Co-registration

In the case of multiple scans per acquisition, such as in brain activation imaging and fMRI, the realignment process allows correction for slight movement between timepoint images with the same contrast, while co-registration allows the superimposition of images with differing contrasts from different sequences or different imaging modalities such as PET and MRI. These processes are not necessary if the analysis involves only a single scan per subject.

Normalization

The anatomical standardization of SPM is a mathematical method that allows the subject

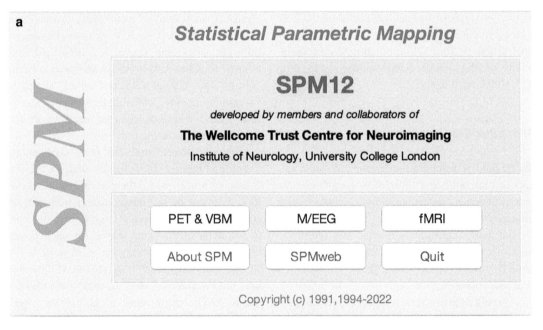

Fig. 13.1 The screen at SPM12 startup (**a**) and the display screen (**b**) for analysis of the target FDG-PET image in SPM12

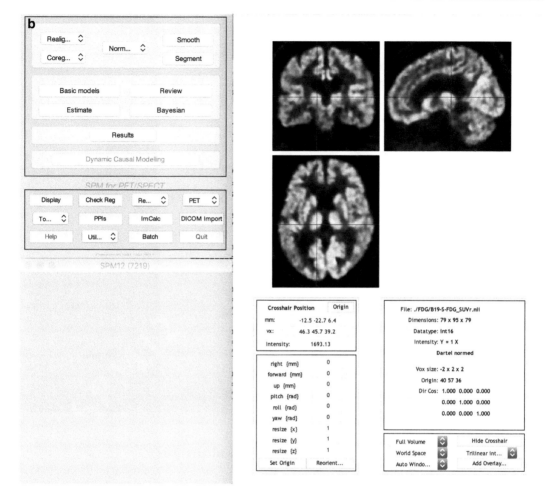

Fig. 13.1 (continued)

images to be translated and warped to fit the geometry of a pre-defined template. The subject's 3D brain image is warped to fit a template in the defined coordinate space of the Montreal Neurological Institute (MNI) atlas (Fig. 13.2).

Fig. 13.2 The tissue probability map (TPM) template of SPM12

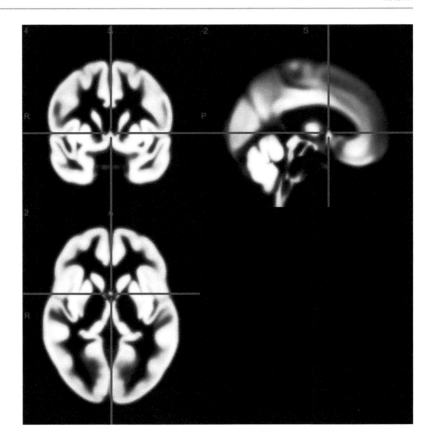

Smoothing

After normalization, the SPM procedure usually involves smoothing to reduce the individual differences in brain gyri and improve the signal-to-noise ratio. This process also brings the voxel value distribution closer to the normal distribution, which is the premise of statistical processing.

Statistical analysis

The statistical principles of SPM are based on the normal distribution and the general linear model. The statistical results are displayed as shown in Fig. 13.3.

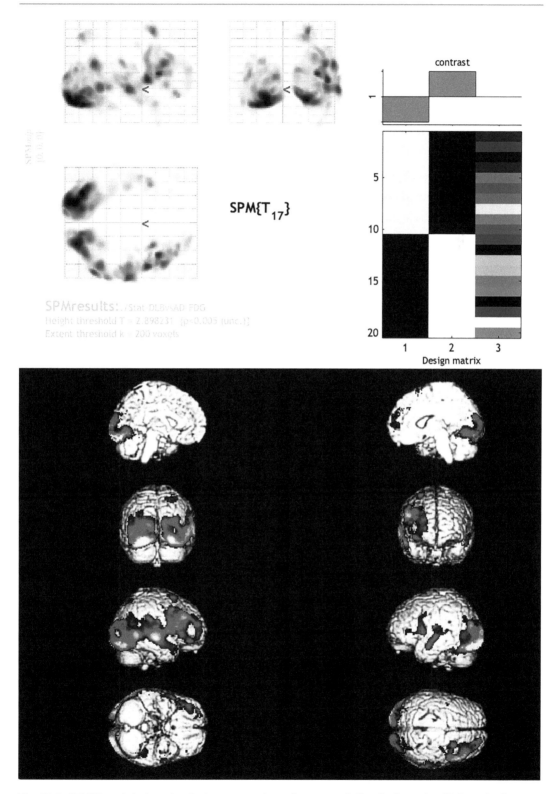

Fig. 13.3 SPM12 statistical results display screen: the glass brain projection map and overlap with the MRI rendered image, which demonstrate significantly decreased glucose metabolism in dementia with Lewy bodies compared to Alzheimer disease

3D-SSP (Three-Dimensional Stereotactic Surface Projections)

3D-SSP is a procedure in NEUROSTAT, a suite of statistical imaging analysis packages developed by Minoshima et al. [3, 4]. A characteristic of 3D-SSP is that it was developed not only for research, but also for diagnostic applications.

The 3D-SSP procedure is as follows. After correcting PET/SPECT brain images for tilt during scanning, four reference points are searched for on a sagittal cross-section of a template image realigned to the Talairach standard atlas, and the brain size is adjusted by linear deformation to fit the reference plane of the anterior commissure–posterior commissure line. In the current version, this transformation is performed using mutual information. The next procedure in the 3D-SSP processing pipeline is anatomical standardization by warping, which involves a nonlinear transformation that aligns the individual brain to the template as much as possible. The next process, the extraction of brain surface data, is the most important feature of 3D-SSP. This is performed by extracting the pixel with the maximum value within a depth of 6 pixels (2.25 mm × 6) perpendicular to the surface of the brain cortex on the

anatomically-standardized image. These values are then displayed as two-dimensional brain surface images viewed from eight directions. The values can be absolute values (cerebral glucose consumption, cerebral blood flow) or relative values normalized by the values of the whole brain, cerebellum, thalamus, pons, or primary sensorimotor cortex. This method compensates for deviations within subjects where the anatomically-standardized image does not completely match with the standard brain, such as in cases with an enlarged longitudinal fissure. Needless to say, this method does not correct for decreased values caused by partial volume effects. The above process can also be applied to brain images of normal subjects (or controls) to build a database, which allows the creation of a statistical image comparing the brain surface image of an individual patient with those in the database (Fig. 13.4). Such statistical comparison images can be used in clinical practice, e.g., as a diagnostic aid by creating a z-score map for each subject to determine brain areas where metabolism and blood flow are significantly lower than in normal subjects.

The z-score is calculated using the following formula:

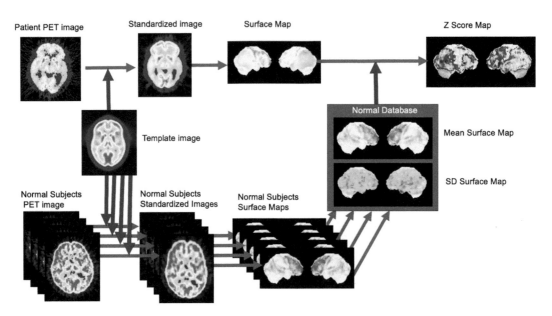

Fig. 13.4 The process for creating a statistical z-score image in 3D-SSP

$$z - score = (\text{normal group mean value} - \text{individual value}) / \text{normal group standard deviation}$$

The z-score is calculated for each pixel and the disease is diagnosed on the basis of the distribution pattern of the scores.

In addition, 3D-SSP can perform group comparisons between normal and disease groups, with corresponding t-tests performed on a voxel-by-voxel basis.

Voxel-Based Analysis for Interpretation of Medical Images

Although SPM and 3D-SSP were originally used as analysis tools in research, they are now also being developed as diagnostic aids and tools for clinical applications, and pharmaceutical companies are working together with the developers to improve and develop the packages into easy-to-use software for clinical use, examples of which are now distributed as freeware.

For 3D-SSP, the software iSSP is specialized for diagnostic assistance, and is distributed free of charge by Nihon Medi-Physics, Inc. in cooperation with Minoshima et al. This software has been widely used for image analysis and diagnostic assistance in Alzheimer's disease (AD) and other degenerative dementias (Fig. 13.5).

In another example, following anatomical standardization using SPM, z-score maps can be superimposed on the MRI template image to assist in diagnosis. This method is applied in the software eZIS [5], which was developed by Matsuda et al. and PDR Pharma Co.

The statistical analysis images so created can be used as aids in medical image interpretation and to improve diagnostic accuracy. For physicians, not only beginners but also experts, the use of statistical images as a supplemental diagnostic aid can be more effective than the use of axial images alone.

A further step involves the development of an automated diagnostic system for neurodegenerative disease such as AD using FDG-PET and 3D-SSP. The technique is based on regions of interest in which metabolism and blood flow are specifically reduced in AD, with this statistical-based imaging system allowing comparisons between patients with AD and normal subject groups. The summed z-scores within volumes of interest (VOIs) are calculated for each individual subject, and if the total summed score exceeds a threshold, a diagnosis of AD is made. This method has demonstrated diagnostic performance comparable with that of expert nuclear medicine physicians, and its combined use with conventional manual analysis can improve diagnostic performance [6]. The technique has been applied to differential diagnosis of AD and dementia with Lewy bodies [7] using FDG-PET imaging, and also to analysis of perfusion SPECT imaging [8]. A similar method using summed t values produced with SPM [9] is also provided in the form of the PMOD Alzheimer's Discrimination Tool (PALZ) (Fig. 13.6) by PMOD Technologies LLC.

These statistical image analysis methods are very useful as aids to image interpretation, but caution needs to be exercised in making the diagnosis because:

(a) if the normal database is not obtained with the same PET scanner and imaging protocol as that used in clinical practice, an incorrect statistical image may be produced,

(b) there is a risk of incorrect anatomical standardization (and thus incorrect z-scores) in cases with high levels of atrophy or large infarcts.

Therefore, when interpreting FDG-PET images or perfusion SPECT images, the diagnosis should never be made solely on the basis of statistical images. First, the original axial, coronal, and sagittal images should be interpreted, including a search for regionally decreased metabolic/perfusion regions and lesions, then the statistical image can be observed to reveal whether the regions show significant decreases compared with the normal database. It should then be verified that the results of the visual inspection and statistical images are consistent. If the results of the visual inspection and statistical images differ, it is important to rereview the original images to check for artifacts in the statistical image before making the final diagnosis.

Brugnolo et al. investigated the differentiation of patients with prodromal AD from controls on FDG-PET, and compared diagnostic performance between three SPM-based approaches,

another voxel-based tool, and a volumetric region of interest support vector machine (VROI-SVM)-based approach. They reported that the automated VROI-SVM performed better than the other voxel-based methods [10], but that this finding was limited to the differential diagnosis of prodromal AD, and therefore voxel-based methods are still useful in the diagnosis of mild cognitive impairment (MCI) or early AD, and a combination of visual inspection and voxel-based analysis aids is recommended for the clinical

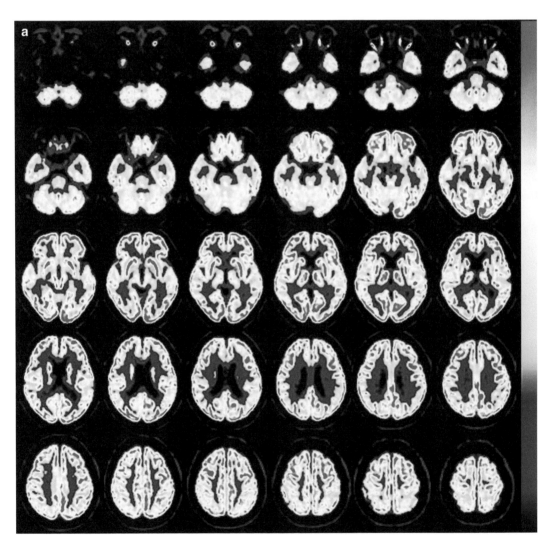

Fig. 13.5 A representative case of mild cognitive impairment due to AD. Original FDG-PET imaging demonstrates an AD-specific pattern of reduced metabolism (**a**).

The z-score map allows easier detection of regions showing decreased metabolism (**b**)

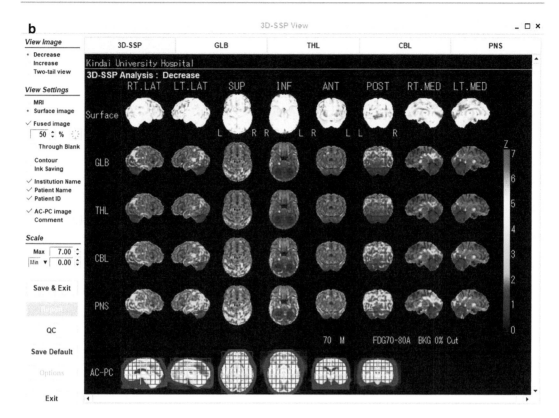

Fig. 13.5 (continued)

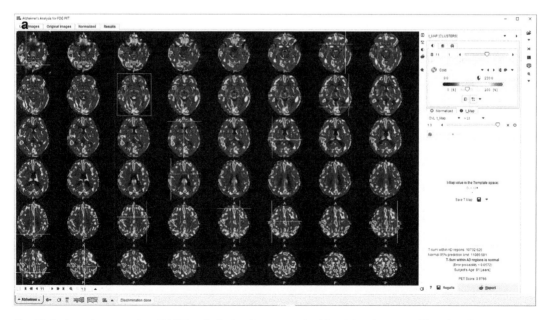

Fig. 13.6 A results screen from PALZ analysis showing a normal subject (**a**) and a severe AD patient (**b**)

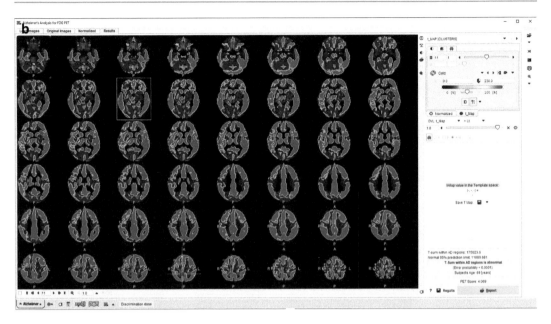

Fig. 13.6 (continued)

diagnosis of early-stage neurodegenerative disorders.

Although the recent development of deep learning methods has improved the diagnostic performance of FDG-PET interpretation of neurodegenerative diseases [11, 12], the basis of interpretation is still visual inspection, and voxel-based statistical methods based on 3D-SSP or SPM should be utilized only as a means of assisting interpretation.

Measurement of SUVR on Molecular Images

Although visual inspection is clinically used for the interpretation of amyloid PET images, the standardized uptake value ratio (SUVR), a semi-quantitative value, may be used as an interpretation aid. Such semi-quantitative measurements are reported to show good correlation with visual interpretations [13], and the SUVR and regional counts relative to reference counts are commonly used in quantitative analysis of amyloid PET. The SUVR is calculated as the ratio of cortical-to-cerebellar counts. In amyloid PET imaging,

counts should be measured within a volume of interest (VOI) set up on a standard brain template for each region being analyzed. To do this, each subject's amyloid PET image is spatially normalized to a standard brain. This anatomical standardization can be performed directly on the amyloid PET imaging alone [14] or with the use of corresponding MRI [15].

It should also be noted that the SUVRs of amyloid PET images differ for each tracer, and there have therefore been attempts to standardize them. One is the Centiloid Project, which involves a 100-point scale called the "Centiloid"; this has a mean of 0 for "highly probable" amyloid-negative subjects and a mean of 100 for "typical" AD subjects [16]. Calibration to the centroid scale allows for easier comparisons of units across sites. All data used in the Centiloid Project and the VOI set are available for download (Fig. 13.7) from the URL (https://www.gaain.org/centiloid-project). Tools have also been devised for SUVR measurement using SPM, conversion to the Centiloid Project format, and creation of z-score images, and they are expected to be applied clinically in the near future [17].

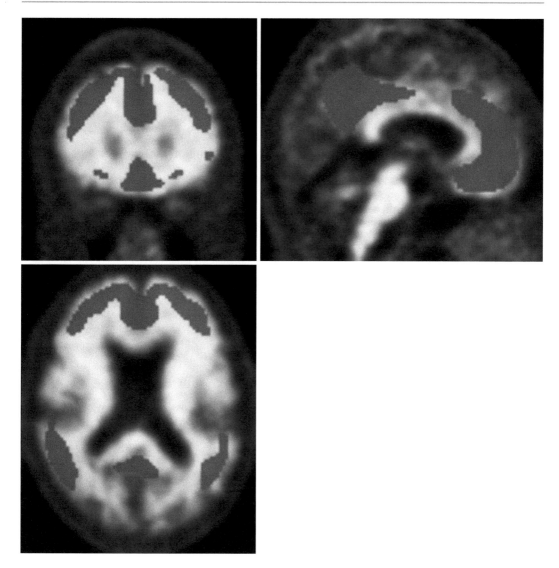

Fig. 13.7 VOIs of cerebral cortices defined in the Centiloid Project

Conclusion

Statistical image analysis using 3D-SSP or SPM is a very useful aid in the interpretation of molecular imaging of the brain. These methods involve converting the individual brain into standard space with anatomical standardization, voxel-by-voxel statistical analysis, and the production of z-score images that can then be used as aids in clinical diagnosis.

References

1. Friston KJ, Frith CD, Liddle PF, Frackowiak RS. Comparing functional (PET) images: the assessment of significant change. J Cereb Blood Flow Metab. 1991;11:690–9.
2. Ashburner J, Friston KJ. Voxel-based morphometry—the methods. NeuroImage. 2000;11:805–21.
3. Minoshima S, Koeppe RA, Frey KA, Ishihara M, Kuhl DE. Stereotactic PET atlas of the human brain: aid for visual interpretation of functional brain images. J Nucl Med. 1994;35:949–54.

4. Minoshima S, Frey KA, Koeppe RA, Foster NL, Kuhl DE. A diagnostic approach in Alzheimer's disease using three-dimensional stereotactic surface projections of fluorine-18-FDG PET. J Nucl Med. 1995;36:1238–48.

5. Matsuda H, Mizumura S, Nagao T, et al. An easy Z-score imaging system for discrimination between very early Alzheimer's disease and controls using brain perfusion SPECT in a multicentre study. Nucl Med Commun. 2007;28:199–205.

6. Ishii K, Kono AK, Sasaki H, et al. Fully automatic diagnostic system for early- and late-onset mild Alzheimer's disease using FDG PET and 3D-SSP. Eur J Nucl Med Mol Imaging. 2006;33:575–83.

7. Kono AK, Ishii K, Sofue K, Miyamoto N, Sakamoto S, Mori E. Fully automatic differential diagnosis system for dementia with Lewy bodies and Alzheimer's disease using FDG-PET and 3D-SSP. Eur J Nucl Med Mol Imaging. 2007;34:1490–7.

8. Ishii K, Ito K, Nakanishi A, Kitamura S, Terashima A. Computer-assisted system for diagnosing degenerative dementia using cerebral blood flow SPECT and 3D-SSP: a multicenter study. Jpn J Radiol. 2014;32:383–90.

9. Herholz K, Salmon E, Perani D, et al. Discrimination between Alzheimer dementia and controls by automated analysis of multicenter FDG PET. NeuroImage. 2002;17:302–16.

10. Brugnolo A, De Carli F, Pagani M, et al. Head-to-head comparison among semi-quantification tools of brain FDG-PET to aid the diagnosis of prodromal Alzheimer's disease. J Alzheimers Dis. 2019;68:383–94.

11. Ding Y, Sohn JH, Kawczynski MG, et al. A deep learning model to predict a diagnosis of Alzheimer disease by using (18)F-FDG PET of the brain. Radiology. 2019;290:456–64.

12. Kim S, Lee P, Oh KT, et al. Deep learning-based amyloid PET positivity classification model in the Alzheimer's disease continuum by using 2-[(18)F] FDG PET. EJNMMI Res. 2021;11:56.

13. Yamane T, Ishii K, Sakata M, et al. Inter-rater variability of visual interpretation and comparison with quantitative evaluation of (11)C-PiB PET amyloid images of the Japanese Alzheimer's disease neuroimaging initiative (J-ADNI) multicenter study. Eur J Nucl Med Mol Imaging. 2017;44:850–7.

14. Akamatsu G, Ikari Y, Ohnishi A, et al. Automated PET-only quantification of amyloid deposition with adaptive template and empirically pre-defined ROI. Phys Med Biol. 2016;61:5768–80.

15. Ishii K, Yamada T, Hanaoka K, et al. Regional gray matter-dedicated SUVR with 3D-MRI detects positive amyloid deposits in equivocal amyloid PET images. Ann Nucl Med. 2020;34:856–63.

16. Klunk WE, Koeppe RA, Price JC, et al. The centiloid project: standardizing quantitative amyloid plaque estimation by PET. Alzheimers Dement. 2015;11(1–15):e11–4.

17. Matsuda H, Yamao T. Software development for quantitative analysis of brain amyloid PET. Brain Behav. 2022;12:e2499.

Greg Zaharchuk

Key Points

- AI is posed to revolutionize neuroimaging broadly and has many applications for molecular imaging.
- AI approaches cover a wide spectrum of applications, including image acquisition improvement, cross-modality image translation, and prediction of current and future biomarkers and disease states.
- Challenges with AI adoption include the lack of large, publicly-available datasets, generalizability issues, bias in predictions, and explainability.

Introduction

The past 10 years have been described as a golden era for artificial intelligence (AI) research [1]. We have seen the rise of deep learning and convolutional neural networks as well as large foundational models that demonstrate ever increasing performance. These advances are beginning to pervade the medical domain, which tend to lag other fields due to the lack of large, shared datasets and conservative nature of medicine. In this chapter, we will discuss the application of modern AI techniques to structural and quantitative

neuroimaging for the purposes of improving the care of patients with neurodegenerative disease. Potential applications span the spectrum of care, starting with improved quality and reduced cost of neuroimaging and extending to the prediction of current and future dementia biomarkers. However, there remain significant challenges with these techniques, including their generalizability and potential bias, which must be considered and addressed to realize the promise of these exciting new technologies.

AI in Medicine

What do we mean when we talk about AI as a tool in clinical medicine? Technology has gone hand in hand with advances in medicine for decades if not centuries. AI is often described as a device or algorithm that can perform a task that is thought to be uniquely human [2]. As such, this definition has changed over time, and would encompass applications as diverse as the abacus and AlphaFold [3], a computer program capable of deciphering the 3D structures of all known proteins. Into this category fall many post-processing algorithms that are used routinely in medical imaging, from physics-based reconstruction to rules-based segmentation tools.

Increasingly, when we speak of AI, we are referring specifically to machine learning methods where computers learn patterns in data with-

G. Zaharchuk (✉)
Stanford University, Stanford, CA, USA
e-mail: gregz@stanford.edu

out explicit programming of rules. As such, they "let the data speak for itself" and therefore are sometimes called "data-driven" algorithms. Many of these still require humans to identify the most salient features in the data. At the simplest end of the spectrum is multivariate linear regression, in which human-defined features are associated and combined with weights so as to minimize the error in the prediction of an output variable of interest. More complex versions of this basic approach include increasingly complex algorithms meant to minimize the errors in prediction and overcome the assumptions of linearity in data, which is not always present. These include techniques such as principal component analysis, support vector machines, and tree-based decision systems such as random forest.

All of these methods share the requirement that humans must define the input features of interest for the model. Such models have been successful, but an important assumption is that the chosen features are relevant and important for predicting the output. The identification of appropriate features has often been performed by biomedical scientists using their domain knowledge, usually relying on an underlying, mechanistic hypothesis of the underlying biology. However, this can be problematic. Informative features might not be known or might be excluded from models due to bias or lack of understanding. Or there may be complex inter-relationships that we as humans cannot identify. One approach to circumvent this need to define features manually has been to use radiomics approaches which return thousands of features, at least some of

which are hoped to be relevant to predicting the output variables of interest [4]. For these reasons, such feature-driven algorithms have inherent limitations.

It is only in the last 10 years that we have developed robust tools to solve these problems without making assumptions about the relevant features. The meteoric rise of deep learning has been due to a confluence of several factors, including big datasets, improved software algorithms, and reduced cost of computational hardware such as GPUs that significantly reduce the time for training [5, 6]. Deep learning builds on the success of neural network architectures that bear some resemblance to those seen in biological systems. These networks can be self-trained, with the "deep" in the name referring to multiple hidden layers of neurons that allow them to represent even complex features. When applied to images, computational efficiency favors the use of convolutional neural networks (CNNs), which when combined into multiple layers can represent different size scales of features in a location-invariant way. This turns out to be advantageous for processing images, where the location of important features cannot generally be predicted in advance. A typical deep neural network is shown schematically in Fig. 14.1.

There are several important advantages of deep CNNs. One is that they are largely agnostic to inputs and outputs, which can be swapped in and out easily to perform new tasks. This facilitates the rapid testing of many hypotheses without wholesale changes in network architecture. The second is that the features are derived through the

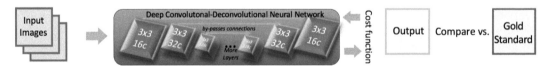

Fig. 14.1 Schematic of a deep convolutional neural network using a supervised learning framework. Input images are fed into an algorithm that performs multiple stages of non-linear filtering, usually with small convolutional kernels (3 by 3 in this example) that serve as filter weights. Multiple kernels create multiple channels that typically increase in number as the network gets deeper. Application of these filters produces an output, which is

then compared to the true output, usually a gold standard of some sort. The difference between true and predicted outcomes, operationalized in terms of a mathematical estimate of error known as the cost function, is used to iteratively adjust the weights of the non-linear filter banks to improve future predictions. Through this process, the network is trained and can then be applied to new, unseen inputs

Table 14.1 Overview of upstream and downstream AI

	Upstream	Downstream
Common tasks	• Image quality improvement • Scan time reduction • Cross-modality image synthesis • Prediction of future imaging appearance	• Prediction of presence/absence of disease • Classification into different disease groups (or normal) • Prediction of an imaging biomarker • Prediction of future disease (prognosis, survival)
Inputs	• Images • Raw sensor data (k-space, sinograms, etc.)	• Images • Demographics • Clinical information • Genetics
Outputs	• Images • Segmentations (lesion/not-lesion) • Anatomic regions • future images	• Disease class • Biomarkers • Future biomarkers, disease class
Example applications	• Faster imaging (MRI, PET) • Lower dose imaging (CT, PET) • MR attenuation correction for PET • Fracture detection on MRI	• Diagnosing presence/absence of Alzheimer's disease • Predicting fast and slow disease progressors

training of the network when multiple examples of available inputs and desired outputs are provided to the algorithm. A loss function representing the error in the prediction for an individual training example can be back-propagated through the network to change the weights that connect the neurons slightly during every iteration to improve the prediction of the model. With enough training data, the network weights will converge to identify meaningful features in the data without human guidance. This process can be quite time-consuming. However, once the model training is complete, the weights between the neurons in all the layers are fixed. This means when a new input example in an independent test set is given to the model, the inference process can rapidly produce the predicted outcome, which can be compared with the ground truth to assess the performance of the model. As such deep learning models have advantages over traditional iterative methods in neuroimaging that are plagued by long reconstruction times [7].

This chapter will focus on deep learning applications to modern neuroimaging. These can be applied at multiple levels in the radiology value chain, starting with image reconstruction, encompassing data post-processing, and extending to biomarker measurements and clinical classifica-

tion of patients into different disease states (Table 14.1). One exciting potential application is the use of historical datasets to predict disease trajectories and prognoses.

Upstream AI for Neuroimaging of Neurodegenerative Disease

Faster Imaging and Reconstruction

Imaging is one of the most important advances in medicine over the past several decades but there remain multiple challenges [8, 9]. It still often involves radiation, which can cause secondary malignancies. For example, the estimated added risk of cancer from the radiation in a standard PET/CT has been estimated to be 0.5–0.6% [10]. While this might be acceptable in patients with terminal primary malignancies, it is suboptimal if molecular imaging with PET is to be extended to patients with non-terminal conditions or those in which life expectancy may still be measured in decades, for example, neurodegenerative diseases. In fact, radiation (along with cost) is a limiting factor when discussing screening programs, as could be envisioned for early diagnosis of dementia.

Another problem with imaging is its high cost. This is multifactorial, but one reason that advanced imaging methods such as PET and MRI are expensive is because of the limited number of patients that can be scanned per day. Despite advances in MRI over the past 30 years, the average length of an exam in the USA has not changed significantly [9]. Faster imaging techniques have been proposed, and are often utilized, but additional contrasts have been added to extract more value from the MR examination. Finally, the volume of medical imaging continues to increase [11], due in part to the recognition of the central role of imaging in patient diagnosis and expeditious triage. For all these reasons, methods to reduce the cost and risks of imaging are desirable.

It took several years after the explosion of interest in computer vision using neural networks as evidenced by the success of AlexNet in the 2012 ImageNet Challenge before it was realized that neural networks would be transformative for medical imaging reconstruction [12]. Initial applications were the use of AI for the denoising of medical images that required multiple repetitions for signal averaging, such as arterial spin labeling [13]. Other approaches used iterative methods on raw MRI data to replace simple rules-based compressed sensing type acquisitions with neural network regularizers [14, 15]. Another popular application was image super-resolution, in which faster, low-resolution images could be transformed into higher resolution based on a deep learning framework [16]. Multiple start-up companies and established scanner vendors have obtained FDA clearance for products that provide faster imaging with minimal to no degradation of image quality [17].

Advantages for PET Imaging

Beyond MRI, other medical imaging reconstruction problems proved amenable to deep learning. AutoMAP, a sequence initially developed for MRI which learned the mapping between raw scanner acquisitions and image space, was shown to applicable to other imaging modalities such as CT and PET [18]. There was a proliferation of papers showing that MR-based attenuation correction for PET could be learned by neural networks trained on pairs of MR and co-registered CT images [19–21]. PET reconstruction from sinograms was also shown to be equivalent to the typical iterative reconstruction methods, usually with better performance and massively-reduced reconstruction times [7].

Since PET scanners are essentially cameras for gamma rays, the advantages provided by deep learning can be translated to either reduced bed times, reduced radiotracer dose, or a combination of the two. These can be traded off against each other depending on the application. For example, a patient who cannot tolerate lying still for a standard PET study could receive a faster scan. Additionally, reduced time of the exam could translate into more availability at a particular imaging site to accommodate more patients without increasing hours of operation or paying for additional technologist support. In the long term, this could lead to lower costs to perform PET imaging, which is one of the most expensive imaging modalities. Alternatively, the increased sensitivity afforded by deep learning could be used to image reduced radiotracer dose. This might be used in a setting where a patient arrives late and the dose has decayed. Or it might be preferred in a patient in whom the risk of secondary malignancy is a concern, such as in young patients expected to survive their acute condition. Other opportunities include the ability to do more frequent longitudinal follow-up studies or to perform multiple radiotracer studies. Many of the benefits due to low dose are relevant to patients undergoing PET for neurodegenerative disease diagnosis, treatment, and monitoring [22].

Finally, from an accessibility aspect, PET scanners remain concentrated in major metropolitan areas and are not available to patients who live in rural locations without significant travel and disruptions. Partly this is due to the cost of PET, but another important issue is that radiotracer delivery is not possible in many rural locations, because of the logistics of transporting doses over long distances. The ability to image at significantly lower dose would enable transport of doses over much longer distances, making PET studies feasible in a much wider area. Such applications show that AI for PET can improve health equity.

A recent prospective, multicenter study has shown the potential to perform PET at four-fold dose reduction, with equivalent diagnostic performance for whole body FDG cancer interpretation [23]. By combining low-dose PET with simultaneously acquired MRI, it was shown that amyloid imaging could be performed at 1–2% of standard dose, both through the use of simulations and with actual reduced dose [24, 25] (Fig. 14.2). Finally, a study evaluated the use in patients with lymphoma to show that simulated

reduced dose of up to 50% could be used without changing scan interpretation or patient triage [26]. Such methods are also FDA cleared and have entered the routine workflow in many sites in the US and Europe.

Cross-Modality Image Synthesis

Due to the flexible nature of neural network architecture, it is possible to swap in different modalities at the input and output of the network. This application essentially aims to synthesize one modality from another (Fig. 14.3). This has advantages if the synthesized modality is expen-

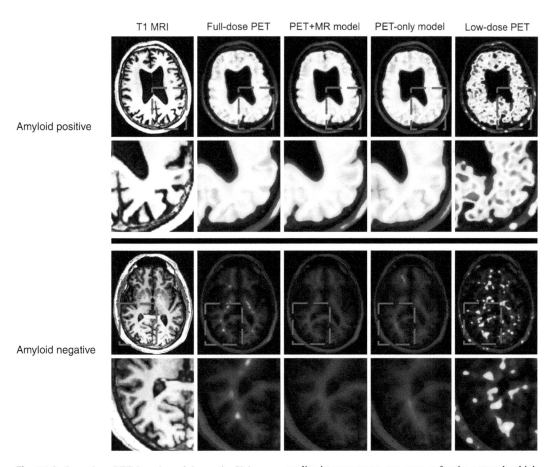

Fig. 14.2 Low-dose PET imaging of dementia. Using a deep learning network to enhance low-dose 18F-florbetaben (amyloid) PET imaging improves image quality. In this case, simulations of 1% dose in an amyloid positive and negative patient are shown. While image quality improvements are present for the network which only took the ultralow-dose PET images as input, better image quality can be achieved if the inputs also include MRI structural images (T1, T2 FLAIR)

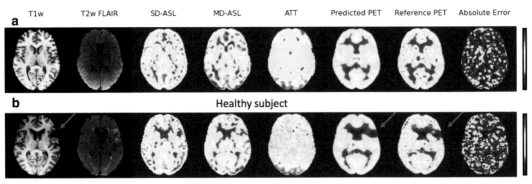

T1w   T2w FLAIR   SD-ASL   MD-ASL   ATT   Predicted PET   Reference PET   Absolute Error

Healthy subject

Patient with chronic infarct

Fig. 14.3 Cross-modality image synthesis with deep learning. In this case, a deep learning model using MR images as input (including both structural and functional [i.e., arterial spin label] images) were used to predict gold standard cerebral blood flow maps created from oxygen-15 water PET in (**a**) a healthy subject and (**b**) a patient with a chronic infarct (red arrows)

sive, risky, or not available for the patient. One example of this is the use of MRI to predict CT, obviating the need for radiation or extra scan cost [27–29]. This has been shown possible for the diagnosis of some conditions that have traditionally been CT-based, such as evaluating the pediatric cranial structures without radiation [30]. Another example is the prediction of gold standard oxygen-15 water PET cerebral blood flow from simultaneously acquired MR imaging, using structural and perfusion MR. [31] More recent work has shown the potential to synthesize FDG brain PET from MRI alone, which may find value in the imaging of patients with or at risk of dementia in a radiation-free manner [32]. The presumption in cross-modality synthesis is that the relevant information exists in the input scans to predict the second modality, even if it is not immediately obvious to the trained radiologist. Importantly, this is something that can be tested easily using standard AI methodology.

Classification of Disease with AI

Downstream AI can be defined as classifying images based on patient characteristics or disease states. This use of AI is most similar to many computer vision challenges, such as the ImageNet challenge, in which the task is to define the mean-

ingful content of a natural image. While it is natural to apply such approaches to medical images, there are important differences between natural and medical images. For example, the natural imaging task often has a central object that has good contrast with the background, but this is often not the case for medical images, where small changes in signal intensity or shape either focally or diffusely may convey the crucial evidence of disease presence or absence (Fig. 14.4). Another difference between nature image prediction and medical image disease diagnosis is the relatively small size of medical imaging datasets. For example, one of the largest datasets put together for classification of brain tumors includes 40,000 cases [33]; this is 350 times smaller than the number of examples in ImageNet (14 M). Finally, disease prevalence is low for many conditions; this is very relevant for real-life use, since in a low prevalence environment, very high sensitivity and especially specificity are required for the algorithm to add clinical value. For these reasons, predicting disease on medical images is substantially more challenging. Several recent review articles give a nice overview, focusing primarily on neurodegenerative disease [34, 35].

Despite this, there have been scores of efforts to perform disease diagnosis from medical imaging datasets. The most studied area for tomo-

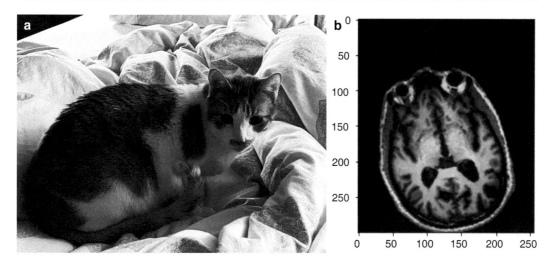

Fig. 14.4 Challenges of classifying medical images. (**a**) Typical ImageNet example, with a dominant object in the foreground of the image. (**b**) Typical medical imaging example, where subtle global atrophy is the defining feature of this patient with Alzheimer's disease

graphic studies has been the detection of critical abnormalities on non-contrast CT. The largest study to date has been the study from Chilamkurthy et al., who trained a network using 313,318 head CTs to predict five different types of brain hemorrhage, calvarial fracture, midline shift, and mass effect [36]. They reported their performance on a dataset of 500 cases selected to have a broad distribution of the abovementioned entities drawn from two different centers, using a gold standard of consensus of three radiologists. Using their high sensitivity threshold, they showed sensitivities ranging between 0.91 and 0.95. Specificity was much lower, between 0.67 and 0.89. Therefore, for entities with low prevalence, most of the positive predictions will be false positives. An example of this difference in real-world versus test set performance was seen by Arbabshirani et al. [37], who developed an algorithm specifically for identifying intracranial hemorrhage. In the retrospective test dataset, the area-under-the-curve (AUC) performance was 0.85. When applied to a prospective cohort, ICH was flagged in 94 of 347 studies, of which 60 were in agreement with radiologist reports. The rest (34 out of 94, 36%) were false positives. Of note, 9% of radiologist-determined ICH was missed by the algorithm. It is likely that most environments in which an ICH detector would be helpful would have much lower prevalence even than this study (25%), which would increase the number of false positives. Such issues are important to consider to fully understand the challenge of disease diagnosis tasks and their potential value in the clinical setting.

Predicting Along the Alzheimer's Disease Continuum

So far, the most common applications in the neurodegenerative space have been focused on the detection and classification of dementia, primarily Alzheimer's disease (AD). There are several reasons for this, including the fact that AD is the most common cause of dementia. Another is the existence of the large, public Alzheimer's Disease Neuroimaging Initiative (ADNI) dataset, which has proven to be a prescient and invaluable resource for AI studies that require big data. Particularly valuable has been the longitudinal data, sometimes over 10 years, which enables the development of prognostic models.

The simplest task is to predict the presence or absence of AD, or to further classify into finer groups, such as normal, mild cognitive impairment (MCI), and AD. Another interesting task is to separate out patients with MCI into those who are stable versus those who progress to AD within a pre-defined time period. One early example is the work of Liu et al. [38], who used an autoencoder with MRI as an input to classify 311 subjects drawn from ADNI. They presented good results for distinguishing healthy controls from AD, with an accuracy of 88%. This fell to 77% for distinguishing MCI patients from healthy controls, as might be expected. For separating their four classes (further separating MCI into stable and progressive forms), predictive accuracy fell to 47%, highlighting that it is easier to predict two widely separated classes (i.e., healthy control and AD) than more relevant clinical tasks such as predicting MCI or different progression within the MCI class. Some groups have tried to add clinical and genetic information to imaging to improve predictions. For example, Venugopalan et al. studied different models (deep vs. conventional machine learning) and different combinations of clinical, genetic, and MR imaging data to distinguish AD, MCI, and control patients in ADNI [39]. They found that the best performance for distinguishing these three classes was using all three sources of data using a deep learning model, measuring an accuracy of 78% in their external test dataset. Therefore, it appears that performance for this task using historical data has reasonable accuracy, though it remains debatable whether 80% accuracy is sufficient for clinical use.

Application to Non-Alzheimer's Disease Conditions

Often, the relevant question is not whether patients have dementia, but whether it reflects AD or some other neurodegenerative condition. To this end, several authors have examined the question of distinguishing AD from non-AD dementias. These studies tend to be more recent and involve smaller numbers of patients. Wada et al. examined whether it would be possible to distinguish dementia with Lewy bodies (DLB), AD, and healthy controls using a deep learning

framework examining the MR connectome as derived from resting-state functional MRI in a relatively small cohort [40]. They found an accuracy of 73% for this classification task, and interestingly predicted the relative probability/contribution of these three "components" in each patient. This is particularly interesting since it is known that patients can have more than one cause for dementia. Another article addressed this question by using data from single photon emission computed tomography (SPECT) using 99Tc-ethyl cysteinate dimer (ECD), a blood flow agent [41]. They found excellent performance of 94–95% accuracy for distinguishing either of the dementia conditions from the healthy controls, but unsurprisingly found separating AD from DLB more challenging, with an accuracy of 74%. Interestingly, they used 18F-FDG images from ADNI to pre-train the network, which was then fine-tuned on their own data.

Another relevant task is separating AD from frontotemporal dementia (FTD). 18F-FDG imaging has high diagnostic performance for this task [42]. Sadeghi et al. proposed the use of a decision tree algorithm that relies on FDG imaging to make this classification [43]. Using activity based on stereographic surface projections in 48 patients with AD or FTD, they found a range of accuracies between 67 and 94% for different parameterizations of the model. This was similar to the accuracy of six neurologists on this dataset (89%). Since regional atrophy is known finding that can help with diagnosis of these two entities, it is possible also to use T1-weighted MRI for this classification [44]. Using a dataset composed of cases from ADNI and the Frontotemporal Lobar Degeneration Neuroimaging Initiative, they found an accuracy of 93% for distinguishing the two conditions using a deep CNN architecture.

Future Prediction of Neurodegenerative Disease Trajectories

While the last section detailed how AI can be used to classify disease based on neuroimaging, the methods used can be easily modified to take on the question of prognosis. This can range from predicting events (e.g., survival, toxicity), a classification task, to predicting future biomarkers (regression task) and even future imaging studies (image transformation). From a methodological perspective, training such models is straightforward if longitudinal data is available. In this case, imaging or demographic data from a prior point in time can be used as input to the models, while the output is the variable of interest at a later time point. Once trained, when applied to data acquired in the present, the model can make a prediction about the future.

Identification of patients with more or less aggressive disease course is valuable, not least of all for the patient's expectation and resource planning. Another key value add is the potential to stratify patients with different future disease course. For example, patients with more aggressive disease courses might be offered treatments that are accompanied by a higher degree of risk or toxicity. At minimum, such methods could help inform patient-physician decision making in a more personalized manner.

Another compelling benefit of AI-based future disease course prediction would be for clinical trial patient selection. It is well documented that the cost of clinical trials is an impediment to the development of novel therapeutics. Two large drivers of cost of clinical trials are their size and duration. If AI could be used to select patients who are likely to have severe disease and who are likely to progress quickly, the number of patients required to show a positive effect of the therapy can be reduced. Furthermore, if they progress faster than the average patient, it is possible that the length of the clinical trial can be reduced. There are challenges with any metrics that are used to select patients, since the performance of the drug in a larger, unselected population cannot be assessed. However, once proof of efficacy of a treatment is established, it de-risks subsequent studies on a broader population.

Finally, AI can be applied retrospectively to already completed clinical trials to understand the difference between treatment and non-treatment (or between two different treatments) at the individual level. The basic idea is that two

prognostic models can be developed, one in the patients in the treatment arm and one in the placebo arm [45, 46]. Assuming the populations are drawn from the same representative sample, the output of the two different models should give an estimate of how the patient will progress with and without treatment. Patients in whom there is not much difference between the two arms might be able to avoid the treatment, which could reduce their risk and cost of care. Patients in whom the model-predicted poorer outcome could be actively steered away from the treatment. Finally, patients who have a better model-predicted outcome would be ideal patients to treat. In this way, patients can act as their own virtual controls, leading to a maximally personalized treatment plan that is based on the historical data.

Several studies have used this basic premise, using neuroimaging to predict future outcomes and biomarkers. For example, Ding et al. trained a network using the ADNI dataset to predict the presence of AD from FDG PET brain imaging [47]. They then applied this to a small external cohort of patients with clinical diagnoses documented an average of 6–7 years after the imaging, demonstrating 82% sensitivity and 100% specificity to classify patients into AD versus non-AD. Such a model could in theory be used as a screening tool for patients to predict the presence or absence of disease in the future. If a pharmaceutical was being developed to prevent the development of AD, a clinical trial might consider only enrolling patients who were predicted to have AD in the future without treatment, reducing the enrollment of patients who will not progress regardless of the efficacy of the treatment.

Instead of predicting an outcome, another option is to predict a biomarker. This may be more objective than predicting an outcome, and the quantitative range of the biomarker might provide more information to the model during training than compared to a less-informative classification approach. One example here is the work of Reith et al., who also used the ADNI dataset to predict the change in amyloid burden as measured by the SUVR value within a composite cortical region on 18F-florbetapir PET imaging [48]. The input to the model was the current florbetapir image and several clinical, demographic, and genetic features; the output to the model was the SUVR change over a 2–8 year period. Deep features for the amyloid imaging were obtained by predicting current amyloid SUVR from the images [49]. These were then combined with the non-imaging features using a gradient-boosted decision tree machine learning method to make a final prediction of the SUVR change. Using this strategy, it was shown that it was possible to better select the fastest progressing patients (defined as the top 10% of patients with the highest SUVR increase) by almost fourfold over random selection. Such an approach could be used as entry criteria to a clinical trial to enrich the population of fast progressors with the goal of shortening the length of a clinical trial.

Remaining Challenges

While there is much to be optimistic about given the current advances in AI for neuroimaging, multiple challenges remain (Table 14.2). AI benefits immensely from very large datasets; one unexpected attribute of deep learning, for example, is its ability to continue to improve as data sizes increase. Therefore, the full benefit of these technologies may not be realized due to the sequestration of imaging data amongst different institutions due to concerns about patient privacy. Another increasingly obvious barrier to sharing is also that institutions are beginning to realize the value of the data that they possess and want to either reserve it for their own researchers or monetize it. Larson et al. suggest an ethical framework that once clinical data is used for its intended use of treating the patient, it should be available as a public good [50]. The fact that much of the research that occurs is funded by taxpayer dollars implies that such data should be freely available. For molecular imaging of neurodegenerative disease, ADNI itself is an excellent example of the value of broad sharing and has been the focus of many AI studies. Federated learning, in which models are shared between institutions rather than

Table 14.2 Outstanding challenges in the application of AI to medical imaging

Problem	Example	Mitigation
Lack of availability of large-shared datasets	Training a classification algorithm is challenging without enough training examples	• Improving sharing culture of radiology • Sharing model weights rather than data (federated learning) • Unsupervised and semi-supervised learning • Models optimized for small datasets
Generalization	Algorithms developed at one institution may work poorly in other settings	• Training on multi-institutional datasets • Periodic reassessment and re-calibration
Bias	Methods developed using non-representative training sets may not perform well in less represented classes	• Testing on representative populations • Broadly representative training (if required)
Fair evaluation	An image enhancement algorithm fails to capture an important clinical detail	• Multi-reader studies • Performance on automated tasks (segmentation, biomarkers, etc.)

data, can avoid the need to share patient data and potentially mitigate privacy issues [51]. However, such collaboration between institutions is somewhat limiting, as only one or a few models and questions can be explored. In this author's opinion, open sharing of neuroimaging datasets is less limiting and a more democratic way of enabling larger and more diverse populations. This better promotes collaboration with our colleagues outside of imaging (i.e., computer science, data science), allowing them to participate fully in the development of AI-assisted technologies, and as such should be encouraged. It is heartening to see that the National Institutes of Health will begin to require data sharing more broadly for awards submitted in 2023 [52]; it will be important that such requirements are enforced in a meaningful way.

Another challenge is that of data drift. Standardization of imaging data is challenging. Each scanner and each institution may have different scanners and acquire images in slightly different ways. If disease prevalence is different at different institutions, AI algorithms may rely on statistical correlations or shortcuts to make their predictions based on an identification of site or scanner [53]. Furthermore, imaging scientists are keenly aware that technologies change over time. It is likely that algorithm performance may be significantly influenced using new data input with different underlying characteristics, even if it is of nominally better quality. Non-imaging factors may also change over time, such as prevalence of disease or the effects of new treatments. It is likely that some sort of continuous learning or periodic re-certification of AI algorithms may be needed to address these issues. One unsolved problem is determining when this is necessary and who will pay for these evaluations. It should be noted that most algorithms currently used in radiology suffer from similar issues and no requirements exist for them to be periodically re-certified or modified.

The last challenge to be aware of is that of bias. AI that has been trained on historical datasets has been shown to replicate any pre-existing biases [54]. While we may believe that imaging data is more objective, it is known that algorithms can determine patient sex and even ethnicity from imaging data. This should not be too surprising, given that different national organizations have developed separate brain templates that more faithfully represent the characteristics of their populations [55]. As such, it is possible that AI outputs could use such intermediate steps as shortcuts for predicting disease or response to treatment in inappropriate manners. Training data for models may under-represent certain protected groups, as the demographics of patients who receive advanced imaging does not match the demographics of the community as a whole.

Possibly because of this, performance of algorithms may differ by protected group status, which is obviously undesirable. Attention to these issues is somewhat new for the imaging community but are important to make sure that algorithms are maximally fair to different protected groups.

Summary

AI holds much promise for neuroimaging applications, particularly those involving molecular imaging and applied to neurodegenerative disease. We are still in early days in terms of harnessing these technologies. Deep learning in particular enables a data-driven way to combine imaging and non-imaging data without the need for human feature selection and will likely dominate in terms of applications for the immediate future. Applications span a wide range, from image acquisition, to segmentation and post-processing, all the way to disease classification and biomarker prediction. Using historical longitudinal data offers the unique ability to make statements about future disease and personalize treatment. While some challenges and potential pitfalls of AI technology need to be considered, it is likely that we are only seeing the beginning of what these technologies are capable and their potential to benefit patients with neurological disease.

References

1. Kaynak O. The golden age of artificial intelligence. Discov Artif Intell. 2021;1:1–7.
2. Moore A. Carnegie Mellon dean of computer science on the future of AI. Forbes Magazine. Accessed 30 Oct 2017.
3. Jumper J, Evans R, Pritzel A, Green T, Figurnov M, Ronneberger O, Tunyasuvunakool K, Bates R, Zidek A, Potapenko A, Bridgland A, Meyer C, Kohl SAA, Ballard AJ, Cowie A, Romera-Paredes B, Nikolov S, et al. Highly accurate protein structure prediction with Alphafold. Nature. 2021;596:583–9.
4. Gillies R, Kinahan P, Hricak H. Radiomics: images are more than pictures, they are data. Radiology. 2016;278:563–77.
5. LeCun Y, Bengio Y, Hinton G. Deep learning. Nature. 2015;521:436–44.

6. Zaharchuk G, Gong E, Wintermark M, Rubin D, Langlotz CP. Deep learning in neuroradiology. AJNR Am J Neuroradiol. 2018;39:1776–84.

7. Haggstrom I, Schmidtlein CR, Campanella G, Fuchs TJ. Deeppet: a deep encoder-decoder network for directly solving the PET image reconstruction inverse problem. Med Image Anal. 2019;54:253–62.

8. Fuchs V, Sox H Jr. Physicians views of the relative importance of thirty medical innovations. Health Aff. 2001;20:30–42.

9. Edelstein WA, Mahesh M, Carrino JA. MRI: Time is dose—and money and versatility. J Am Coll Radiol. 2010;7:650–2.

10. Huang B, Law MW, Khong PL. Whole-body PET/CT scanning: estimation of radiation dose and cancer risk. Radiology. 2009;251:166–74.

11. Smith-Bindman R, Kwan ML, Marlow EC, Theis MK, Bolch W, Cheng SY, Bowles EJA, Duncan JR, Greenlee RT, Kushi LH, Pole JD, Rahm AK, Stout NK, Weinmann S, Miglioretti DL. Trends in use of medical imaging in US health care systems and in Ontario, Canada, 2000-2016. JAMA. 2019;322:843–56.

12. Krizhevsky A, Sutskever I, Hinton G. Image net classification with deep convolutional neural networks. In: Advances neural information processing systems. Cambridge: The MIT Press; 2012. p. 25.

13. Gong E, Pauly J, Zaharchuk G. Boosting SNR and/or resolution of arterial spin label (ASL) imaging using multi-contrast approaches with multi-lateral guided filter and deep networks, vol. 3938. Honolulu: Proceedings of ISMRM; 2017.

14. Mardani M, Gong E, Cheng J, Vasanawala S, Zaharchuk G, Xing L, Pauly J. Deep generative adversarial networks for compressed sensing MRI. IEEE Trans Med Imaging. 2019;38:167–79.

15. Hammernik K, Klatzer T, Kobler E, Recht MP, Sodickson DK, Pock T, Knoll F. Learning a variational network for reconstruction of accelerated MRI data. Magn Reson Med. 2018;79:3055–71.

16. Chaudhari AS, Fang Z, Kogan F, Wood J, Stevens KJ, Gibbons EK, Lee JH, Gold GE, Hargreaves BA. Super-resolution musculoskeletal MRI using deep learning. Magn Reson Med. 2018;80:2139–54.

17. US FDA. Artificial intelligence and machine learning (AI/ML)-enabled medical devices, vol. 2022. White Oak: US FDA; 2021.

18. Zhu B, Liu JZ, Cauley SF, Rosen BR, Rosen MS. Image reconstruction by domain-transform manifold learning. Nature. 2018;555:487–92.

19. Liu F, Jang H, Kijowski R, Zhao G, Bradshaw T, McMillan AB. A deep learning approach for (18) F-FDG PET attenuation correction. EJNMMI Phys. 2018;5:24.

20. Liu F, Jang H, Kijowski R, Bradshaw T, McMillan AB. Deep learning MR imaging-based attenuation correction for PET/MR imaging. Radiology. 2018;286:676–84.

21. Bradshaw TJ, Zhao G, Jang H, Liu F, McMillan AB. Feasibility of deep learning-based PET/MR attenuation correction in the pelvis using only diagnostic MR images. Tomography. 2018;4:138–47.

22. Zaharchuk G. Next generation research applications for hybrid PET/MR and PET/CT imaging using deep learning. Eur J Nucl Med Mol Imaging. 2019;46:2700–7.

23. Chaudhari AS, Mittra E, Davidzon GA, Gulaka P, Gandhi H, Brown A, Zhang T, Srinivas S, Gong E, Zaharchuk G, Jadvar H. Low-count whole-body PET with deep learning in a multicenter and externally validated study. NPJ Digit Med. 2021;4:127.

24. Chen KT, Gong E, de Carvalho Macruz FB, Xu J, Boumis A, Khalighi M, Poston KL, Sha SJ, Greicius MD, Mormino E, Pauly JM, Srinivas S, Zaharchuk G. Ultra-low-dose (18)F-florbetaben amyloid PET imaging using deep learning with multi-contrast MRI inputs. Radiology. 2019;290:649–56.

25. Chen KT, Toueg TN, Koran MEI, Davidzon G, Zeineh M, Holley D, Gandhi H, Halbert K, Boumis A, Kennedy G, Mormino E, Khalighi M, Zaharchuk G. True ultra-low-dose amyloid PET/MRI enhanced with deep learning for clinical interpretation. Eur J Nucl Med Mol Imaging. 2021;48:2416.

26. Theruvath AJ, Siedek F, Yerneni K, Muehe AM, Spunt SL, Pribnow A, Moseley M, Lu Y, Zhao Q, Gulaka P, Chaudhari A, Daldrup-Link HE. Validation of deep learning-based augmentation for reduced (18)F-FDG dose for PET/MRI in children and young adults with lymphoma. Radiol Artif Intell. 2021;3:e200232.

27. Jans LBO, Chen M, Elewaut D, Van den Bosch F, Carron P, Jacques P, Wittoek R, Jaremko JL, Herregods N. MRI-based synthetic CT in the detection of structural lesions in patients with suspected sacroiliitis: comparison with MRI. Radiology. 2021;298:343–9.

28. Yang H, Sun J, Carass A, Zhao C, Lee J, Prince JL, Xu Z. Unsupervised MR-to-CT synthesis using structure-constrained CycleGAN. IEEE Trans Med Imaging. 2020;39:4249–61.

29. Florkow MC, Zijlstra F, Willemsen K, Maspero M, van den Berg CAT, Kerkmeijer LGW, Castelein RM, Weinans H, Viergever MA, van Stralen M, Seevinck PR. Deep learning-based MR-to-CT synthesis: the influence of varying gradient echo-based MR images as input channels. Magn Reson Med. 2020;83:1429–41.

30. Eshraghi Boroojeni P, Chen Y, Commean PK, Eldeniz C, Skolnick GB, Merrill C, Patel KB, An H. Deep-learning synthesized pseudo-CT for MR high-resolution pediatric cranial bone imaging (MR-HIPCB). Magn Reson Med. 2022;88:2285–97.

31. Guo J, Gong E, Fan AP, Goubran M, Khalighi MM, Zaharchuk G. Predicting (15)O-water PET cerebral blood flow maps from multi-contrast MRI using a deep convolutional neural network with evaluation of training cohort bias. J Cereb Blood Flow Metab. 2019;40:2240–53.

32. Ouyang J, Chen K, Zaharchuk G. Zero-dose PET reconstruction with missing input by U-net with attention modules. Proceedings 33rd conference on neural

information processing systems (NeurIPS 2019). 2019.

33. Gao P, Shan W, Guo Y, Wang Y, Sun R, Cai J, Li H, Chan WS, Liu P, Yi L, Zhang S, Li W, Jiang T, He K, Wu Z. Development and validation of a deep learning model for brain tumor diagnosis and classification using magnetic resonance imaging. JAMA Netw Open. 2022;5:e2225608.

34. Silva-Spinola A, Baldeiras I, Arrais JP, Santana I. The road to personalized medicine in Alzheimer's disease: the use of artificial intelligence. Biomedicine. 2022;10:10.

35. Battineni G, Chintalapudi N, Hossain MA, Losco G, Ruocco C, Sagaro GG, Traini E, Nittari G, Amenta F. Artificial intelligence models in the diagnosis of adult-onset dementia disorders: a review. Bioengineering (Basel). 2022;9:9.

36. Chilamkurthy S, Ghosh R, Tanamala S, Biviji M, Campeau NG, Venugopal VK, Mahajan V, Rao P, Warier P. Deep learning algorithms for detection of critical findings in head CT scans: a retrospective study. Lancet. 2018;392:2388–96.

37. Arbabshirani MR, Fornwalt BK, Mongelluzzo GJ, Suever JD, Geise BD, Patel AA, Moore GJ. Advanced machine learning in action: identification of intracranial hemorrhage on computed tomography scans of the head with clinical workflow integration. NPJ Digit Med. 2018;1:9.

38. Liu S, Liu S, Cai W, Pujol S, Kikinis R, Feng D. Early diagnosis of Alzheimer's disease with deep learning. Proceedings 2014 IEEE 11th International Symposium on Biomedical Imaging (ISBI). Beijing: IEEE; 2014. p. 1015–8.

39. Venugopalan J, Tong L, Hassanzadeh HR, Wang MD. Multimodal deep learning models for early detection of Alzheimer's disease stage. Sci Rep. 2021;11:3254.

40. Wada A, Tsuruta K, Irie R, Kamagata K, Maekawa T, Fujita S, Koshino S, Kumamaru K, Suzuki M, Nakanishi A, Hori M, Aoki S. Differentiating Alzheimer's disease from dementia with Lewy bodies using a deep learning technique based on structural brain connectivity. Magn Reson Med Sci. 2019;18:219–24.

41. Ni YC, Tseng FP, Pai MC, Hsiao IT, Lin KJ, Lin ZK, Lin CY, Chiu PY, Hung GU, Chang CC, Chang YT, Chuang KS. The feasibility of differentiating Lewy body dementia and Alzheimer's disease by deep learning using ECD SPECT images. Diagnostics. 2021;11:11.

42. Foster NL, Heidebrink JL, Clark CM, Jagust WJ, Arnold SE, Barbas NR, DeCarli CS, Turner RS, Koeppe RA, Higdon R, Minoshima S. FDG-PET improves accuracy in distinguishing frontotemporal dementia and Alzheimer's disease. Brain. 2007;130:2616–35.

43. Sadeghi N, Foster N, Wang A, Minoshima S, Lieberman A, Tasdizen T. Automatic classification of Alzheimer's disease vs. frontotemporal dementia: a spatial decision tree approach with FDG-PET. In:

Proceedings 5th IEEE International Symposium on Biomedical Imaging: From Nano to Macro. Paris: IEEE; 2008. p. 408–11.

44. Hu J, Qing Z, Liu R, Zhang X, Lv P, Wang M, Wang Y, He K, Gao Y, Zhang B. Deep learning-based classification and voxel-based visualization of frontotemporal dementia and Alzheimer's disease. Front Neurosci. 2020;14:626154.

45. Nielsen A, Hansen MB, Tietze A, Mouridsen K. Prediction of tissue outcome and assessment of treatment effect in acute ischemic stroke using deep learning. Stroke. 2018;49:1394–401.

46. Yu Y, Xie Y, Thamm T, Gong E, Ouyang J, Christensen S, Marks M, Lansberg M, Albers G, Zaharchuk G. Tissue at-risk and ischemic core estimation using deep learning in acute stroke. Am J Neuroradiol. 2021;42:1030–7.

47. Ding Y, Sohn JH, Kawczynski MG, Trivedi H, Harnish R, Jenkins NW, Lituiev D, Copeland TP, Aboian MS, Mari Aparici C, Behr SC, Flavell RR, Huang SY, Zalocusky KA, Nardo L, Seo Y, Hawkins RA, et al. A deep learning model to predict a diagnosis of Alzheimer disease by using (18)F-FDG PET of the brain. Radiology. 2019;290:456–64.

48. Reith FH, Mormino EC, Zaharchuk G. Predicting future amyloid biomarkers in dementia patients with machine learning to improve clinical trial patient selection. Alzheimers Dement. 2021;7:e12212.

49. Reith F, Koran M, Davidzon G, Zaharchuk G. Application of deep learning to predict standardized uptake value ratio and amyloid status on 18F-florbetapir PET using ADNI data. Am J Neuroradiol. 2020;41:980–6.

50. Larson DB, Magnus DC, Lungren MP, Shah NH, Langlotz CP. Ethics of using and sharing clinical imaging data for artificial intelligence: a proposed framework. Radiology. 2020;295:675–82.

51. Sheller MJ, Edwards B, Reina GA, Martin J, Pati S, Kotrotsou A, Milchenko M, Xu W, Marcus D, Colen RR, Bakas S. Federated learning in medicine: facilitating multi-institutional collaborations without sharing patient data. Sci Rep. 2020;10:12598.

52. Lauer M. Introducing NIH's new scientific data sharing website. https://nexus.od.nih.gov/all/2022/04/05/introducing-nihs-new-scientific-data-sharing-website/. Accessed 19 Sept 2022.

53. Zech JR, Badgeley MA, Liu M, Costa AB, Titano JJ, Oermann EK. Variable generalization performance of a deep learning model to detect pneumonia in chest radiographs: a cross-sectional study. PLoS Med. 2018;15:e1002683.

54. Panch T, Mattie H, Atun R. Artificial intelligence and algorithmic bias: implications for health systems. J Glob Health. 2019;9:010318.

55. Lee JS, Lee DS, Kim J, Kim YK, Kang E, Kang H, Kang KW, Lee JM, Kim JJ, Park HJ, Kwon JS, Kim SI, Yoo TW, Chang KH, Lee MC. Development of Korean standard brain templates. J Korean Med Sci. 2005;20:483–8.

Harry T. Chugani

Why Has Molecular Neuroimaging of Neurodegenerative Disorders Lagged in Children?

In general, neuroimaging in children has been considered cumbersome for several reasons, the most important being that young children typically move during the procedure and therefore need to be sedated. However, compared to MRI scans, the period of sedation at least for 2-deoxy-2(^{18}F)fluoro-D-glucose (FDG) PET scans is actually quite short. Indeed, current high-resolution high-sensitivity PET scanners require sedation for less than 20 min to acquire static glucose metabolism images. During the "uptake" period of 30–40 min, the child actually needs to be awake in a separate quiet room. Furthermore, some movement by the child during image acquisition can be corrected using software tools.

Excessive radiation exposure has often been cited as an obstacle when applying molecular imaging in children, but the actual exposure is minimal and has been accepted by radiation safety agencies for more than three decades in clinical studies on children with refractory epilepsy. Since many hospitals now have good access to PET scanners for oncology imaging and the ^{18}FDG radiotracer for studies of glucose

metabolism is purchased (around US\$120 per dose) and delivered on the same day as the scheduled scan, access to PET scanners should no longer be considered an obstacle. Therefore, although children remain admittedly more difficult to study than adults, with relatively minimal additional effort they should not be denied the benefits of molecular neuroimaging.

Importance of Molecular Imaging biomarkers in Pediatric Neurodegenerative Disorders

MRI scans remain the first line neuroimaging test and may assist in the initial diagnosis of neurodegenerative disorders. However, with few exceptions, MRI does not provide useful biomarkers to assess *disease progression* or *response to treatment*. In contrast, molecular neuroimaging allows biochemical/physiological changes to be quantified thus providing a more accurate window of the *rate* of neurodegeneration through serial studies. It is timely to discuss this advantage because current advances in precision medicine are introducing new treatments for some of the rare neurodegenerative disorders in children. At present, although some molecular imaging biomarkers appear to be sensitive to progression, the numbers of patients studied thus far are small.

This concept is well illustrated in the case of Dravet syndrome, an epileptic channelopathy

H. T. Chugani (✉)
Department of Neurology, NYU School of Medicine, New York, NY, USA
e-mail: Harry.Chugani@nyulangone.org

Fig. 15.1 FDG PET images in a child with Dravet syndrome (SCN1A pathogenic mutation) at 2 time points. At age 1 year, glucose metabolism appears normal, whereas at age 5 years there is severe hypometabolism in frontal, parietal and temporal cortex, and thalamus with relative sparing of the occipital cortex and basal ganglia

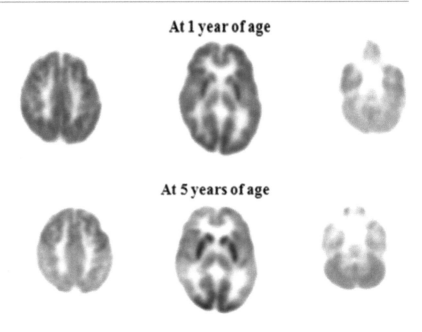

caused in 70–80% of cases by a pathogenic mutation in the SCN1A gene. Other gene alterations also resulting in Dravet syndrome include PCDH19, GABARG2, SCN1B, and probably others. MRI scans in these children typically show normal findings in the early stages and, eventually, nonspecific brain atrophy.

In contrast, FDG PET is far more useful clinically. In 4 of 8 children with Dravet syndrome, Ferrie et al. [1] reported PET abnormalities (unilateral, bilateral, diffuse hypometabolism) in brain regions suspected to be abnormal based on seizure semiology. In our longitudinal molecular imaging study on three children with Dravet syndrome (documented SCN1A gene mutations), we reported a normal pattern of glucose metabolism when the children were 1 year of age or younger [2]. However, when studied again at 4 years of age or later, all three children had developed bilateral glucose hypometabolism, most pronounced in frontal, parietal, and temporal cortex and thalamus without significant focal features (Fig. 15.1). These findings are further supported by Haginoya et al. [3] who similarly evaluated eight children with Dravet syndrome with a single PET scan after the late infantile period and reported extensive cortical hypometabolism. Thus, FDG PET provides a unique tool to study

the dynamic course of Dravet syndrome. An important question to be asked is whether the PET changes are reversible (or can be altogether prevented) with treatment and could thus serve as a biomarker. This question becomes extremely relevant now that new pharmacological treatments (e.g., fenfluramine, cannabis) have been introduced for the treatment of Dravet syndrome [4].

This illustration in Dravet syndrome will be the central theme of this chapter in which we will explore the same principles in a number of pediatric neurodegenerative disorders in which PET has been performed. We analyze its contributory role toward diagnosis and clinical management including the search for molecular imaging biomarkers as new treatments become available.

Inborn Errors of Metabolism

Inborn errors of metabolism form a large class of genetic diseases the majority of which are due to defects of single genes that code for enzymes which facilitate conversion of various substrates into other chemicals. Failure of this conversion results in accumulation of various substances and neurotoxicity.

Most of the case reports and small series on PET imaging in the inborn errors of metabolism have come from King Faisal Specialist Hospital in Saudi Arabia. The high incidence of parental consanguinity in Saudi Arabia, together with the rich resources in medical technology, make this country an ideal setting to investigate a number of rare inherited neurodegenerative disorders, which often arise from consanguineous union. Not surprisingly, brain glucose metabolism has been studied in Saudi children with diverse inborn errors of metabolism using PET. Although the numbers of children studied are small, and sometimes described in case reports, the potential of PET scanning to further our understanding of pathophysiology, and to monitor disease progression and response to new treatments is emphasized repeatedly in these publications.

Al-Essa et al. [5] studied eight patients with *glutaric aciduria type 1*, an organic aciduria where the body is unable to metabolize the amino acids lysine, hydroxylysine, and tryptophan. Excessive levels of these amino acids and their intermediate breakdown products are neurotoxic, particularly to the basal ganglia. Both MRI and PET showed involvement of the putamina in all eight subjects studied. The PET scans demonstrated hypometabolism in the head of the caudate nuclei in all of the patients. Brain atrophy and the "open" Sylvian fissures were better demonstrated by MRI, whereas the cerebral cortex and thalami appeared structurally normal in all patients. PET showed decreased FDG uptake in the cerebral cortex in seven, and in the thalami in three patients. The authors concluded that both PET and MRI are clinically useful when evaluating children with *glutaric aciduria type 1*.

Al-Essa et al. [6] also performed PET studies in four patients with *3-methylglutaconic aciduria*, another organic aciduria which consists of at least five metabolic disorders impairing energy production in the mitochondria, leading to the build-up of 3-methylglutaconic acid and 3-methylglutaric acid. These investigators found three patterns of abnormality which allowed them to classify the progression of the disorder into three stages (Fig. 15.2). In stage I, there was absent uptake in the heads of the caudate, accompanied by mildly decreased thalamic and cerebellar metabolism. In stage II, there was absent uptake in the anterior half and posterior quarter of the putamina, in addition to mild-moderate hypometabolism in the cerebral cortex especially in the parieto-temporal region and with continued progression of thalamic and cerebellar hypometabolism. The characteristic feature of stage III was a total absence of metabolic activity in the putamina and severe hypometabolism of the cerebral cortex and cerebellum consistent with brain atrophy seen on MRI. This study demonstrates that PET could identify useful molecular imaging biomarkers to allow staging of the disease, and these patterns can be used to monitor disease progression. However, it should be noted that the disorder itself is heterogeneous (at least five subtypes) and therefore it is conceivable that different subtypes were being studied. Clearly, much more remains to be done in order to sort out disease progression through serial studies in the same patient.

Indeed, *serial* MRI and PET scans of brain glucose metabolism were performed by Al-Essa et al. [7] in five children with *proprionic acidemia*, an organic aciduria in which mutations in the *PCCA* or *PCCB* gene disrupt the function of the enzyme propionyl-CoA carboxylase thus preventing the normal breakdown of certain proteins and fats. These investigators found early PET and MRI scans to be normal. As the disease progressed, MRI showed atrophy and abnormal signal in caudate and putamen with normal thalami, whereas PET showed *increased* uptake in basal ganglia and thalami with further progression to *decreased* uptake in basal ganglia. The serial studies uncovered a period of *transient hypermetabolism* in the basal ganglia demonstrating that the neurodegeneration process in this disorder follows a dynamic course characterized by molecular signals visible on neuroimaging. This very important study allows various hypotheses to be formulated, including clinical staging, halting progression or even reversing the molecular signals with treatment.

There have also been a number of case reports of FDG PET scanning in various other inborn errors of metabolism. A 2-year-old boy with *eth-*

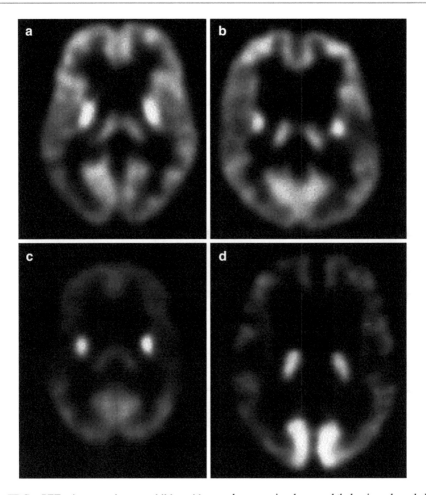

Fig. 15.2 FDG PET images in a child with 3-methylglutaconic aciduria. (**a**) Stage I: absent [18]FDG uptake in the head of the caudate, mild decreased thalamic and cerebellar metabolism. (**b, c**) Stage II: absent uptake in the anterior half and posterior quarter of the putamina, the heads of the caudate, decreased uptake in the cerebral cortex more prominently in the parieto-temporal lobes, and progressive decreased thalamic and cerebellar uptake. (**d**) Stage III: absent uptake in the putamen and heads of the caudate, and severe decreased cortical uptake consistent with brain atrophy. There was further decreased cerebellar uptake. The thalamic activity seems to increase (at least relatively) as compared with cortical activity. (Reprinted with permission from Elsevier from [6])

ylmalonic aciduria (an inborn error of short chain fatty acid β-oxidation) showed a normal MRI scan but bilateral intense *hypermetabolism* in the caudate and putamen on PET (Fig. 15.3). One year later, PET showed bilateral hypometabolism in the putamen, caudate head, and frontal cortex, whereas MRI showed atrophy and infarcts in the basal ganglia [8]. These findings are consistent with the selective vulnerability of the basal ganglia in this disorder. An obvious issue to be addressed here is the timing of the hypermetabolism and its relation to the clinical course.

It can be seen from above that various inborn errors of metabolism show somewhat different patterns of abnormality in glucose metabolism, depending upon which areas of the brain are most affected (or selectively vulnerable) to the accumulated toxins. These patterns of abnormality provide important clues toward our understanding of the pathophysiologic processes involved in injury to the brain from the metabolic errors. However, to identify precise biomarkers in these disorders will require larger numbers of patients to be studied, perhaps in multicenter collabora-

Fig. 15.3 (**a, b**) FDG PET images in a 6 months-old-infant with ethylmalonic aciduria showing intense bilateral hypermetabolism in the caudate nucleus and putamen and mild frontal cortex hypometabolism. (**a, b**): Repeat PET at 20 months of age showed evolution to hypometabolism in caudate and putamen reflecting progressive basal ganglia degeneration. The frontal lobe hypometabolism has also worsened. Reprinted with permission from Elsevier from [8]

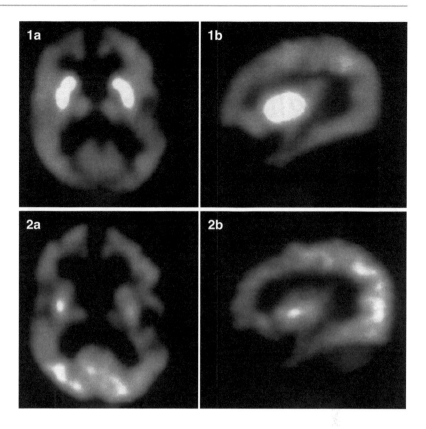

tions due to the rarity of these disorders or perhaps in countries where certain of these disorders are more prevalent. An exciting and clinically translatable aspect of this research is to determine whether the PET abnormalities described above for various inborn errors of metabolism might show an improvement (or even normalize) following treatment interventions but, unfortunately, to date there have been no such published studies.

- There are many inborn errors of metabolism other than the organic acidurias described above. "Pediatric neurotransmitter disease" includes a group of genetic disorders affecting the synthesis, metabolism, and catabolism of neurotransmitters in children. These inborn errors of metabolism affect the central nervous system in children and if left untreated can lead to severe neurological abnormalities.

Succinic semialdehyde dehydrogenase (SSADH) deficiency is an autosomal recessive inborn error of metabolism caused by mutations in the ALDH5A1 gene. This disorder is also known as *4-hydroxybutyric aciduria*. The mutation results in a failure to break down the neurotransmitter GABA and, as a result, there is accumulation and toxicity from excess GABA and a related chemical gamma hydroxybutyrate (GHB). The symptoms are variable and may include intellectual disability, seizures, ataxia, hypotonia, and nystagmus. MRI scan in these children may show atrophy of the cerebellar vermis. Indeed, FDG PET in one such child revealed a marked decrease in cerebellar metabolism [9].

Since molecular imaging of GABA neurotransmission is available, Pearl et al. [10] measured GABA$_A$ receptor binding using the radiotracer ^{11}C-flumazenil in seven patients with SSADH deficiency. Reduced binding was observed in amygdala, hippocampus, cerebellar vermis, frontal, parietal, and occipital cortex in patients with SSADH deficiency compared to healthy controls (Fig. 15.4). These findings were interpreted as a downregulation of GABA$_A$ recep-

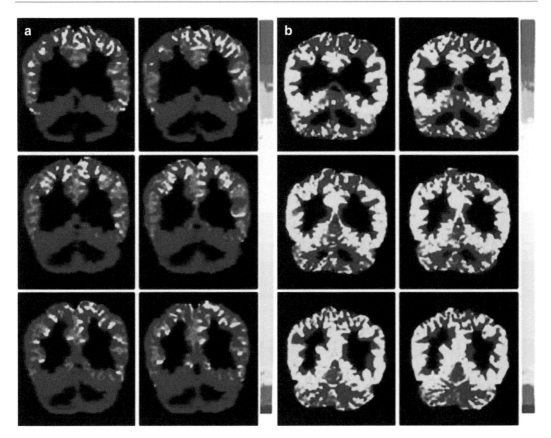

Fig. 15.4 ^{11}C-flumazenil PET scans in a patient with succinic semialdehyde dehydrogenase (SSADH) deficiency (**a**) and in a control subject (**b**). Note the severe reduction of GABA$_A$ receptor binding involving multiple regions in the patient. (Reprinted with permission from Wolters Kluwer Health, Inc. from [10])

tors in response to the high endogenous brain GABA levels. Further studies using transcranial magnetic stimulation and murine genetic models of mutations in the ALDH5A1 gene have led to therapeutic trials where ^{11}C-flumazenil PET scanning might provide an important measure of treatment response [11].

Neuronal Ceroid Lipofuscinosis (NCL)

At least 20 pathogenic gene alterations are associated with the various neuronal ceroid lipofuscinoses (NCL, sometimes called Batten disease), which were previously classified only according to age of onset. Symptoms vary widely depending on the specific type of NCL, and may include mental regression, blindness, epilepsy, ataxia, and

various neuromuscular features ranging from decreased to increased muscle tone. Up until recently, management strategies consisted only of palliative care and attention to quality of life [12]. Even now, there is only one FDA-approved drug for NCL (Brineura), which is a cerebrospinal fluid administered enzyme replacement therapy with the active ingredient being cerliponase alfa [13]. Brineura is a recombinant form of human TPP$_1$, the enzyme deficient in patients with the CLN$_2$ type of NCL and, therefore, applicable only to this NCL subtype. Since MRI scans are poorly sensitive to disease stages in NCL, showing only nonspecific brain atrophy which gradually worsens, reliable biomarkers of disease progression could be incorporated immediately into the management of CLN$_2$ and treatment with Brineura.

The first molecular neuroimaging study on NCL was performed by De Volder et al. [14] on four siblings with NCL. FDG PET showed hypo-metabolism in gray matter structures, most pro-nounced in thalamus and posterior association cortex. There was a positive relationship between severity of hypometabolism and the degree of clinical impairment in these four children. Subsequently, our group described a similar pat-tern of glucose hypometabolism in seven unrelated subjects with Spielmeyer-Vogt disease, which is associated with mutations in the CLN$_3$ gene [15]. Five of the seven patients showed a distinctive age-related progression with hypome-tabolism starting in the calcarine cortex and pro-gressing rostrally to involve the entire cerebral cortex. In the advanced stages of the disease, glu-cose metabolism remained only in the basal gan-glia and brainstem with little to no FDG uptake in the cerebral cortex (Fig. 15.5), consistent with

the classic findings of an isoelectric (flat) electro-encephalogram (EEG) at this stage. These find-ings have been replicated by others [16, 17], but there have been no large studies to further develop and validate this unusual pattern of glucose metabolism as a clinical tool or biomarker.

Molecular imaging of neurotransmitters has also been attempted in NCL. For example, imaging of dopamine receptors in NCL has shown only nonspecific findings consisting of a mild decrease of D1 receptor binding with no change in D2 binding compared to controls [18]. We suggest focusing on a systematic serial FDG PET study on the various subtypes of NCL to determine "metabolic staging" and subse-quently incorporating FDG PET into clinical tri-als (e.g., Brineura trial) as they become available.

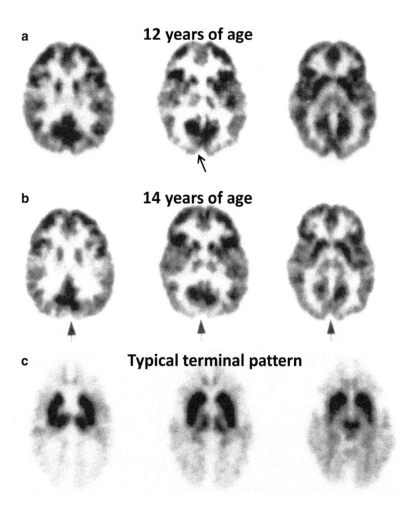

Fig. 15.5 (a) PET images of glucose metabolism in a 12-year-old child with NCL, showing only very mild calcarine cortex hypometabolism (arrow); (b) Two years later, there has been progression of posterior cortex hypometabolism (arrowheads) with sparing of the frontal lobes; (c) hypometabolism is widespread in the advanced stages of the disease in a different child with activity remaining only in the striatum, brainstem and to some extent the thalamus

Niemann-Pick Type C Disease

Niemann-Pick type C (NPC), sometimes referred to as "Childhood Alzheimer's," is a lysosomal storage disease associated with mutations in NPC1 and NPC2 genes. NPC affects an estimated 1:150,000 people. Approximately, 50% of cases present before 10 years of age, but often the diagnosis is missed until much later. Clinical features are broad, including progressive intellectual deterioration, hepatosplenomegaly, cerebellar ataxia, cataplexy, neuromuscular, and psychiatric symptoms. The first PET study of glucose metabolism in NMC was performed on identical 4-year-old twin girls and this revealed mild diffuse cortical hypometabolism, particularly in the medial frontal cortex (Fig. 15.6a) [19]. When studied again at age 6 years, there had been dramatic progression in both twins to severe hypometabolism in medial and inferior frontal cortex, thalamus, as well as parietal (medial and lateral

portions) and temporal cortex (Fig. 15.6b); the MRI scan remained normal (Fig. 15.6c). This unusual pattern of glucose hypometabolism had not been reported in other pediatric disorders and, therefore, sparked interest in using PET as a tool toward earlier diagnosis of NMC and, perhaps to monitor disease progression and response to new interventions. As mentioned above, new treatments are emerging (albeit slowly) for the various pediatric neurodegenerative disorders and, for NMC, miglustat (Zavesca, Actelion Pharmaceuticals, Allschwil, Switzerland) is now in use [20]. This is a small iminosugar molecule which reversibly inhibits glycosphingolipid synthesis. Longitudinal FDG PET studies in both treated and untreated patients will be of immense value in tracking disease progression.

This notion is supported by the study of Benussi et al. [21], who reported monozygotic twins with NMC, one of who was severely affected while the other had only very mild

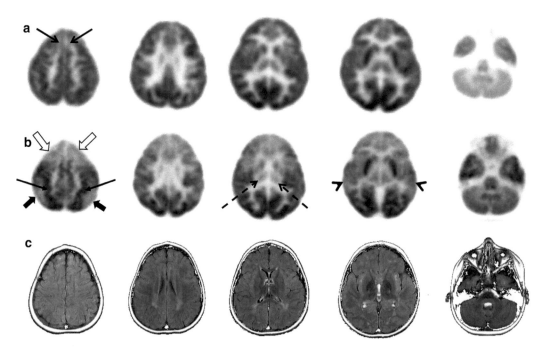

Fig. 15.6 (a) PET images showing glucose hypometabolism in medial frontal cortex (arrows) at age 4 years in one of the twins with Niemann-Pick C disease. (b) At age 6 years, with clinical progression, there is now also metabolic progression to include most of the frontal cortex (hollow arrows), thalamus (dotted arrows), temporal (arrowheads) and parietal cortex (thick short arrows). The deeper layers of the parietal cortex show relatively higher metabolism (long thin arrows). The pattern of hypometabolism in parietal cortex is unique and has not been reported in other disorders of childhood. (c) Normal MRI scan

impairment. PET scans in both twins showed frontal and temporal cortex hypometabolism, but the abnormality was more pronounced in the more affected twin. In addition, Huang et al. [22] reported MRI, MRS, and glucose metabolism PET findings in a 22-year-old male with NMC, showing progressive (age 19 and 22 years) cerebral atrophy particularly in the frontal regions and white matter changes posteriorly. No major findings were seen on MRS, but the PET at 22 years showed hypometabolism in the bilateral prefrontal cortex and dorsomedial thalamus.

There has been much recent interest in the molecular imaging of inflammation in the brain, since so many of the neurodegenerative disorders (both in adults and in children) are mediated by primary or secondary neuroinflammation. Various radiotracers that bind to the protein TSPO in the mitochondria of microglia have been developed. TSPO binding is upregulated when microglia are activated such as during inflammation. We studied a patient with NMC using PET with ^{11}C-PK11195 (a first generation TSPO-binding agent) and reported increased uptake in and around the deep gray matter structures (Fig. 15.7) [23]. TSPO PET could be a very useful clinical biomarker to monitor disease progression and treatment response in neurological disorders associated with neuroinflammation. More sensitive second and third generation

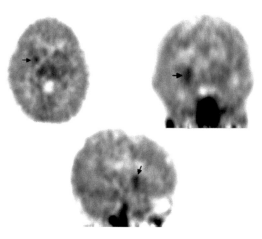

Fig. 15.7 PET scan using ^{11}C-PK11195 in a child with Niemann-Pick C showing inflammation in and around the deep gray matter structures (arrows)

TSPO-binding radiotracers have been developed since our study and will likely significantly impact the management of these disorders. In the case of NMC, both glucose metabolism PET as well as TSPO PET could prove to be useful in monitoring efficacy of treatment with miglustat in children. There are a number of studies using PET in the adult form of NMC, discussed elsewhere in this volume.

Juvenile Huntington's Disease

Even prior to brain atrophy on structural neuroimaging, FDG PET studies show hypometabolism in the caudate nuclei of adult patients with Huntington's disease (HD) [24]. An in-depth discussion of molecular neuroimaging in adults with HD is provided elsewhere in this volume.

There have been far fewer PET studies on children with HD, also referred to as juvenile HD, which has a different phenotype than the adult form. De Volder et al. [25] found markedly decreased glucose metabolism in caudate nuclei with sparing of the cerebral cortex in two children with juvenile HD. This pattern of hypometabolism is identical to that seen in adult HD subjects even though the phenotypes show distinct differences. Adult HD patients typically present with cognitive difficulties followed by gait disturbances and chorea, whereas juvenile HD patients are more likely to manifest epilepsy, muscle stiffness, and less often chorea. Our own studies have also found striking caudate nuclei hypometabolism in juvenile HD (Fig. 15.8), but Matthews et al. [26] found additional hypometabolism in the posterior thalamus. More recently, Zhou et al. [27] performed a dual PET study on a 16-year-old boy with juvenile HD using both FDG and ^{18}F-dihydrotetrabenazine (DTBZ, a measure of vesicular-monoamine-transporter-type 2 [VMAT2] binding). They reported hypometabolism and decreased ^{18}F-DTBZ binding in the striatum.

Of some relevance is the study of Diggle et al. [28], who reported germline PDE10A mutations in eight individuals from two families that manifested early-onset hyperkinetic movement disor-

Fig. 15.8 FDG PET images from a child with juvenile Huntington's disease showing marked hypometabolism in the caudate nuclei (arrows)

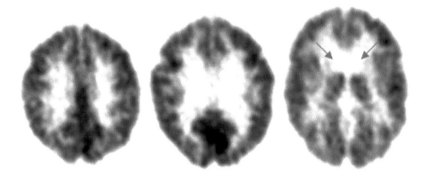

der. PDE10A is a key regulator of striatal circuitry. One of the affected individuals had a PET scan using [^{11}C]IMA107 to image PDE10A activity and this showed a significant decrease of PDE10A signal in the striatum, which appeared normal on MRI. Thus, [^{11}C]IMA107 PET may be a useful new tool to investigate both adult and juvenile HD.

There has been little success in pharmacological treatments for HD. However, there is considerable effort in developing gene therapy, including antisense oligonucleotides, small interfering RNAs, and gene editing for treating HD and, therefore, PET biomarkers will likely be integral to upcoming clinical trials.

Dystonia

Dystonia is a symptom rather than a disease per se and can be caused by a number of progressive and non-progressive disorders. In children, the most common conditions manifesting with dystonia include the inherited dystonias (mutations in DYT1, DYT6, DYT11, and other genes), metabolic disorders, toxins, some medications, autoimmune disorders, and hypoxic-ischemic brain injury. Several studies have used PET methodology to investigate dystonia in children. Szyszko et al. [29] performed FDG PET scans in 15 children with primary (inherited) dystonia and 12 dystonic children who had neurodegeneration with brain iron accumulation (NBIA, a metabolic disease). No major abnormalities could be appreciated in either group upon visual inspection of the images. However, quantitative analysis

showed higher uptake in posterior cingulate and posterior putamina, but lower uptake in occipital cortex and cerebellum in the NBIA subjects compared to those with primary dystonia. A major confounding factor in this study was that the two groups of children did not show the same degree of dystonia, which was more severe in the NBIA group. These investigators proposed that the more severe dystonia in the NBIA group may be related to higher activity in the putamen and lower activity in cerebellum and that perhaps the putamen/cerebellum ratio of glucose metabolism might serve as a useful biomarker to monitor severity of dystonia.

The most common form of dystonia in children is dystonic cerebral palsy, also known as athetoid cerebral palsy or dyskinetic cerebral palsy, which follows the "near-total" type of hypoxic-ischemic injury (HIE) during birth, such as with placental abruption, uterine rupture or umbilical cord prolapse. The dystonia in these children is static rather than progressive. We have reported an acute transient "hypermetabolism" on FDG PET in the basal ganglia followed by a unique pattern of severe hypometabolism in the lenticular nuclei and thalami when studied in the chronic stages and having developed dystonic cerebral palsy [30] (Fig. 15.9). This chronic pattern on FDG PET was reported earlier by our group in five children with dystonic cerebral palsy [31] and is a reliable biomarker of the "near-total" type of HIE during birth, distinct from the "partial prolonged" asphyxia. Acute hypermetabolism in the basal ganglia supports the long-held notion of selective vulnerability of this region to "near-total" neonatal asphyxia, per-

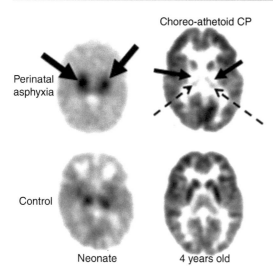

Choreo-athetoid CP

Perinatal
asphyxia

Control

Neonate   4 years old

Fig. 15.9 FDG PET scan of a child who suffered hypoxic-ischemic encephalopathy at birth and later developed dystonic/choreoathetoid cerebral palsy. The left image from the newborn period showed intense hypermetabolism in the basal ganglia (solid arrows) compared to control. The right image at 5 years of age showed severe hypometabolism in the lenticular nuclei (solid arrows) and thalami (dotted arrows). Note the relative preservation of metabolism in the cerebral cortex

haps related to the transient excess of glutamate receptors seen in the newborn basal ganglia compared to older children and adults [32]. We have suggested that the transition from hypermetabolism to hypometabolism indicates the culmination of the brain injury due to excitotoxic mechanisms, which are mediated by glutamatergic neurotransmission. Furthermore, the in-depth study of these FDG patterns in new treatments of newborn HIE, such as brain or total body cooling, may provide important insights into understanding cerebral palsy associated with HIE.

Since pharmacological manipulation of the dopamine system is widely used to treat dystonia, it seems logical to perform PET scans of dopamine neurotransmission in dystonic subjects. Indeed, Rinne et al. [33] evaluated three aspects of the dopaminergic system (dopamine transporter, D1 and D2 receptors) using PET and specific dopamine radiotracers. Their study population consisted of seven patients who suffered from dopa-responsive dystonia, a diverse group of inherited dystonias which improve dra-

matically with levodopa treatment. All seven patients underwent the three PET studies of the dopamine system. Increased D2 receptor binding in putamen and caudate nucleus were seen in the patients compared to controls, but no changes were seen in D1 receptor or dopamine transporter binding. Thus, monitoring of D2 receptor binding with PET may be useful in assessing the various types of dystonia.

Gene therapy is being developed for some disorders that manifest dystonia. Recently, Onuki et al. [34] evaluated eight children who underwent gene therapy for aromatic l-amino acid decarboxylase (AADC) deficiency. Using PET with 6-[^{18}F]fluoro-l-m-tyrosine (FMT), a specific AADC tracer, they were able to show a gradual increase of FMT uptake in the putamen. This is just one example of how molecular imaging will play an important role in gene therapy for pediatric neurodegenerative disorders.

Mitochondrial Disorders

Leigh syndrome and MELAS syndrome (mitochondrial encephalomyopathy, lactic acidosis, and stroke-like episodes) are two of the most frequent mitochondrial diseases of childhood. Both are severe and disabling without cure, but various vitamins and supplements may offer some relief and slowing of the degenerative course. These include various combinations (mitochondrial cocktails) of coenzyme Q10, alpha lipoic acid, riboflavin, arginine (for stroke-like events), folinic acid, and L-carnitine.

PET methodology allows the study of mitochondrial function and dynamics, as well as stoichiometry. Brain clearance of ^{11}C-pyruvate was measured in two patients with mitochondrial encephalomyopathy and one with Leigh disease using PET [35]. These investigators reported increased uptake of the radiotracer in cerebral cortex, basal ganglia, and thalamus, as well as slower brain clearance of the ^{11}C-pyruvate compared to patients with epilepsy who served as a control group.

In another study, Yokoi et al. [36] examined pyruvate turnover from brain and epicranial muscles using ^{11}C-pyruvate PET in six patients with mitochondrial encephalomyopathy. The time-activity curve for ^{11}C in both brain and muscle for both normal subjects and patients consisted of a fast and a slow component, likely representing the aerobic (mitochondrial) and anaerobic (glycolytic) metabolism of pyruvate, respectively. In the brain and muscle of patients, the aerobic component was smaller whereas the anaerobic component was larger compared to the normal subjects. In general, the extent of this abnormality correlated with the severity of disease. A milder abnormality for [^{11}C]pyruvate turnover was also seen in the brains of presymptomatic patients. Collectively, these very important studies provide evidence that ^{11}C-pyruvate PET may be useful for the evaluation of brain mitochondrial energy metabolism in mitochondrial disorders and could be applied to monitor disease progression and response to treatments.

Using a different PET approach, Shishido et al. [37] measured cerebral blood flow (CBF), oxygen metabolism (CMRO2), and glucose metabolism (CMRGlc) in five patients with mitochondrial encephalomyopathy. The molar ratio between the oxygen and glucose consumptions was reduced diffusely, as CMRO2 was markedly decreased (due to impaired oxidative metabolism) and CMRGlc was slightly reduced (anaerobic glycolysis relatively stimulated). There were no major changes in CBF.

Another interesting study [38] combined proton magnetic resonance spectroscopy (^{1}H MRS) and FDG PET to evaluate brain energetics in two children with congenital lactic acidosis, which is often seen in pediatric mitochondrial disorders. A massive increase of glycolysis was seen, likely due to the high demand of energy consumption in the developing brain [39], resulting in lactate accumulation/acidosis.

Haginoya et al. [40] performed FDG PET in five children with Leigh syndrome, 4 of who had reported gene mutations in their mitochondrial DNA. Hypometabolism was noted in the basal ganglia and cerebellum of the patients compared to controls, likely related to the dystonia and ataxia in the patients.

In summary, PET with various selected radiotracers is a potentially powerful tool to calculate the stoichiometry of mitochondrial function in children with mitochondrial disorders and monitor progression of the disease. A better understanding of brain energetics will lead to new interventions for mitochondrial disorders. In this regard, combined PET/MRI data acquisitions using new hybrid PET/MR scanners provide a powerful clinical approach since both PET and MR datasets can be acquired in the same session and the child is sedated (if necessary) only once.

Rett Syndrome

Rett syndrome is a neurodegenerative disorder that primarily affects girls. In the first 6–18 months, development appears to be normal, then developmental progress is halted, followed by the rapid loss of previously acquired language and motor skills. Repetitive stereotypic hand movements, autistic features, apnea or hyperpnea, gait ataxia, apraxia, and seizures may also be seen. Classic Rett syndrome is caused by mutations in the MECP2 gene, although atypical forms associated with other mutations are also seen. Despite various treatments that have been attempted for symptom control, there is no cure for Rett syndrome.

Naidu et al. [41] performed a multimodal neuroimaging study on a number of subjects with Rett syndrome (unclear how many patients were studied). The tests included MRI volumetry, magnetic resonance spectroscopy (MRS), diffusion tensor imaging (DTI), cerebral blood flow measurements with MRI, and FDG PET. Brain volumetry showed reductions in both gray and white matter. The frontal lobe in Rett syndrome appeared particularly vulnerable as it showed a preferential reduction of blood flow on MRI, increased choline and reduced n-acetyl aspartate (NAA) on MRS, and *hypermetabolism* on FDG PET, which the authors attributed to increased glutamate cycling in synapses.

Studies evaluating nigrostriatal function in Rett syndrome have also been performed. Using PET in nine patients with Rett syndrome, Dunn et al. [42] found reduced fluorodopa uptake in caudate and putamen, but increased dopamine D2 receptor binding in the same regions. These observations suggested a mild presynaptic deficit of nigrostriatal activity. Further studies showed that D2 receptor density was significantly reduced in the striatum of women with Rett syndrome compared to control subjects and, moreover, dopaminergic dysfunction was also present in the MECP2-deficient mouse model of the disease [43]. These findings should be explored further and may lead to discovery of useful clinical biomarkers as treatments become available for Rett syndrome. Finally, a recent review [44] provides an excellent summary of new radiotracers being developed preclinically that could be applied in the clinical arena for Rett syndrome.

Lysosomal Storage Diseases

There are over 70 rare inherited metabolic disorders resulting from defects in lysosomal function; collectively, these are known as lysosomal storage diseases. Lysosomes are cellular organelles containing enzymes which digest large molecules and allow the fragments to be recycled within the cell. When one of the enzymes is defective due to a pathogenic mutation, the large molecules are not metabolized and will be "stored" in the cell resulting in toxicity and cell death. Because these are rare disorders, molecular imaging studies have been limited to case reports. Even so, some interesting observations have emerged. Again, these have been from populations with high parental consanguinity.

FDG PET in a 2-year-old Saudi boy with *infantile GM1 gangliosidosis* revealed a mild hypometabolism in the basal ganglia, moderate to severe hypometabolism in thalamus and visual cortex, and a hypermetabolic focus in the left frontal lobe, presumed to be an epileptic focus [45]. Since the EEG was not monitored during the FDG uptake period, it is not clear whether the hypermetabolism was related to ictal activity versus some other process related to brain toxicity.

The MRI scan showed only nonspecific findings of mild diffuse brain atrophy and dysmyelination/demyelination.

The pattern of injury is totally different in a patient with *juvenile GM2 gangliosidosis* where MRI at ages 2, 4, and 6 years revealed progressive brain atrophy, particularly affecting the thalamus. FDG PET at age 6 years showed diffuse hypometabolism, also particularly involving thalamus (Fig. 15.10) [46]. Thus, selectively vulnerable brain regions are dependent upon the type of unmetabolized molecule, in at least the gangliosidoses and probably also in other lysosomal storage disorders. If confirmed in larger studies, these metabolic features on PET scanning may be useful as diagnostic aids as well as biomarkers.

In a 2-year-old Saudi boy with *infantile Krabbe's disease*, MRI revealed nonspecific findings of mild brain atrophy and white matter disease mainly in the centrum semiovale. In contrast, FDG PET showed marked hypometabolism in the left cerebral cortex and no uptake in the caudate heads, but the thalami, lentiform nuclei, and cerebellum appeared normal [47]. The severe hypometabolism in the heads of the caudate nuclei may be related to the neuromuscular features of this disorder and could be useful in monitoring disease progression.

Increased understanding of the genetics and molecular biological mechanisms contributing to the pathophysiology of the lysosomal storage diseases have led to active investigations in search for new treatment approaches, such as enzyme replacement therapy and gene therapy [48]. For example, preliminary studies in *Krabbe's disease* suggest that hematopoietic stem cell transplantation (umbilical cord blood stem cells) may be an effective treatment in affected babies who are presymtomatic and in older people with a milder form of the disease. Molecular neuroimaging with PET may provide much needed biomarkers in the lysosomal storage disorders to monitor the natural history as well as the effects of emerging treatments.

Fig. 15.10 MRI and
FDG PET scans in a
child with juvenile GM2
gangliosidosis. The MRI
scans at ages 3 (**a**), 4 (**b**)
and 6 (**c**) years showed
progressive cerebral
atrophy, particularly
involving thalamus.
Glucose metabolism
PET scan at age 6 years
(**a, b**) showed diffuse
cerebral
hypometabolism, also
particularly involving
thalamus. Note relative
sparing of basal ganglia.
(Reprinted with
permission from
Springer Nature from
[46])

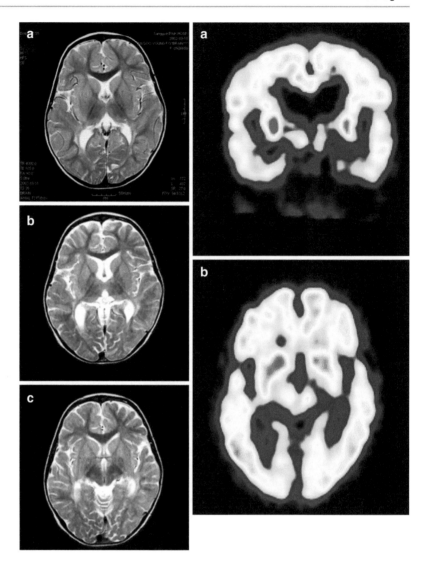

Dysmyelinating Disorders

Dysmyelination refers to the abnormal formation of myelin which, as a result, functions abnormally. This is distinct from demyelination, where normal myelin formation has occurred but then, due to a disease process (often autoimmune), the myelin is broken down and functions abnormally. In children, dysmyelinating disorders are typically neurogenetic, resulting from various pathogenic mutations. There is considerable overlap among these neurogenetic disorders so that a specific disease may be classified into more than on category. For example, Krabbe disease

(discussed above) is classified as a lysosomal disorder but can also be classified as a dysmyelinating disorder.

Molecular neuroimaging with PET has been applied to several progressive *dysmyelinating* disorders in children. Sawaishi et al. [49] studied a 13-year-old boy with *juvenile Alexander disease* (an autosomal dominant leukodystrophy caused by GFAP gene mutation) using FDG PET, which showed hypometabolism in the frontal white matter corresponding to leukodystrophic regions, with preserved glucose metabolism in the overlying gray matter.

Salsano et al. [50] performed FDG PET on 12 subjects with adrenoleukodystrophy. The adrenoleukodystrophy patients showed relative hypermetabolism in frontal lobes compared to cerebellum and temporal lobes. These findings are consistent with those from a number of case reports published earlier. It cannot be determined from visual inspection of the images whether there is an "absolute" hypermetabolism in the frontal lobes versus an appearance of hypermetabolism due to the hypometabolism in posterior brain regions.

Our group [51] used ^{11}C-PK11195 PET to study neuroinflammation in a single child with X-linked adrenoleukodystrophy. Increased tracer binding (i.e., inflammation) was seen in the occipital, parietal, and posterior temporal white matter, corpus callosum genu, bilateral posterior thalami, internal capsule posterior limb, bilateral cerebral peduncles, and brainstem (Fig. 15.11). There was only minimal ^{11}C-PK11195 PET

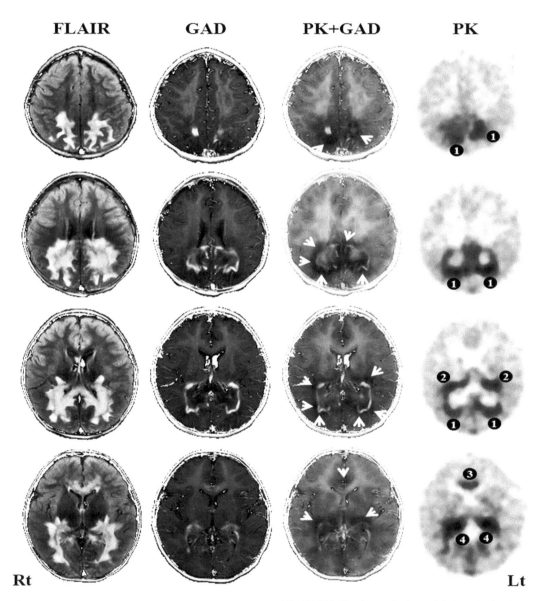

Fig. 15.11 FLAIR MRI, gadolinium enhanced T1-weighted MRI, ^{11}C-PK11195 PET images superimposed on gadolinium enhanced T1-weighted MR images (small white arrows) and ^{11}C-PK11195 PET images in child with X-linked adrenoleukodystrophy. Increased ^{11}C-PK11195 binding is seen in the occipital, parietal and posterior temporal white matter (*1*), posterior limb of internal capsule (*2*), genu of corpus callosum (*3*), bilateral posterior thalami (*4*), bilateral cerebral peduncles and brain stem (not shown here)

uptake in the cerebellum (i.e., minimal inflammation), despite previous observations of cerebellar hypometabolism. Therefore, FDG PET seems to be much less useful than ^{11}C-PK11195 PET in this disorder. We believe that ^{11}C-PK11195 PET may be a powerful tool to evaluate the inflammatory burden, disease evolution and response to novel therapeutic interventions for X-linked adrenoleukodystrophy.

Glucose Transporter Glut1 Deficiency

In Glut1 deficiency syndrome, transport of glucose across the blood–brain barrier is impeded due to a mutation in the SLC2A1 gene. Affected children may have developmental delay, intellectual disability, microcephaly, spasticity, ataxia, epilepsy, and involuntary eye movements. Although there is no cure for Glut1 deficiency syndrome, treatment with the ketogenic diet can lead to significant improvement.

Pascual et al. [52] performed FDG PET scans on 14 patients with the Glut1 deficiency syndrome based on genetic testing. Other than microcephaly, the MRI scans showed normal findings. In contrast, the PET scans showed diffuse hypometabolism in the cerebral cortex, particularly medial temporal regions and thalami, whereas the basal ganglia appeared normal. The authors suggested that this pattern of glucose metabolism may be a radiological "signature" and aid in diagnosis of this disorder. Recently, however, Natsume et al. [53] reported that the age-adjusted lenticular nuclei/thalami radioactivity ratio on PET may be a more accurate measure in diagnosing patients with Glut1 deficiency syndrome.

Lesch-Nyhan Disease

Lesch-Nyhan disease is an X-linked recessive genetic disorder that affects almost exclusively males. This disorder is caused by mutations in the gene coding for the enzyme hypoxanthine-guanine phosphoribosyltransferase (HPRT), leading to deficient enzyme activity. As a result,

there is often a marked increase in the production of uric acid and hyperuricemia.

The main symptoms are impaired kidney function, acute gouty arthritis, dystonia, and self-mutilating behaviors such as lip and finger biting and/or head banging. A deficit in basal ganglia dopamine, homovanillic acid, and dopa decarboxylase has been found in postmortem studies and further shown by PET studies. Using PET with the presynaptic radiotracer ^{18}F-fluorodopa in 12 patients with Lesch-Nyhan disease, Ernst et al. [54] reported decreased uptake in putamen (31% of control values), caudate nucleus (39%), frontal cortex (44%), and ventral tegmental complex (substantia nigra and ventral tegmentum; 57%) in the patients compared to uptake in 15 healthy control subjects. In another study, which used the PET radiotracer ^{11}C-WIN-35,428 to image dopamine transporters, Wong et al. [55] found 50–63% reduced binding in the caudate, and 64–75% reduced binding in the putamen of Lesch-Nyhan patients compared to a normal control group.

Currently, there is no specific treatment for the nervous system manifestations of Lesch-Nyhan disease. However, recent attempts using deep brain stimulation of the globus pallidi internus have shown promising results [56]. PET studies of dopamine function may provide useful biomarkers to monitor not only the disease course, but also response to treatment.

"Biomarkers" in Search of a Disease

FDG PET scans are increasingly being performed clinically on children with poorly controlled epilepsy in search for an epileptic focus for surgical treatment. For example, children with uncontrolled infantile spasms often undergo FDG PET scans as part of their surgical evaluation [57]. In performing such studies, we have observed a pattern of bitemporal hypometabolism with a consistent phenotype which included autism. These patients are not surgical candidates. We followed 18 such subjects with bilateral temporal hypometabolism for up to 10 years. Analysis of outcome in 14 of the 18 subjects revealed a relatively homogeneous phenotype: (1) all had severe developmental delay; (2) language development had been minimal or absent; (3) 10 of the 14 met the DSM-IV criteria for autistic disorder. Therefore, in patients with infantile spasms, we can offer a likely prognosis based on the FDG PET pattern even without a specific etiology for their spasms [58].

In another study, we searched for children in our FDG PET database who had any type of epilepsy and showed a more diffuse pattern of cortical hypometabolism [59]. Many of these children have developmental delay, and some have neurodegenerative conditions. All had failed to show an epileptic focus on PET. We found 31 patients showing *severe* bilateral diffuse cortical hypome-

tabolism. Of these, 14 patients were lost to follow-up and 1 patient was deceased. The remaining 16 patients (9 males) were contacted (follow-up period: 15 ± 4.8 years). MRI was normal in 12 and showed nonspecific changes in 4, not providing diagnostic information. Four of the 16 patients had a specific diagnosis, consisting of Mecp2 gene duplication, Lafora disease, 4 MB deletion of mitochondrial genome, and Sanfillipo's disease. Not surprisingly, 14 of the 16 patients continued to have seizures, likely due to patient selection bias in an epilepsy center. Twelve patients remained without an etiology. Analysis of the PET scans showed six patterns of glucose hypometabolism (Fig. 15.12).

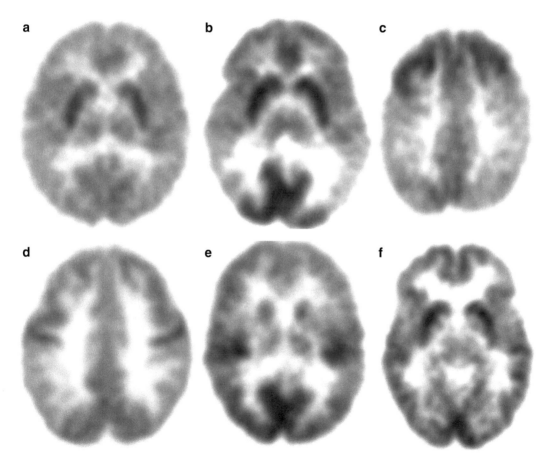

Fig. 15.12 Different patterns of bilateral diffuse glucose hypometabolism on PET scans. (**a**) Diffuse hypometabolism involving all the lobes. (**b**) Diffuse hypometabolism sparing medial occipital cortex. (**c**) Diffuse hypometabolism sparing portions of frontal cortex. (**d**) Diffuse hypo- metabolism sparing motor cortex. (**e**) Diffuse hypometabolism sparing auditory and occipital cortex. (**f**) Diffuse hypometabolism sparing medial frontal and medial occipital cortices

Unfortunately, in both of the above studies, advanced genetic testing was not available, most often due to insurance denial and, therefore, a correlation between genotype and PET phenotype could not be made. Because of the symmetric or diffuse patterns of hypometabolism on PET, it is unlikely that these diffuse and bitemporal groups of patients have underling structural brain lesions (supported by negative MRI) and are, therefore, ideal subjects for the genetic studies. These PET patterns of abnormalities may be hidden biomarkers "in search of a disease." We believe that next generation sequencing studies together with FDG PET on such patients will uncover useful biomarkers that may assist in diagnosis, clinical management, and prognosis.

Reimbursement for PET scans in Children

Unlike in adults, at present the only type of brain PET scans in children that are reimbursed by insurance carriers are for epilepsy surgery evaluation and for some brain tumors. Progressive cognitive deterioration (i.e., dementia), while reimbursed in adults, is not reimbursed for children in the USA. In other words, most of the conditions discussed in this chapter would not meet reimbursement criteria for a PET scan. One reason is that most of these pediatric neurodegenerative disorders are relatively rare and, therefore, large scale validation studies are not possible, unlike in adults with dementia. Therefore, reimbursement in children will never occur if one were to rely only on large scale validation studies. We believe that this policy is unethical since there are already a number of "potential" PET biomarkers which have been suggested in various small series or case reports of children with neurodegenerative disorders. Furthermore, these PET biomarkers, at least for FDG studies, have diagnostic and management value, not to mention the monitoring of new treatments already in place and on the horizon. The criteria for reimbursement must be modified for children for FDG PET. We agree that more specific PET scans to evaluate neurotransmitter and enzyme func-

tion, at least for now, should be assessed on a case-by-case basis, and should remain at a research level.

From a practical perspective, FDG PET imaging in children for neurodegenerative disorders is both less cumbersome and less expensive than the reimbursed studies for intractable epilepsy because concurrent electroencephalogram (EEG) monitoring during the tracer "uptake" period is not necessary for most children with neurodegenerative disorders, whereas ictal activity is typically monitored with EEG in epileptic children since it can affect image interpretation. In conclusion, the time has come to revise the guidelines for reimbursement in children and to include FDG PET imaging for neurodegenerative disorders. We believe that many of these unfortunate children will benefit from FDG PET evaluation.

References

1. Ferrie CD, Maisey M, Cox T, Polkey C, Barrington SF, Panayiotopoulos CP, Robinson RO. Focal abnormalities detected by 18FDG PET in epileptic encephalopathies. Arch Dis Child. 1996;75:102–7.
2. Kumar A, Juhász C, Luat A, Govil-Dalela T, Behen ME, Hicks MA, Chugani HT. Evolution of brain glucose metabolic abnormalities in children with epilepsy and SCN1A gene variants. J Child Neurol. 2018;33:832–6.
3. Haginoya K, Togashi N, Kantea T, et al. [^{18}F] fluorodeoxyglucose-positron emission tomography study of genetically confirmed patients with Dravet syndrome. Epilepsy Res. 2018;147:9–14.
4. Lagae L. Dravet syndrome. Curr Opin Neurol. 2021;34:213–8.
5. Al-Essa M, Bakheet S, Patay Z, Al-Watban J, Powe J, Joshi S, Ozand PT. Fluoro-2-deoxyglucose (18FDG) PET scan of the brain in glutaric aciduria type 1: clinical and MRI correlations. Brain Dev. 1998;20:295–301.
6. Al-Essa M, Bakheet S, Al-Shamsan L, Patay Z, Powe J, Ozand PT. 18Fluoro-2-deoxyglucose (18FDG) PET scan of the brain in type IV 3-methylglutaconic aciduria: clinical and MRI correlations. Brain Dev. 1999;21:24–9.
7. Al-Essa M, Bakheet S, Patay Z, Al-Shamsan L, Al-Sonbul A, Al-Watban J, Powe J, Ozand PT. 18Fluoro-2-deoxyglucose (18FDG) PET scan of the brain in propionic acidemia: clinical and MRI correlations. Brain Dev. 1999;21:312–7.
8. Al-Essa MA, al-Shamsan LA, Ozand PT. Clinical and brain 18fluoro-2-deoxyglucose positron emis-

sion tomographic findings in ethylmalonic aciduria, a progressive neurometabolic disease. Eur J Paediatr Neurol. 1999;3:125–7.

9. Al-Essa MA, Bakheet SM, Patay ZJ, Powe JE, Ozand PT. Clinical, fluorine-18 labeled 2-fluoro-2-deoxyglucose positron emission tomography (FDG PET), MRI of the brain and biochemical observations in a patient with 4-hydroxybutyric aciduria; a progressive neurometabolic disease. Brain Dev. 2000;22:127–31.

10. Pearl PL, Gibson KM, Quezado Z, et al. Decreased GABA-A binding on FMZ-PET in succinic semialdehyde dehydrogenase deficiency. Neurology. 2009;73:423–9.

11. Pearl PL, Parviz M, Vogel K, Schreiber J, Theodore WH, Gibson KM. Inherited disorders of gamma-aminobutyric acid metabolism and advances in ALDH5A1 mutation identification. Dev Med Child Neurol. 2015;57:611–7.

12. Williams RE, Adams HR, Blohm M, et al. Management strategies for CLN2 disease. Pediatr Neurol. 2017;69:102–12.

13. Mole SE, Anderson G, Band HA, et al. Clinical challenges and future therapeutic approaches for neuronal ceroid lipofuscinosis. Lancet Neurol. 2019;18:107–16.

14. De Volder AG, Cirelli S, de Barsy T, Brucher JM, Bol A, Michel C, Goffinet AM. Neuronal ceroid-lipofuscinosis: preferential metabolic alterations in thalamus and posterior association cortex demonstrated by PET. J Neurol Neurosurg Psychiatry. 1990;53:1063–7.

15. Philippart M, Messa C, Chugani HT. Spielmeyer-Vogt (batten, Spielmeyer-Sjogren) disease. Distinctive patterns of cerebral glucose utilization. Brain. 1994;117:1085–92.

16. Iannetti P, Messa C, Spalice A, Lucignani G, Fazio F. Positron emission tomography in neuronal ceroid lipofuscinosis (Jansky-Bielschowsky disease): a case report. Brain Dev. 1994;16:459–62.

17. Philippart M, da Silva E, Chugani HT. The value of positron emission tomography in the diagnosis and monitoring of late infantile and juvenile lipopigment storage disorders (so-called Batten or neuronal ceroid lipofuscinoses). Neuropediatrics. 1997;28:74–6.

18. Rinne JO, Ruottinen HM, Nagren K, Aberg LE, Santavuori P. Positron emission tomography shows reduced striatal D1 but not D2 receptors in juvenile neuronal ceroid lipofuscinosis. Neuropediatrics. 2002;33:138–41.

19. Kumar A, Chugani HT. Niemann-pick disease type C: unique 2-deoxy-2[^{18}F] fluoro-D-glucose PET abnormality. Pediatr Neurol. 2011;44:57–60.

20. Mengel E, Patterson MC, Da Riol RM, Del Toro M, Deodato F, Gautschi M, et al. Efficacy and safety of arimoclomol in Nieman-pick disease type C: results from a double-blind, ramdomised, placebo-controlled, multinational phase 2/3 trial of a novel treatment. J Inherit Metab Dis. 2021;44(6):1463–80.

21. Benussi A, Alberici A, Premi E, et al. Phenotypic heterogeneity of Niemann-pick disease type C in monozygotic twins. J Neurol. 2015;262:642–7.

22. Huang JY, Peng SF, Yang CC, Yen KY, Tzen KY, Yen RF. Neuroimaging findings in a brain with Niemann-pick type C disease. J Formos Med Assoc. 2011;110:537–42.

23. Kumar A, Chugani HT, Muzik O, Chakraborty P. [C-11]PK-11195 as a positron emission tomography biomarker of brain inflammation in children with Niemann-pick disease type-C. J Nucl Med. 2009;50(supp-2):96P.

24. Hayden MR, Martin WR, Stoessl AJ, et al. Positron emission tomography in the early diagnosis of Huntington's disease. Neurology. 1986;36:888–94.

25. De Volder A, Bol A, Michel C, Cogneau M, Evrard P, Lyon G, Goffinet AM. Brain glucose utilization in childhood Huntington's disease studied with positron emission tomography (PET). Brain Dev. 1988;10:47–50.

26. Matthews PM, Evans AC, Andermann F, Hakim AM. Regional cerebral glucose metabolism differs in adult and rigid juvenile forms of Huntington disease. Pediatr Neurol. 1989;5:353–6.

27. Zhou X-Y, Lu J-Y, Zuo C-T, Wang J, Sun Y-M. Juvenile onset hypokinetic-rigid Huntington's disease: a case with dual-tracer positron emission tomography. Quant Imaging Med Surg. 2021;11:479–82.

28. Diggle CP, Rizzo SJS, Popiolek M, et al. Biallelic mutations in PDE10A lead to loss of striatal PDE10A and a hyperkinetic movement disorder with onset in infancy. Am J Hum Genet. 2016;98:735–43.

29. Szyszko TA, Dunn JT, O'Doherty MJ, Reed L, Lin JP. Role of ^{18}F-FDG PET imaging in paediatric primary dystonia and dystonia arising from neurodegeneration with brain iron accumulation. Nucl Med Commun. 2015;36:469–76.

30. Batista CE, Chugani HT, Juhász C, Behen ME, Shankaran S. Transient hypermetabolism of the basal ganglia following perinatal hypoxia. Pediatr Neurol. 2007;36:330–3.

31. Kerrigan JF, Chugani HT, Phelps ME. Regional cerebral glucose metabolism in clinical subtypes of cerebral palsy. Pediatr Neurol. 1991;7:415–25.

32. Greenamyre T, Penney JB, Young AB, Hudson C, Silverstein FS, Johnston MV. Evidence for transient perinatal glutamatergic innervation of globus pallidus. J Neurosci. 1987;7:1022–30.

33. Rinne JO, Iivanainen M, Metsähonkala L, Vainionpää L, Pääkkönen L, Någren K, Helenius H. Striatal dopaminergic system in dopa-responsive dystonia: a multi-tracer PET study shows increased D2 receptors. J Neural Transm (Vienna). 2004;111:59–67.

34. Onuki Y, Ono S, Nakajima T, Kojima K, Taga N, Ikeda T, Kuwajima M, Kurokawa Y, Kato M, Kawai K, Osaka H, Sato T, Muramatsu S-I, Yamagata T. Dopaminergic restoration of prefrontal cortico-putaminal network in gene therapy for aromatic l-amino acid decarboxylase deficiency. Brain Commun. 2021;3:fcab078. https://doi.org/10.1093/braincomms/fcab078.

35. Toyoda M, Sakuragawa N, Arai Y, Yoshikawa H, Sugai K, Arima M, Hara T, Iio M, Satoyoshi E. Positron emission tomography using pyruvate-1-11C in two cases of mitochondrial encephalomyopathy. Ann Nucl Med. 1989;3:103–9.

36. Yokoi F, Hara T, Iio M, Nonaka I, Satoyoshi E. 1-[11C]pyruvate turnover in brain and muscle of patients with mitochondrial encephalomyopathy. A study with positron emission tomography (PET). J Neurol Sci. 1990;99:339–48.

37. Shishido F, Uemura K, Inugami A, Tomura N, Higano S, Fujita H, Sasaki H, Kanno I, Murakami M, Watahiki Y, Nagata K. Cerebral oxygen and glucose metabolism and blood flow in mitochondrial encephalomyopathy: a PET study. Neuroradiology. 1996;38:102–7.

38. Duncan DB, Herholz K, Kugel H, Roth B, Ruitenbeek W, Heindel W, Wienhard K, Heiss WD. Positron emission tomography and magnetic resonance spectroscopy of cerebral glycolysis in children with congenital lactic acidosis. Ann Neurol. 1995;37:351–8.

39. Chugani HT, Phelps ME, Mazziotta JC. Positron emission tomography study of human brain functional development. Ann Neurol. 1987;22:487–97.

40. Haginoya K, Kaneta T, Togashi N, et al. FDG-PET study of patients with Leigh syndrome. J Neurol Sci. 2016;362:309–13.

41. Naidu S, Kaufmann WE, Abrams MT, Pearlson GD, Lanham DC, Fredericksen KA, et al. Neuroimaging studies in Rett syndrome. Brain Dev. 2001;23(Suppl 1):S62–71.

42. Dunn HG, Stoessl AJ, Ho HH, MacLeod PM, Poskitt KJ, Doudet DJ, et al. Rett syndrome: investigation of nine patients, including PET scan. Can J Neurol Sci. 2002;29:345–57.

43. Wong DF, Blue ME, Brašić JR, Nandi A, Valentine H, Stansfield KH, et al. Are dopamine receptor and transporter changes in Rett syndrome reflected in Mecp2-deficient mice? Exp Neurol. 2018;307:74–81.

44. Kong Y, Li Q-B, Yuan C-H, Jiang X-F, Zhang G-Q, Cheng N, Dang N. Multimodal neuroimaging in Rett syndrome with MECP2 mutation. Front Neurol. 2022;13:838206. (published online).

45. Al-Essa MA, Bakheet SM, Patay ZJ, Nounou RM, Ozand PT. Cerebral fluorine-18 labeled 2-fluoro-2-deoxyglucose positron emission tomography (FDG PET), MRI, and clinical observations in a patient with infantile G(M1) gangliosidosis. Brain Dev. 1999;21:559–62.

46. Lee SM, Lee MJ, Lee JS, Kim HD, Lee JS, Kim J, et al. Newly observed thalamic involvement and mutations of the HEXA gene in a Korean patient with juvenile GM2 gangliosidosis. Metab Brain Dis. 2008;23:235–42.

47. Al-Essa MA, Bakheet SM, Patay ZJ, Powe JE, Ozand PT. Clinical and cerebral FDG PET scan in a patient with Krabbe's disease. Pediatr Neurol. 2000;22:44–7.

48. Biffi A. Gene therapy for lysosomal storage disorders: a good start. Hum Mol Genet. 2016;25(R1):R65–75.

49. Sawaishi Y, Hatazawa J, Ochi N, Hirono H, Yano T, Watanabe Y, Okudera T, Takada G. Positron emission tomography in juvenile Alexander disease. J Neurol Sci. 1999;165:116–20.

50. Salsano E, Marotta G, Manfredi V, Giovagnoli AR, Farina L, Savoiardo M, Pareyson D, Benti R, Uziel G. Brain fluorodeoxyglucose PET in adrenoleukodystrophy. Neurology. 2014;83:981–9.

51. Kumar A, Chugani HT, Chakraborty P, Huq AH. Evaluation of neuroinflammation in X-linked adrenoleukodystrophy. Pediatr Neurol. 2011;44:143–6.

52. Pascual JM, Van Heertum RL, Wang D, Engelstad K, De Vivo DC. Imaging the metabolic footprint of Glut1 deficiency on the brain. Ann Neurol. 2002;52:458–64.

53. Natsume J, Ishihara N, Azuma Y, Nakata T, Takeuchi T, Tanaka M, Sakaguchi Y, Okai Y, Ito Y, Yamamoto H, Ohno A, Kidokoro H, Hattori A, Nabatame S, Kato K. Lenticular nuclei to thalamic ration PET is useful for diagnosis of GLUT1 deficiency syndrome. Brain Dev. 2021;43:69–77.

54. Ernst M, Zametkin AJ, Matochik JA, Pascualvaca D, Jons PH, Hardy K, Hankerson JG, Doudet DJ, Cohen RM. Presynaptic dopaminergic deficits in Lesch-Nyhan disease. N Engl J Med. 1996;334:1568–72.

55. Wong DF, Harris JC, Naidu S, et al. Dopamine transporters are markedly reduced in Lesch-Nyhan disease in vivo. Proc Natl Acad Sci U S A. 1996;93:5539–43.

56. Tambirajoo K, Furlanetti L, Hasegawa H, Rasian A, Gomeno H, Lin J-P, Selway R, Ashkan K. Deep brain stimulation of the internal pallidum in Lesch-Nyhan syndrome: clinical outcomes and connectivity analysis. Neuromodulation. 2021;24:380–91.

57. Chugani HT, Ilyas M, Kumar A, Juhász C, Kupsky WJ, Sood S, Asano E. Surgical treatment for refractory epileptic spasms: the Detroit series. Epilepsia. 2015;56:1941–9.

58. Chugani HT, da Silva EA, Chugani DC. Infantile spasms: III. Prognostic implications of bitemporal hypometabolism on positron emission tomography. Ann Neurol. 1996;39:643–9.

59. Shandal V, Veenstra AL, Behen M, Sundaram S, Chugani H. Long-term outcome in children with intractable epilepsy showing bilateral diffuse cortical glucose hypometabolism pattern on positron emission tomography. J Child Neurol. 2012;27:39–45.

Simultaneous PET/MR Imaging of Dementia

Ciprian Catana

Introduction

As discussed in detail in the other chapters, positron emission tomography (PET) is extensively used for research and clinical applications in dementia, including in the assessment of cerebral glucose metabolism, amyloid and tau deposition, microglia activation, synaptic density, status of neurotransmitter systems, etc. Magnetic resonance (MR) provides complementary information about changes in anatomy, function, metabolism using techniques such as MRI volumetry, diffusion tensor imaging, functional MR imaging, MR spectroscopy, etc. While the PET and MR data can be obtained separately, some of the opportunities enabled by the simultaneous acquisition using the integrated clinical PET/MR imaging scanners developed over the last 15 years will be discussed in this chapter. Of particular interest to imaging of dementia, the simultaneously acquired MRI data can be used to improve the PET data quality, an approach termed MR-assisted PET data optimization. Specifically, examples of standard and machine learning methods developed for using MR-derived information for PET attenuation and motion correc-

tions, image enhancement, and non-invasive radiotracer arterial input function estimation will be presented, particularly focusing on those that were applied to imaging of neurodegeneration. Finally, research and clinical applications that benefit from the simultaneous nature of the data collected using integrated PET/MRI scanners will be briefly discussed.

Integrated PET/MR Imaging Hardware

The first human scanner capable of simultaneous PET and MRI data acquisition was the BrainPET prototype (Siemens Healthineers, Erlangen, Germany). This avalanche photodiode-based PET insert was designed to fit in the bore of a standard 3-Tesla MRI scanner [1]. Subsequently, three whole-body integrated PET/MR scanners capable of simultaneous data acquisition were introduced: Biograph mMR (Siemens Healthineers, Erlangen, Germany) [2], SIGNA TOF PET/MRI (General Electric Healthcare, Waukesha, WI, USA) [3], and uPMR790 (United Imaging Healthcare, Shanghai, China) [4]. The last two devices use silicon photomultipliers as the photon detector. All three whole-body devices are currently approved for clinical use by the FDA. The axial field of view of the PET component of these scanners is at least 25 cm, which allows the imaging of the whole brain in one bed

C. Catana (✉)
Department of Radiology, Athinoula A. Martinos Center for Biomedical Imaging, Massachusetts General Hospital and Harvard Medical School, Charlestown, MA, USA
e-mail: ccatana@mgh.harvard.edu

position. Their spatial resolution at the center of the field of view is in the 2.72–4.3 mm range, with the uPMR790 having the best performance. Their sensitivity is in the 1.5–2.3% range, with the Signa PET/MRI having the best performance.

In addition, several efforts are ongoing around the world to develop MR-compatible PET inserts for brain imaging [5]. For example, a 7-Tesla MR compatible BrainPET with an order of magnitude higher sensitivity is currently developed by investigators from the Martinos Center, Siemens Healthineers, Hamamatsu Photonics, University of Tübingen, Complutense University of Madrid, University of Texas at Arlington, Boston University, and McLean Hospital. A spherical geometry was chosen for this device to achieve solid angle coverage of 71% and the expected sensitivity is 25% (without considering the time-of-flight sensitivity amplifier effect that is expected to contribute another factor of 2). While the primary goal of this project is to dramatically improve the temporal resolution of PET, the substantially higher sensitivity compared to existing devices will also lead to increased signal-to-noise ratio in the images, which can be traded to enable substantially higher spatial resolution PET imaging. This will also make it one the highest spatial resolution scanners for human brain imaging, which will allow imaging of small structures such as thalamic and brainstem nuclei, midbrain structures (e.g., periaqueductal gray), hippocampal subfields, raphe nucleus, and locus coeruleus.

Methodological Opportunities

Attenuation Correction

The 511 keV annihilation photons can interact with the subject before reaching the PET detectors, leading to biased quantification, image artifacts, and increased noise. Obtaining the data needed for attenuation correction is particularly difficult in integrated PET/MRI scanners because the MR signal is related to proton density and tissue relaxation times and not to electron density. One of the key factors that must be considered for

implementing an accurate MR-based head attenuation correction is the need to accurately account for bone tissue. Countless approaches have been proposed over the years to generate head attenuation maps starting from the data acquired with conventional and dedicated (e.g., ultra-short or zero echo time) MR sequences using segmentation or atlas-based techniques [6]. Eleven of these approaches have been tested in a multicenter setting using data from patients and healthy volunteers who were scanned on the Biograph mMR and subsequently underwent low-dose computed tomography (CT) examinations. The cohort of subjects also included 201 patients with mild cognitive impairment (MCI), Alzheimer's disease (AD) or clinical dementia who were scanned with [18F]FDG, [11C]PiB or [18F]-florbetapir. MR-based attenuation maps for a representative subject are shown in Fig. 16.1. Across all subjects, the average bias in the estimation of the radiotracer concentration in relevant brain regions was within ±5% of the values obtained using the standard CT-based approach for most of the MR-based approaches methods included in the analysis. The authors cautiously concluded "that the challenge of improving the accuracy of MR-[attenuation correction] in adult brains with normal anatomy has been solved to a quantitatively acceptable degree, which is smaller than the quantification reproducibility in PET imaging" [7].

More recently, deep learning methods have been used successfully for this purpose. For instance, an auto-encoder network was trained using 30 datasets to segment air, bone, and soft tissue from the high spatial resolution morphological MRI data. The average bias in the PET data was less than 1% in most brain regions, which was significantly lower than that observed for the Dixon- or CT-based template registration approaches [8]. Another method based on a 3D convolutional neural network (CNN) was trained and tested using a larger cohort of patients. The authors also investigated the qualitative and quantitative effects of using different MR sequence as input, training cohort size, and transfer learning after a software upgrade. The attenuation maps generated from the Dixon, T1-weighted and ultra-short echo time data were

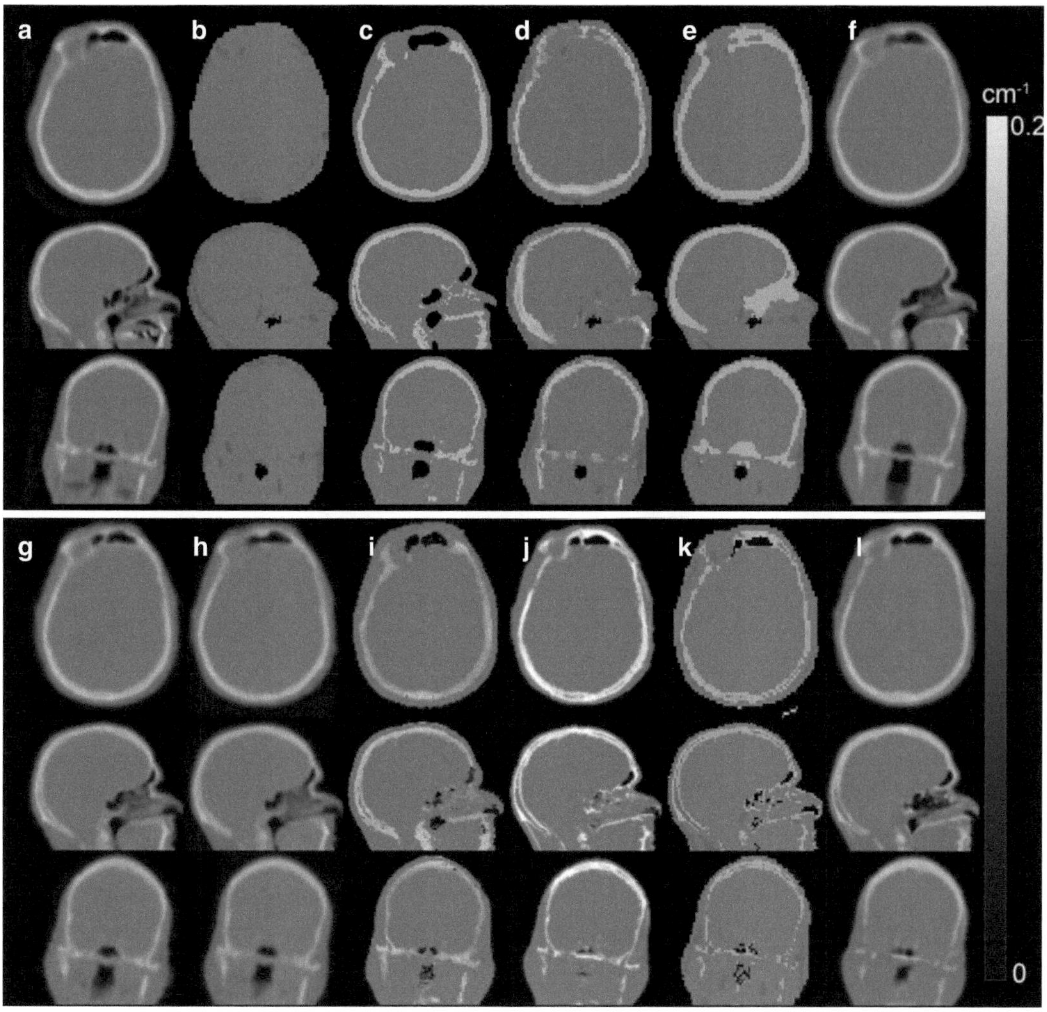

Fig. 16.1 Head attenuation map generation: (**a**) CT-based attenuation map (**b–l**) MR-based attenuation maps generated using the 11 methods tested. The selected patient minimizes the difference of the overall brain error to the median error across all methods. (Figure originally published in NeuroImage [7])

of excellent quality, even in the skull based and nasal cavities, regions that have been particularly challenging for MR-based approaches. Increasing the group size decreased the blurring and increased the image contrast and overall detail level in the attenuation maps. A total of 100 subjects were required to outperform one of the conventional methods that performed the best in the multicenter comparison mentioned above. There was a clear correlation between group size and model performance in terms of outliers at the 3% FDG PET error-level. Fine-tuning after a major software upgrade was necessary, but as few as ten subjects were sufficient for convergence, and

incremental improvements were noted with increasing group sizes [9].

Nevertheless, it is still very difficult to qualify PET/MRI scanners for multicenter clinical trials, primarily because of lingering concerns about the accuracy of MR-based head attenuation correction methods. The additional challenge is that a PET/MRI scanner cannot be qualified in the same manner adopted for hybrid PET/CT devices because the attenuation properties of conventional PET phantoms cannot be obtained from the MR data. A solution recently proposed is to separate the head attenuation correction from the other factors that affect PET data quantification and use a *patient as a phantom* to assess the former. Guidelines for data acquisition, image reconstruction and analysis were proposed in a consensus paper, and the approach was successfully tested using data collected with the Biograph mMR and Signa TOF PET/MRI scanners [10].

Motion Correction

Head motion is difficult to avoid in PET studies given the relatively long acquisition times (i.e., minutes to hours) needed to collect enough coincidence events to reconstruct good quality images. This leads to blurring of the PET images, emission-attenuation data mismatch, and overall biased quantification. An opportunity opened by the simultaneous acquisition is to characterize the head motion using the MR information. Numerous MR-based head motion tracking approaches have been developed and the resulting motion estimates can be used to correct the simultaneously acquired PET data in integrated PET/MRI scanners.

Proof-of-principle studies were performed using the BrainPET prototype more than a decade ago [11]. The motion estimates were obtained from high temporal resolution navigators embedded in several MR sequences or by registering echo planar imaging volumes acquired simultaneously every 3 s. The motion was accounted for by applying the MR-derived rigid-body transformers to the lines-of-response joining the pairs of crystals in which the 511 keV photons were detected. After further optimization, this algorithm was tested in dementia subjects. The variability in PET measurements was reduced after motion correction, especially in the group of subjects that exhibited high motion during the scan, highlighting the need to perform motion correction in the case of less-compliant subjects [12].

As an alternative to modifying the MR sequences that are part of the standard protocol, motion navigators can be acquired between these sequences, which is practical but provides a limited number of motion estimates [13]. An even more straightforward approach consists of deriving the motion estimates from the morphological MR images/volumes (e.g., T1-weighted, T2-weighted,

echo planar imaging, diffusion weighted imaging, arterial spin labeling, etc.) [14]. Both approaches have the disadvantage that intra-sequence motion cannot be characterized and accounted for.

Recognizing the potential clinical impact of head motion correction, the equipment manufacturers implemented their own versions. The algorithm provided by Siemens for the Biograph mMR scanner, called BrainCOMPASS, uses a PACE-based navigators [15]. Motion is estimated each time its amplitude exceeds a threshold, and the rigid-body transformers are used to align the PET volumes corresponding to the motion-free frames. Alternatively, the correction can be accounted for before image reconstruction using a rebinning algorithm that applies the correction to the lines-of-response [16].

Image Enhancement

The spatial resolution of PET is inferior to that of MR due to factors related to positron emission and annihilation physics (i.e., positron range and the non-collinearity of the annihilation photons), the performance of the detectors used to record the annihilation photons, and of the image reconstruction algorithms. These and other factors contribute to the partial volume effects that lead to an underestimation of the activity concentration in structures that are smaller than 2–3 times the spatial resolution of the scanner (spill-out effect) and an apparent increase in the activity concentration in adjacent structures (spill-in effect). While partial volume effects need to be considered in neurological studies in general given the size of the structures of interest (e.g., the thickness of the cortical gray matter is approximately 1–2 mm), they are exacerbated in the case of dementia patients when brain atrophy is also present. Even before integrated PET/MRI scanners were developed, the high-resolution morphological information derived from MRI was used to account for these effects. The hardware registration enabled by the simultaneous acquisition eliminates the need for software registration.

In a recent study, the impact of partial volume effects correction in 216 symptomatic individuals on the AD continuum was investigated. Higher changes in [18F]-florbetapir standardized uptake value ratios (SUVR) and a better correlation between SUVR longitudinal changes and Mini Mental State Examination score decreases were observed after correction, suggesting the β-amyloid buildup curve in AD should be reshaped [17]. This correction is also relevant in other neurodegenerative disorders. For instance, in premanifest Huntington disease gene-expansion carriers, the influence of the correction was the largest in objects with the smaller absolute MRI volumes [18]. In another example, patients with corticobasal syndrome showed higher differences in [18F]GE-180 SUV after partial volume effects correction and smaller volumes compared to healthy controls [19].

The morphological information derived from MR can also be incorporated directly in the PET image reconstruction. An approach for anatomy-aided reconstruction uses kernel features that are extracted directly from the MRI images without having to segment the structures of interest [20]. When this method and motion correction were applied to [18F]FDG PET data, the signal-to-noise ratio increased and the coefficients of variation were lowered in a composite cortical region consisting of areas with preserved metabolism in dementia patients. The contrast between hypo-metabolic and preserved regions in each population assessed using the Cohen's d metric as a surrogate of the physician's ability to separate these regions was also higher [21]. As shown in Fig. 16.2 for a representative subject, all the

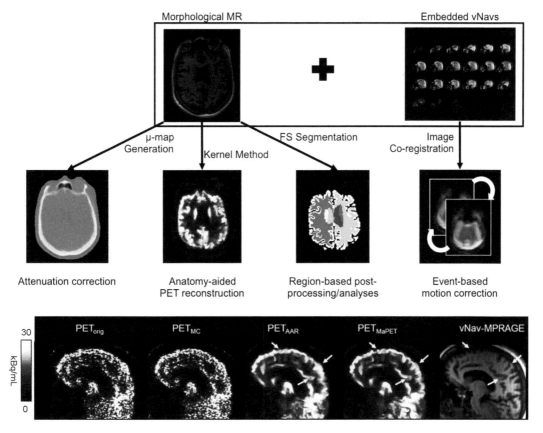

Fig. 16.2 MR-assisted PET data optimization. The MR information obtained using a morphological MR sequence with embedded motion navigators is used for attenuation and motion corrections, anatomy-aided reconstruction, region-based post-processing and analyses. The PET and MR images for a subject who moved during the examination are shown in the lower panel: before (PET$_{orig}$) and after (PET$_{MC}$) motion correction, after anatomy-aided reconstruction (PET$_{AAR}$), and after applying all the corrections (PET$_{MaPET}$). The arrows point to the areas that showed the most improvement in the visualization of anatomical structures after data optimization. (Figure originally published in The Journal of Nuclear Medicine [21])

information required for performing the above-mentioned corrections as well as ROI-based analysis was derived from the data acquired in ~6 min using a single morphological MR sequence with embedded motion navigators. Alternatively, the anatomical information can be incorporated in image space using a deep learning approach, which has the advantage of not requiring modifications to the image reconstruction algorithm or access to the raw data [22].

A closely related group of methods are aimed at generating high- from low-resolution images with deep learning. Using two coupled generative adversarial networks, a self-supervised technique has been implemented to generate higher spatial resolution PET images using as inputs a low-resolution PET image, a high-resolution MR image, the axial and radial coordinates (needed to account for the spatially variant nature of the point spread function), and a high-dimensional feature set extracted from an auxiliary CNN which is separately-trained in a supervised manner using paired simulation datasets. The deep learning approach outperformed the partial volume effects correction techniques [23].

Finally, one of the most popular topics in the image enhancement field is the generation of high-quality images from low-count data. For example, a CNN was trained to generate high-quality [18F]-florbetaben PET images from multiple MR and the low-count PET images. The synthesized PET images showed significantly reduced noise compared with the low-count PET images [24]. When generalized, this method can be applied to data acquired with different hardware and protocols [25], which allows the model to be shared between different institutions to be trained on local datasets (Fig. 16.3). Eliminating the data sharing concerns addresses one of the biggest challenges in deep learning—the need for large training datasets.

Non-invasive Radiotracer Arterial Input Function Estimation

Accurate quantification in PET requires an input function (i.e., the radiotracer plasma time-activity curve) to the compartment models used for estimating parameters of interest. The "gold standard" method for measuring the input function is arterial blood sampling. As this procedure requires catheterization of the radial artery, its usefulness in routine clinical PET studies is limited. Instead, this information could be obtained non-invasively from a region of interest placed

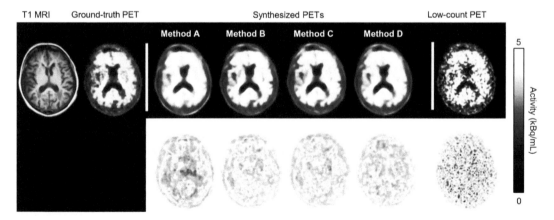

Fig. 16.3 Ultra-low dose PET amyloid imaging. The ground-truth PET and reference T1-weighted MR images for an amyloid-positive subject are shown in the first two columns. The difference images between the ground-truth and the other images are shown in the lower row. Compared to the low-count PET images shown in the last column, the images synthesized using the deep learning models had reduced noise. The images obtained by directly using a network trained with data from another site (Method A) are blurrier than those obtained with networks that were fine-tuned (Method B) or trained from scratch (Methods C and D). (Figure originally published in the European Journal of Nuclear Medicine and Molecular Imaging [25])

across major blood vessels present in the field of view (e.g., carotid arteries in the case brain imaging). The simultaneously acquired morphological MRI data could be used for identifying these vessels and for correcting for confounding effects (e.g., partial volume effects, head motion). Determining the location and size of the vessels of interest can be accomplished using the perfectly registered anatomical images obtained using standard (e.g., those used for acquiring the high-resolution morphological data needed for identifying the brain structures of interest) or dedicated (e.g., time-of-flight angiography) MR sequences. Once the vessels are segmented, the bias introduced by partial volume effects needs to be accounted. Preliminary studies performed using data acquired on the BrainPET prototype demonstrated good correspondence between the [18F]FDG input functions obtained using the image-based and invasive techniques [26, 27]. Similar results were reported using the Biograph mMR in a sheep stroke animal model [28] and in healthy controls [29, 30].

As these techniques require perfect registration of the MR-derived vessel segmentations (that could be inaccurate in the absence of motion correction), a method that uses PET-derived angiograms was also proposed. To address the spill-over problem, the counts obtained from the cervical carotid and vertebral arteries were divided by the MR angiography derived true arterial volume. The spill-in was estimated from the cervical arteries, to minimize the contribution of the brain parenchyma. This method tested using the GE Signa TOF PET/MRI scanner showed reproducible results in gray and white matter structures, with blood flow values consistent with those reported in literature at baseline and after a pharmacological challenge [31].

A semi-automatic software to estimate the input function and perform parametric Patlak mapping was developed to facilitate the use of these methods in routine clinical studies. This comprehensive software, called caliPER (parametric Patlak mapping using PET/MRI input function) was successfully tested in healthy volunteers and frontotemporal dementia patients who underwent [18F]FDG PET/MRI studies

using the Biograph mMR scanner. The net uptake rates and cerebral metabolic rates of glucose obtained non-invasively were within 2% of those obtained using individually-calibrated population-based input functions in relevant brain structures [32].

The input function can also be obtained non-invasively for other radiotracers. For example, the [11C]PiB input functions estimated from the PET and MRI data acquired using the Signa PET/MRI scanner were used to calculate the distribution volumes in patients suspected of early dementia. Excellent correlation was reported between the distribution value ratios obtained using the Logan plot method and the image-derived input function and those calculated using the reference tissue graphical approach. As arterial sampling was not performed in this study, metabolite correction was performed using a Hill-type function applied to the image-derived input function. Another limitation was that only patients without significant head motion during the 70-min scan were included in the analysis [33].

Image-to-Image Translation

Image-to-image translation has been proposed for several tasks. First, synthetic images of less-common radiotracers can be generated from the images obtained with common radiotracers. As an example, deep learning methods have been implemented for predicting [11C]UCB-J PET images of synaptic vesicle protein 2A from [18F]FDG PET data. Using [18F]FDG SUVR and Ki ratio images as the input to the U-Net model provided predictions of [11C]UCB-J SUVR images that were deemed satisfactory visually and quantitatively [34]. Second, image-to-image translation strategies can be used for data harmonization in multi-center trials to minimize the variability when a different radiotracer is used at one of the sites. For example, a network was trained to generate [11C] PiB from [18F]-florbetapir images. The synthetic SUVR images were more similar visually to the real [11C]PiB than the [18F]-florbetapir images [35]. Third, image-to-image translation can be used to replace missing data when performing multimodal analysis. As PET data are missing for many subjects in the ADNI database, a 3D end-to-end generative adversarial network was proposed to synthesize brain PET from MRI images [36].

Applications

Assess the Relationship Between PET- and MRI-Derived Biomarkers

The exact relationship between changes in cerebral glucose metabolism, structural changes/atrophy, and reductions in functional connectivity can be assessed using an integrated PET/MRI scanner. Previous studies using separately acquired data have shown both strong overlap and discrepancy between these biomarkers. Strong atrophy and relatively preserved metabolism have been reported in the hippocampus, a finding that has been discussed to represent regional synaptic compensatory mechanisms, potentially leading to preservation of cognition to some degree. It was also shown that a stronger decrease in hippocampal connectivity is linked with higher metabolism in AD [37].

Simultaneous acquisition has allowed for a direct comparison between the brain's glucose consumption and metrics of intrinsic neural activity. When investigating the relationships between [^{18}F]FDG uptake and several metrics reflecting local and large-scale intrinsic functional connectivity, statistically significant differences in correlation values between the two groups of healthy old individuals and patients were observed, suggesting the presence of bioenergetic coupling in healthy aging but a possible abnormal glucose utilization that differentially impacts neural information transmission in AD [38].

[^{15}O]-water PET is the "gold standard" in measuring cerebral perfusion, but MR-based methods such as arterial spin labeling (ASL) can be used for the same purpose. Using an integrated PET/MRI scanner for cross validating these techniques has the advantage of assessing the flow in the same physiological state, which would be impossible using separately acquired data. Indeed, good agreement in terms of regional hypoperfusion patterns between ^{15}O-water and the ASL methods and a strong correlation between region-based perfusion measurements were reported in frontotemporal dementia (Fig. 16.4) and primary supranuclear palsy

Fig. 16.4 Cross-validation of MR and PET perfusion measurements. Perfusion maps generated by two ASL-MRI methods, and ^{15}O-water PET for one semantic variant frontotemporal dementia patient (top) and the average of all control participants (bottom). (Figure originally published in NeuroImage: Clinical [39])

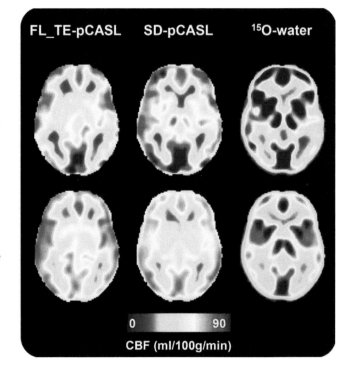

patients who were scanned on the Biograph mMR [39].

Once validated against the gold standard, the correlation between ASL-based perfusion measurements and measures obtained from [18F]FDG PET could be examined. As [18F]FDG uptake reflects perfusion to some extent, it is reasonable to expect and even desirable to obtain similar information with ASL-MRI, a non-invasive technique, as this would allow PET to be used for studies with other radiotracers. When comparing the diagnostic utility of perfusion measurements obtained from ASL-MRI and [18F]FDG PET in ten frontotemporal dementia and healthy controls, similar patterns of abnormalities and a strong correlation were observed between the two modalities. However, the diagnostic accuracy was significantly lower for ASL-MRI [40]. In a similar study performed in AD and MCI patients, there was overlap between hypoperfusion and hypometabolism, but the latter measurements had higher sensitivity in the detection of preclinical AD [41]. Higher performance for [18F] FDG PET compared to ASL-MRI was also reported in patients referred for the diagnosis of dementia who underwent examinations on the GE Signa PET/MRI scanner [42].

Improve Data Acquisition and Processing Workflow

Using an integrated PET/MRI scanner, all the data required for clinical purposes could be acquired in a single examination, which would greatly increase patient comfort, an issue particularly important in the elderly and fragile dementia patients. A "one-stop shop" data acquisition 20-min protocol was suggested to obtain both pathology and neuronal injury biomarkers to support clinical diagnosis of AD [43]. Amyloid load was imaged using [18F]-florbetaben PET, and relative cerebral blood flow using ASL-MRI. A similar protocol was suggested for acquiring the [18F]FDG PET and morphological MRI data needed to identify the most common pathologies. Note that an additional amyloid PET scan was necessary to exclude atypical AD in a patient

diagnosed with semantic dementia [44]. More than 1500 patients with possible cognitive impairment or dementia were examined using a 25-min protocol at a single institution. In addition to obtaining complementary data needed for clinical purposes, integrated PET/MRI demonstrated practical benefits for the patients, caregivers, as well as referring physicians and interpreting radiologists [45]. Combining these streamlined acquisition protocols with the MR-assisted PET data optimization workflow described above, the total scan duration might be reduced even further.

While acquiring dynamic data routinely for clinical purposes is not feasible, amyloid deposition could be assessed from dual time-point PET/MRI data, which has the advantage of removing some of the blood flow dependency of the β-amyloid load estimates. Early images can be obtained from the data acquired between 0 and 10 min after injection, and later images from the data acquired between 90 and 110 min after injection. In addition to parametric images and regional output parameters, two dual time-point metrics can also be obtained. Using this approach, the largest mean differences between amyloid-positive and amyloid-negative patients were observed for the frontal, parietal, insular and occipital lobes. The dual time-point metrics were significantly higher in amyloid-positive patients than in amyloid-negative patients [46].

Increase Diagnostic Certainty

Combining the two sources of evidence was shown to increase the diagnostic certainty in typical patients with AD, semantic dementia, frontotemporal dementia, and posterior cortical atrophy (Fig. 16.5) [43]. When compared to PET/CT, combining the [18F]FDG PET data with information derived from MRI changed the interpretation in a substantial fraction of memory clinic patients [47].

Machine learning approaches could also help in the early diagnosis of AD based on multimodality MR and PET data [48]. For example, a partial least squares method was proposed to

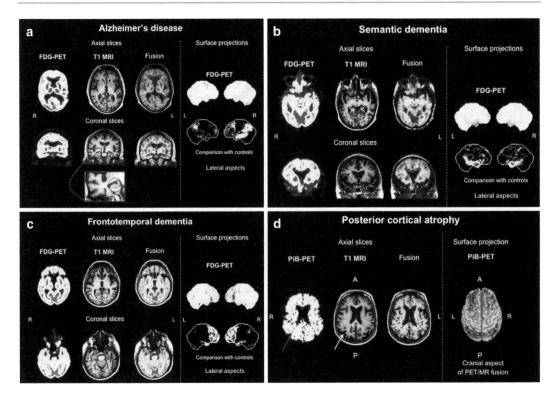

Fig. 16.5 Increased diagnostic certainty using multimodal data in common forms of dementia: (**a**) Alzheimer disease, (**b**) semantic dementia, (**c**) frontotemporal dementia, (**d**) posterior cortical atrophy. (Figure originally published in the Journal of Nuclear Medicine [43])

discriminate MCI converters from MCI non-converters using combined MRI, [18F]FDG PET, and [18F]-florbetapir PET. The tri-modality models had better classification accuracy compared with the single-modality and two-modality models. The performance was even higher when clinical test scores were also considered [49]. AD classification can also be achieved using cascaded CNNs to learn the multi-level and multimodal features of MRI and PET brain images, with higher performance than the MRI- or PET-only approaches [50].

Instead of extracting and fusing features from the two modalities, the actual images could be fused to aid with AD diagnosis. Specifically, the gray matter tissue area of brain MRI and [18F] FDG PET images were fused by registration and mask coding to obtain a new fused modality. The fused images were then used as inputs to CNNs that were trained to perform binary and multi-classification tasks. The model using futures

extracted from the fused images showed superior performance compared to methods relying on unimodal and feature fusion, particularly in the case of the three-classification task [51].

Monitor Treatment Response and Side Effects

Several antibodies that target amyloid-beta have been investigated for the treatment of early AD [52, 53]. The changes in amyloid and tau burden on PET were some of the secondary outcomes in the clinical trials. This suggests PET can provide critical information for patient selection and treatment monitoring. Amyloid-related imaging abnormalities were observed in a substantial fraction of the patients enrolled in these studies, which means MRI needs to be performed serially in patients being treated with these drugs. As longer and larger trials are necessary, PET/MRI provides a perfect solution to the need for repeated MR and PET examinations. Combining two scans into one has a great benefit as patient discomfort and willingness to participate are significant issues in this patient population.

Predict Disease Progression

Numerous studies have used machine learning approaches to predict MCI to AD dementia progression from imaging data [54], using publicly available data from the ADNI database. The most popular classification methods were based on support vector machines and CNNs, with the latter achieving a higher mean accuracy. For example, a CNN was implemented to predict cognitive decline from [^{18}F]FDG and [^{18}F]-florbetapir data [55]. Its sensitivity, specificity, and accuracy for classification between AD and normal controls were 93.5%, 97.8%, and 96.0%, respectively, significantly higher than the values obtained with the support vector machine classifier or the volume of interest-based analyses. Sensitivity, specificity, and accuracy of the CNN-based approach for the prediction of MCI conversion was 81.0%, 87.0%, and 84.2%, respectively. The accuracy of the CNN was significantly higher than volume of interest-based analysis of [^{18}F]FDG PET and the support vector machine classifier. Interestingly, the same systematic review revealed that the approaches combining data from both MRI and PET achieved better results than those relying on a single-modality information [54]. In addition to conversion from MCI to AD dementia, the baseline imaging and clinical data can be used to predict future [^{18}F]-florbetapir SUVR using a gradient-boosted decision tree algorithm [56].

Conclusion

Integrated PET/MRI scanners with performance characteristics similar to the state-of-the-art stand-alone devices are currently commercially available from three equipment manufacturers. Attenuation correction, the most important meth-odological challenge in the early days of PET/MRI, has been adequately addressed for brain imaging. Moreover, many approaches that benefit from the simultaneous nature of the data have been implemented. The perfect spatial registration enabled by the hardware acquisition and the MR-assisted motion correction facilitates the use of conventional and deep learning techniques that utilize the MR-derived information to greatly improve the PET image quality. Simultaneous PET/MRI has been evaluated for numerous research and clinical applications in dementia, including techniques cross-validation, streamlined data acquisition, early diagnosis and predicting disease progression. Very promising results have been obtained with machine learning approaches that extract additional information from the perfectly registered complementary datasets.

References

1. Schlemmer H-PW, Pichler BJ, Schmand M, Burbar Z, Michel C, Ladebeck R, et al. Simultaneous MR/PET imaging of the human brain: feasibility study. Radiology. 2008;248(3):1028–35. https://doi.org/10.1148/radiol.2483071927.
2. Delso G, Furst S, Jakoby B, Ladebeck R, Ganter C, Nekolla SG, et al. Performance measurements of the Siemens mMR integrated whole-body PET/MR scanner. J Nucl Med. 2011;52(12):1914–22.
3. Grant AM, Deller TW, Khalighi MM, Maramraju SH, Delso G, Levin CS. NEMA NU 2-2012 performance studies for the SiPM-based ToF-PET component of the GE SIGNA PET/MR system. Med Phys. 2016;43(5):2334. https://doi.org/10.1118/1.4945416.
4. Chen S, Gu Y, Yu H, Chen X, Cao T, Hu L, et al. NEMA NU2-2012 performance measurements of the united imaging uPMR790: an integrated PET/MR system. Eur J Nucl Med Mol Imaging. 2021;48(6):1726–35.
5. Catana C. Development of dedicated brain PET imaging devices: recent advances and future perspectives. J Nucl Med. 2019;60(8):1044.
6. Catana C. Attenuation correction for human PET/MRI studies. Phys Med Biol. 2020;65(23):23TR02. https://doi.org/10.1088/1361-6560/abb0f8.
7. Ladefoged CNN, Law I, Anazodo U, St Lawrence K, Izquierdo-Garcia D, Catana C, et al. A multi-centre evaluation of eleven clinically feasible brain PET/MRI attenuation correction techniques using a large cohort of patients. Neuroimage. 2016;147:346–59.
8. Liu F, Jang H, Kijowski R, Bradshaw T, McMillan AB. Deep learning MR imaging-based attenua-

tion correction for PET/MR imaging. Radiology. 2018;286(2):676–84.

9. Ladefoged CN, Hansen AE, Henriksen OM, Bruun FJ, Eikenes L, Øen SK, et al. AI-driven attenuation correction for brain PET/MRI: clinical evaluation of a dementia cohort and importance of the training group size. Neuroimage. 2020;222(August):117221. https://doi.org/10.1016/j.neuroimage.2020.117221.

10. Catana C, Laforest R, An H, Boada F, Cao T, Faul D, et al. A path to qualification of PET/MR scanners for multicenter brain imaging studies: evaluation of MR-based attenuation correction methods using a patient phantom. J Nucl Med. 2021;63:615.

11. Catana C, Benner T, Van Der Kouwe A, Byars L, Hamm M, Chonde DB, et al. MRI-assisted PET motion correction for neurologic studies in an integrated MR-PET scanner. J Nucl Med. 2011;52(1):154.

12. Chen KT, Salcedo S, Chonde DB, Izquierdo-Garcia D, Levine MA, Price JC, et al. MR-assisted PET motion correction in simultaneous PET/MRI studies of dementia subjects. J Magn Reson Imaging. 2018;48(5):1288–96.

13. Keller SH, Hansen C, Hansen C, Andersen FL, Ladefoged C, Svarer C, et al. Motion correction in simultaneous PET / MR brain imaging using sparsely sampled MR navigators: a clinically feasible tool. EJNMMI Phys. 2015;2:14. https://doi.org/10.1186/s40658-015-0118-z.

14. Chen Z, Sforazzini F, Baran J, Close T, Shah NJ, Egan GF. MR-PET head motion correction based on co-registration of multicontrast MR images. Hum Brain Mapp. 2019;42:4081. https://doi.org/10.1002/hbm.24497.

15. Thesen S, Heid O, Mueller E, Schad LR. Prospective acquisition correction for head motion with image-based tracking for real-time fMRI. Magn Reson Med. 2000;44(3):457–63.

16. Reilhac A, Merida I, Irace Z, Stephenson MC, Weekes AA, Chen C, et al. Development of a dedicated Rebinner with rigid motion correction for the mMR PET/MR scanner, and validation in a large cohort of 11 C-PIB scans. J Nucl Med. 2018;59(11):1761–7.

17. Rullmann M, McLeod A, Grothe MJ, Sabri O, Barthel H. Reshaping the amyloid buildup curve in alzheimer disease? Partial-volume effect correction of longitudinal amyloid pet data. J Nucl Med. 2020;61(12):1820–4.

18. Hellem MNNN, Vinther-Jensen T, Anderberg L, Budtz-Jørgensen E, Hjermind LE, Larsen VA, et al. Hybrid 2-[18F] FDG PET/MRI in premanifest Huntington's disease gene-expansion carriers: The significance of partial volume correction. PLoS One. 2021;16(6):e0252683.

19. Schuster S, Beyer L, Palleis C, Harris S, Schmitt J, Weidinger E, et al. Impact of partial volume correction on [18F]GE-180 PET quantification in subcortical brain regions of patients with corticobasal syndrome. Brain Sci. 2022;12(2):204.

20. Hutchcroft W, Wang G, Chen KT, Catana C, Qi J. Anatomically-aided PET reconstruction using the kernel method. Phys Med Biol. 2016;61(18):6668.

21. Chen KT, Salcedo S, Gong K, Chonde DB, Izquierdo-Garcia D, Drzezga A, et al. An efficient approach to perform MR-assisted PET data optimization in simultaneous PET/MR neuroimaging studies. J Nucl Med. 2019;60(2):272.

22. Schramm G, Rigie D, Vahle T, Rezaei A, Van Laere K, Shepherd T, et al. Approximating anatomically-guided PET reconstruction in image space using a convolutional neural network. Neuroimage. 2021;224:117399. https://doi.org/10.1016/j.neuroimage.2020.117399.

23. Song TA, Chowdhury SR, Yang F, Dutta J. PET image super-resolution using generative adversarial networks. Neural Netw. 2020;125:83–91. https://doi.org/10.1016/j.neunet.2020.01.029.

24. Chen KT, Gong E, de Carvalho Macruz FB, Xu J, Boumis A, Khalighi M, et al. Ultra-low-dose 18F-florbetaben amyloid PET imaging using deep learning with multi-contrast MRI inputs. Radiology. 2019;290(3):649–56. http://www.ncbi.nlm.nih.gov/pubmed/30526350

25. Chen KT, Schürer M, Ouyang J, Koran MEI, Davidzon G, Mormino E, et al. Generalization of deep learning models for ultra-low-count amyloid PET/MRI using transfer learning. Eur J Nucl Med Mol Imaging. 2020;47(13):2998–3007.

26. Chonde DB. Improved PET data quantification in simultaneous PET/MR neuroimaging. Harvard University; 2014.

27. Chonde DB, Catana C. MR-guided radiotracer input function estimation in simultaneous MR/PET. Melbourne: International Society of Magnetic Resonance in Medicine; 2012.

28. Jochimsen TH, Zeisig V, Schulz J, Werner P, Patt M, Patt J, et al. Fully automated calculation of image-derived input function in simultaneous PET/MRI in a sheep model. EJNMMI Phys. 2016;3(1):2.

29. Sundar LKS, Muzik O, Rischka L, Hahn A, Rausch I, Lanzenberger R, et al. Towards quantitative [18F] FDG-PET/MRI of the brain: automated MR-driven calculation of an image-derived input function for the non-invasive determination of cerebral glucose metabolic rates. J Cereb Blood Flow Metab. 2019;39(8):1516–30.

30. Sari H, Erlandsson K, Law I, Larsson HBW, Ourselin S, Arridge S, et al. Estimation of an image derived input function with MR-defined carotid arteries in FDG-PET human studies using a novel partial volume correction method. J Cereb Blood Flow Metab. 2017;37(4):1398–409.

31. Khalighi MM, Deller TW, Fan AP, Gulaka PK, Shen B, Singh P, et al. Image-derived input function estimation on a TOF-enabled PET/MR for cerebral blood flow mapping. J Cereb Blood Flow Metab. 2018;38(1):126–35.

32. Dassanayake P, Cui L, Finger E, Kewin M, Hadaway J, Soddu A, et al. caliPER: a software for blood-free parametric Patlak mapping using PET/MRI input function. NeuroImage. 2022;256:119261.

33. Okazawa H, Ikawa M, Tsujikawa T, Makino A, Mori T, Kiyono Y, et al. Noninvasive measurement of [11c]

pib distribution volume using integrated pet/mri. Diagnostics. 2020;10(12):993.

34. Wang R, Liu H, Toyonaga T, Shi L, Wu J, Onofrey JA, et al. Generation of synthetic PET images of synaptic density and amyloid from 18F-FDG images using deep learning. Med Phys. 2021;48(9):5115–29.

35. Shah J, Gao F, Li B, Ghisays V, Luo J, Chen Y, et al. Deep residual inception encoder-decoder network for amyloid PET harmonization. Alzheimers Dement. 2022;18(12):2448–57.

36. Zhang J, He X, Qing L, Gao F, Wang B. BPGAN: brain PET synthesis from MRI using generative adversarial network for multi-modal Alzheimer's disease diagnosis. Comput Methods Programs Biomed. 2022;217:106676. https://doi.org/10.1016/j.cmpb.2022.106676.

37. Tahmasian M, Pasquini L, Scherr M, Meng C, Förster S, Mulej Bratec S, et al. The lower hippocampus global connectivity, the higher its local metabolism in Alzheimer disease. Neurology. 2015;84(19):1956–63.

38. Marchitelli R, Aiello M, Cachia A, Quarantelli M, Cavaliere C, Postiglione A, et al. Simultaneous resting-state FDG-PET/fMRI in Alzheimer disease: relationship between glucose metabolism and intrinsic activity. NeuroImage. 2018;176(April):246–58.

39. Ssali T, Narciso L, Hicks J, Liu L, Jesso S, Richardson L, et al. Concordance of regional hypoperfusion by pCASL MRI and 15O-water PET in frontotemporal dementia: Is pCASL an efficacious alternative? Neuroimage Clin. 2022;33:102950. https://doi.org/10.1016/j.nicl.2022.102950.

40. Anazodo UC, Finger E, Kwan BYM, Pavlosky W, Warrington JC, Günther M, et al. Using simultaneous PET/MRI to compare the accuracy of diagnosing frontotemporal dementia by arterial spin labelling MRI and FDG-PET. Neuroimage Clin. 2018;17:405–14.

41. Riederer I, Bohn KP, Preibisch C, Wiedemann E, Zimmer C, Alexopoulos P, et al. Alzheimer disease and mild cognitive impairment: integrated pulsed arterial spin-labeling MRI and (18)F-FDG PET. Radiology. 2018;288(1):198–206.

42. Ceccarini J, Bourgeois S, Van Weehaeghe D, Goffin K, Vandenberghe R, Vandenbulcke M, et al. Direct prospective comparison of (18)F-FDG PET and arterial spin labelling MR using simultaneous PET/MR in patients referred for diagnosis of dementia. Eur J Nucl Med Mol Imaging. 2020;47(9):2142–54.

43. Drzezga A, Barthel H, Minoshima S, Sabri O. Potential clinical applications of PET/MR imaging in neurodegenerative diseases. J Nucl Med. 2014;55(Supplement 2):47S–55S. http://jnm.snmjournals.org/content/55/Supplement_2/47S.abstract

44. Henriksen OM, Marner L, Law I. Clinical PET/MR imaging in dementia and neuro-oncology. PET Clin. 2016;11(4):441–52.

45. Shepherd TM, Nayak GK. Clinical use of integrated positron emission tomography-magnetic resonance Imaging for dementia patients. Top Magn Reson Imaging. 2019;28(6):299–310.

46. Cecchin D, Barthel H, Poggiali D, Cagnin A, Tiepolt S, Zucchetta P, et al. A new integrated dual time-point amyloid PET/MRI data analysis method. Eur J Nucl Med Mol Imaging. 2017;44(12):2060–72.

47. Kaltoft NS, Marner L, Larsen VA, Hasselbalch SG, Law I, Henriksen OM. Hybrid FDG PET/MRI vs. FDG PET and CT in patients with suspected dementia – a comparison of diagnostic yield and propagated influence on clinical diagnosis and patient management. PLoS One. 2019;14(5):1–13.

48. Liu X, Chen K, Wu T, Weidman D, Lure F, Li J. Use of multimodality imaging and artificial intelligence for diagnosis and prognosis of early stages of Alzheimer's disease. Transl Res. 2018;194:56–67.

49. Wang P, Chen K, Yao L, Hu B, Wu X, Zhang J, et al. Multimodal classification of mild cognitive impairment based on partial least squares. J Alzheimers Dis. 2016;54(1):359–71.

50. Liu M, Cheng D, Wang K, Wang Y. Multi-modality cascaded convolutional neural networks for Alzheimer's disease diagnosis. Neuroinformatics. 2018;16(3–4):295–308.

51. Song J, Zheng J, Li P, Lu X, Zhu G, Shen P. An effective multimodal image fusion method Using MRI and PET for Alzheimer's disease diagnosis. Front Digit Health. 2021;3(February):1–12.

52. Sevigny J, Chiao P, Bussiere T, Weinreb PH, Williams L, Maier M, et al. The antibody aducanumab reduces A beta plaques in Alzheimer's disease. Nature. 2016;537(7618):50–6.

53. Mintun MA, Lo AC, Duggan Evans C, Wessels AM, Ardayfio PA, Andersen SW, et al. Donanemab in early Alzheimer's disease. N Engl J Med. 2021;384(18):1691–704.

54. Grueso S, Viejo-Sobera R. Machine learning methods for predicting progression from mild cognitive impairment to Alzheimer's disease dementia: a systematic review. Alzheimers Res Ther. 2021;13(1):162.

55. Choi H, Jin KH. Predicting cognitive decline with deep learning of brain metabolism and amyloid imaging. Behav Brain Res. 2018;344(February):103–9. https://doi.org/10.1016/j.bbr.2018.02.017.

56. Reith FH, Mormino EC, Zaharchuk G. Predicting future amyloid biomarkers in dementia patients with machine learning to improve clinical trial patient selection. Alzheimers Dement (N Y). 2021;7(1):e12212.

Karina Mosci, Tanyaluck Thientunyakit,
Donna J. Cross, Gérard N. Bischof, Javier Arbizu,
and Satoshi Minoshima

Introduction

The brain is the most complex and intriguing part of the human body, and until recently our understanding was confined to what we could learn from post-mortem pathology studies and animal models. The acceleration of neuroscience research and development over the last few decades has given us exciting new technologies to better understand brain function. Imaging modalities have become fundamental tools for the diagnosis and evaluation of brain pathologies as well as to improve our knowledge of normal brain functions.

While conventional imaging, such as CT and MR, provide important structural and anatomic information of the brain, molecular imaging offers the possibility to image and quantify brain function "in vivo," to increase our understanding of normal physiologic and pathologic processes, with the prospect of more personalized patient care.

However, functional imaging interpretation may be challenging and requires an appropriate training. Single-photon emission tomography (SPECT) and positron emission tomography (PET) only detect structures with considerable perfusion, metabolism, protein deposition, or

K. Mosci (✉)
Department of Nuclear Medicine, Hospital das Forças Armadas (HFA), Brasilia, Distrito Federal, Brazil
e-mail: karina.mosci@gruposanta.com.br

T. Thientunyakit
Division of Nuclear Medicine, Department of Radiology, Faculty of Medicine Siriraj Hospital, Mahidol University, Bangkok, Thailand
e-mail: tanyaluck.thi@mahidol.ac.th

D. J. Cross · S. Minoshima
Department of Radiology and Imaging Sciences, University of Utah, Salt Lake City, UT, USA
e-mail: d.cross@utah.edu;
satoshi.minoshima@hsc.utah.edu

G. N. Bischof
Department of Nuclear Medicine, University Hospital Cologne, Cologne, Germany

Molecular Organization of the Brain, Institute for Neuroscience and Medicine (INM-2), Jülich, Germany
e-mail: gerard.bischof@uk-koeln.de

J. Arbizu
Department of Nuclear Medicine, Clínica Universidad de Navarra, Pamplona, Navarra, Spain
e-mail: jarbizu@unav.es

receptor density depending on the radioligand utilized, and possess a lower spatial resolution for identifying brain structures when compared to anatomic imaging methods such as magnetic resonance imaging (MRI). Knowledge of normal radiotracer biodistribution, as well as brain structural and functional anatomy, is fundamental for the recognition of abnormalities. In fact, the identification of specific disease imaging patterns depends not only on the ability to detect the expected abnormalities, but also on an appreciation of the areas, which are usually not affected with specific disease entities. A thorough understanding of neuropathology and the potential association of the observed abnormalities with clinical information can improve the diagnostic accuracy. It is also recognized that the introduction of hybrid technologies with CT or MRI provides correlative anatomic imaging information to the functional imaging, but also requires additional training.

The intent of this chapter is to provide a guide for molecular brain interpretation, which is suitable for all levels of expertise. The content includes a teaching directory with fundamental knowledge, which includes an overview of structural and functional neuroanatomy, and a description of the normal biodistribution of most clinically available radiotracers, as well as physiologic variants and technical artifacts to guide imaging interpretation. The tutorial of systematic imaging analysis is based on visual assessments and aided by semi-quantitate analyses to help improve disease pattern recognition. Suggestions for how to adequately report studies in each molecular imaging modality are presented in case mode. Clinical situations where molecular imaging can aid in the diagnosis of different neurodegenerative pathologies are discussed.

The Fundamentals

Normal Structural and Functional Neuroanatomy for SPECT and PET imaging

In the Appendix, we provide images of cross-sectional neuroanatomy based on MRI and 18F-FDG-PET (FDG-PET), for both beginners and experienced physicians. To learn more about brain anatomy readers should reference existing digital atlases, which are available through neuroimaging software toolsets or provided by independent research groups. Before starting to navigate the three-dimensional brain images, note that the central nervous system (CNS) is organized along the rostrocaudal and dorsoventral axes of the body. The terms for the major anatomical axes within the brain are dorsal–ventral, rostral–caudal, and left–right, equivalent to superior–inferior, anterior–posterior, and left–right, respectively. In addition to these axes, the term lateral–medial is used to describe if a location is near a side edge (lateral) or near the center (medial) of the brain [1] (Fig. 17.1). A short overview of gross brain anatomy and function to promote familiarization with the essential structures is required for a meaningful and accurate interpretation of molecular imaging studies in current clinical applications. For more comprehensive descriptions, readers can also refer to standard texts of neuroanatomy [2–8].

The brain is composed of neurons and glial cells, which provide the underlying substrate for a multitude of brain functions. The cell bodies of neurons constitute the gray matter, which is located in the cortex on the superficial layers, and myelinated axons, located more internally, compose the white matter. There are also "islands" of gray matter within the subcortical white matter, such as the basal ganglia and thalamus, which form nodes that participate in a variety of brain networks [9]. The CNS includes the cerebrum, cerebellum, brain stem, and spinal cord (Fig. 17.2). One approach to a better understanding of the CNS is to conceptualize that it is composed of several functional modules: spinal cord, brainstem, cerebellum, diencephalon, cerebral hemispheres, basal ganglia, and limbic system, and to facilitate molecular imaging interpretation, focus will be given to these various modules (Fig. 17.3). Also noteworthy is the ventricular system, a labyrinth of fluid-filled cavities with supportive and chemical environment regulation functions, which can be very helpful as anatomical landmarks due to their location within each of the seven central nervous system divisions (Fig. 17.4).

BRAIN ORIENTATION

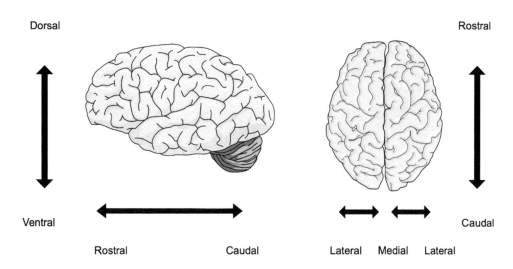

Fig. 17.1 Brain anatomical orientation

Fig. 17.2 Representation of a sagittal view of the central nervous system

CENTRAL NERVOUS SYSTEM

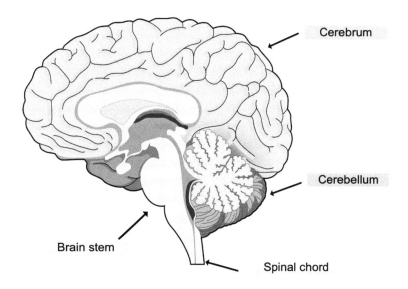

The cerebrum comprises most of the brain. With a highly convoluted surface, which is a result of an evolutionary adaptation to fit a greater surface area into the confined space of the cranial cavity, the cortex on the outer surface contains ridges and grooves, known as gyri and sulci. Brain anatomy is characterized by very deep sulci called fissures [10] (Fig. 17.5).

The cerebrum is divided into left and right hemispheres by a deep longitudinal fissure, known as the interhemispheric fissure. As a general feature, each cerebral hemisphere is divided

CNS FUNCTIONAL MODULES

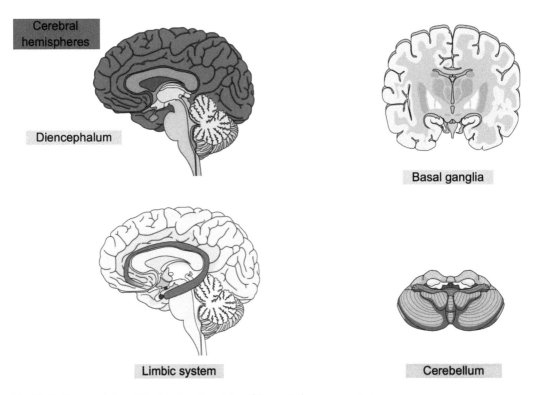

Fig. 17.3 Representation of the functional modules of the central nervous system

into four separate lobes by the central and parieto-occipital sulci, and the lateral fissure. The central sulcus separates the frontal lobe from the parietal lobe and the parieto-occipital sulcus separates the parietal lobe from the occipital lobe. The lateral or Sylvian fissure separates the temporal lobe from the frontal and parietal lobes [11] (Fig. 17.6) (Table 17.1). A full description of all lobe gyri and sulci are beyond the scope of this review, and can be reviewed in standard texts of neuroanatomy [2–8], but we would like to highlight the locations of the precentral, postcentral, and cingulate gyri, as well as the precuneus, which are important structures for imaging interpretation in neurodegeneration (Fig. 17.7).

The two cerebral hemispheres are connected by white matter tracts consisting of nerve fibers or axons, which are collectively referred to as commissures. The corpus callosum is the largest

white matter tract and permits the cerebral cortex to operate as a coordinated structure. The anterior and posterior commissures are smaller bundles of nerve fibers which connect parts of the temporal lobes and midbrain regions. We highlight the importance of these two structures, as they collectively form an important plane for cranial sectional imaging. The anterior commissure/posterior commissure line (AC-PC line), passing through the apex of the anterior and the inferior edge of the posterior commissures, provides reliable anatomic orientation and constitutes a common basis for standardized stereotactic reporting of neuroimaging findings [12] (Fig. 17.8).

The diencephalon is mostly composed of the thalamus and hypothalamus [13]. The thalamus functions as a relay for sensory and motor signals to the cerebral cortex and helps regulate important processes such as consciousness, sleep, and

VENTRICULAR SYSTEM

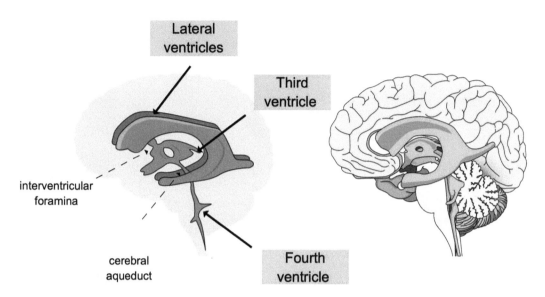

Fig. 17.4 Ventricular system in 3-dimensional representation: Note that each division of the central nervous system (CNS) contains a portion of the ventricular system. The paired lateral ventricles, with components inside frontal, parietal, temporal, and occipital lobes, communicate with the third ventricle in the diencephalon through the interventricular foramina. The third ventricle communicates with the fourth ventricle located in the pons and medulla through the cerebral aqueduct inside the midbrain. The fourth ventricle continues caudally as the central canal of the caudal medulla and spinal cord

alertness [14]. It is easily recognizable in brain imaging, as a midline symmetrical egg-shaped gray matter structure, situated between the cerebral cortex and midbrain, forming the lateral wall of the third ventricle (Figs. 17.3 and 17.9). Note that all the ascending pathways terminate in the thalamic nuclei, and their information is projected with some modifications onto specific regions of the cerebral cortex, on the same side [10]. In fact, the connections between many thalamic nuclei and their projecting cortical areas are so strong that if such a cortical region is destroyed, the neurons in that particular thalamic nucleus subsequently atrophy [14].

The basal ganglia are a subcortical structures buried within the cerebral hemispheres, lateral and anterior to the thalamic nuclei, and include the caudate nucleus, putamen, globus pallidus, and subthalamic nucleus (Fig. 17.9). These nuclei are separated from the cerebral cortex by white matter but are functionally linked to the cerebrum [14]. The basal ganglia are important for motor function, notably the storage and replay of complex motor activities, with cognitive and emotional functions as well [6]. Collectively the putamen and caudate are called the striatum and are continuous in the anterior direction [14]. The putamen combined with the globus pallidus forms the lenticular nucleus, which is wedged between the external capsule and the anterior and posterior limbs of the internal capsule [15]. It is important to note that the internal capsule, comprised of the anterior and posterior limbs, and the genu, is one of the most important components of cerebral white matter. All fibers projecting from the thalami to the cerebral hemispheres pass through the internal capsule, while all fibers leaving the cerebral cortex and going either to the diencephalon, basal nuclei, brain stem, or spinal cord must also pass through these tracts [14].

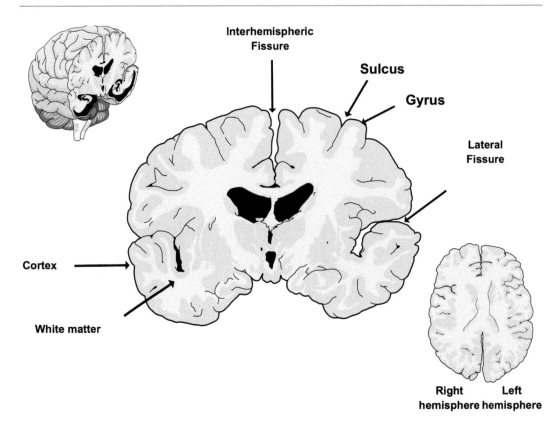

Fig. 17.5 Brain coronal and transaxial slices representation demonstrating the hemispheres, cortex, white matter, sulcus, and gyri

Fig. 17.6 Representation of brain lobes and fissures in lateral view

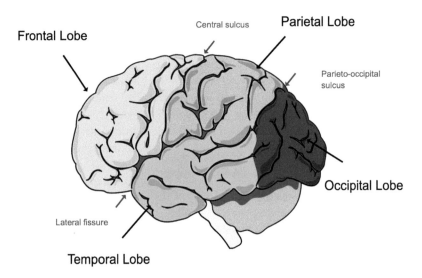

Table 17.1 Brain structures and function

Structure	Function
Frontal lobe	Control of voluntary movement, involved in attention, short-term memory tasks, motivation, planning, speech
Parietal lobe	Integrates proprioceptive and mechanoceptive stimuli; involved in language processing
Temporal lobe	Mediates a variety of sensory functions and participates in memory and emotions
Occipital lobe	Receives and interprets visual input
Insular cortex	Processes and integrates taste sensation, visceral and pain sensation, and vestibular functions
Amygdala	Participates in emotions and helps to coordinate the body's response to stressful and threatening situations
Hippocampus	Critical for the formation of new long-term memories; involved in the voluntary recall of past knowledge and experiences
Basal ganglia	Important for motor function, notably the storage and replay of complex motor programs, and cognitive and emotional functions
Thalamus	Relaying sensory and motor signals to the cerebral cortex; impacts consciousness, sleep, and regulates alertness
Cerebellum	Functions at an subconscious level to coordinate voluntary motor functions; plays a role in higher brain functions, including language, cognition, and emotion

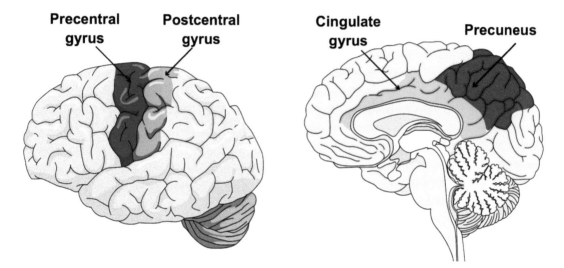

Fig. 17.7 Representation of the precentral gyrus, postcentral gyrus, cingulate gyrus, and precuneus location

The limbic system is a group of structures, which are located along the border between the cerebral cortex and the hypothalamus. These structures are involved in the control of emotions, behavior, and drive, and also may influence memory formation. Anatomically, the limbic structures include the subcallosal, cingulate, and parahippocampal gyri, as well as the hippocampal formation, amygdaloid nucleus, mammillary bodies, and anterior thalamic nucleus (Fig. 17.10). The alveus, fimbria, fornix, mammillothalamic tract, and stria terminalis constitute the connecting pathways to this system [7]. The cingulate passes within the subcortical white matter on the medial surface of the cerebral hemisphere in the cingulate gyrus and connects the subcallosal, medial–frontal, and orbital–frontal cortices with the temporal lobe, occipital, and cingulate cortices [14]. Recognition of the cingulate gyrus is of particular importance due to its early involvement in some neurodegenerative disorders (Figs. 17.7 and 17.10). In fact, the anterior and

Fig. 17.8 Representation of a sagittal view of the CNS showing the anterior commissure/posterior commissure line (AC-PC line), passing through the apex of the anterior and the inferior edge of the posterior commissure, used for standardized stereotactic orientation and reporting of neuroimaging

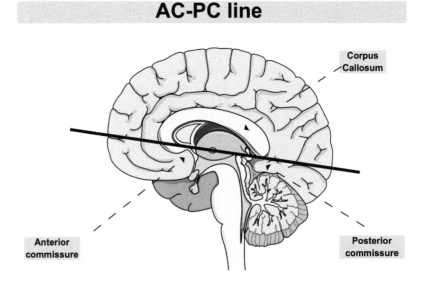

posterior cingulate cortices are distinguished histologically and usually show a distinct pattern of involvement in several neurodegenerative diseases such as Alzheimer disease (AD) and frontotemporal dementia spectrum disorders (FTD). While the anterior cingulum carries information, which is important for attention and volitional control of cognitive and motor function, the posterior cingulate carries information, which plays an integrative role in visuospatial processing and

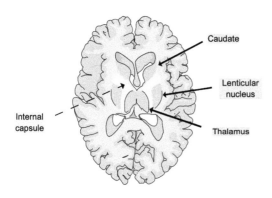

Fig. 17.9 Transaxial representation of brain showing the basal ganglia, composed of the caudate and lenticular nucleus (putamen and globus pallidus), thalamus, and internal capsule

memory [6]. The hippocampus is the posterior part of limbic lobe while frontal part is the amygdala. The hippocampus can be distinguished externally as a layer of densely packed neurons, which curls into S-shaped structure on the edge of temporal lobe [16]. Functionally, anatomically, and cytoarchitecturally, hippocampus is quite different from the cerebral cortex, and is critical for the formation of new long-term memories as well as being involved in voluntary recall of past knowledge and experiences [6]. The amygdala lies dorsally to the hippocampal formation and rostrally to the temporal horn of the lateral ventricle, and not only participates in emotional memory but also helps to coordinate the body's response to stressful and threatening situations [10].

The cerebellum, situated posterior to the brainstem and inferior to the posterior aspects of the cerebral hemispheres, is like a miniature version of the cerebral cortex, having an outer layer of gray matter, which is very highly folded and white matter tracts running within (Fig. 17.11). The white matter tracts provide connections with the rest of the brain, as well as the brainstem. The cerebellum is divided into two lateral hemispheres and the midline is the vermis. It coordinates voluntary motor functions so they occur smoothly

Fig. 17.10 Representation on the limbic system in sagittal view. The limbic structures include the subcallosal, the cingulate, and the parahippocampal gyri, the hippocampal formation, the amygdaloid nucleus, the mammillary bodies, and the anterior thalamic nucleus

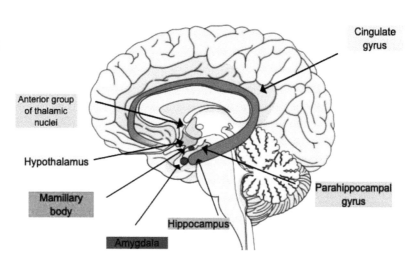

LIMBIC SYSTEM

Cingulate gyrus

Anterior group of thalamic nuclei

Hypothalamus

Mamillary body

Hippocampus

Amygdala

Parahippocampal gyrus

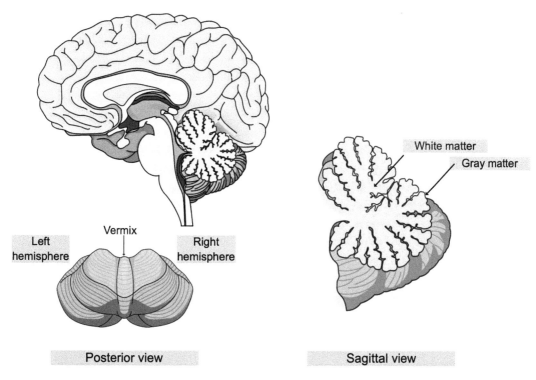

CEREBELLUM

White matter

Gray matter

Vermix

Left hemisphere

Right hemisphere

Posterior view

Sagittal view

Fig. 17.11 Cerebellum representation in sagittal and posterior view

and accurately [14]. In addition, parts of the cerebellum have roles in higher brain functions, including language, cognition, and emotion [10].

The ventricular system is composed of the two lateral ventricles, the third ventricle, the cerebral aqueduct, and the fourth ventricle. Within each cerebral hemisphere the relatively large lateral ventricle is connected to the third ventricle of the diencephalon through the interventricular foramina (of Monro). The third ventricle in turn connects to the fourth ventricle of the pons and medulla through the narrow cerebral aqueduct (of Sylvius) in the midbrain. The fourth ventricle runs caudally as the central canal of the caudal medulla and spinal cord [17]. It is important to note, as previously mentioned, that each division of the CNS contains a portion of the ventricular system, which can provide useful anatomical landmarks (Fig. 17.4).

Functional Areas of the Cerebral Cortex

A simple way to classify the functional areas of the cortex, which is suitable to interpret molecular imaging findings in relation to clinical symptoms/disease presentations, is to assume that the cortical areas are organized into primary, secondary, and associative areas. The primary cortices are responsible for basic motor or sensory processing, while the areas surrounding the primary cortices are the secondary processing regions, which receive afferent projections from the corresponding primary areas as well as the thalamus. The association cortices integrate, process, and analyze the various sensory stimuli, and integrate higher mental functions [18]. Large areas of the cerebral cortex receive input from multiple sensory modalities as well as various secondary regions to create the associations between various kinds of sensory information. These include the multimodal association areas (posterior, anterior, and limbic association areas). The existence of these broad areas with multimodal integration, which combine sensory and motor input with an emotional content, is what makes the human brain so distinctive and complex [14]. Please refer to Fig. 17.12 for the anatomical location of the following areas.

CEREBRAL CORTEX FUNCTIONAL AREAS

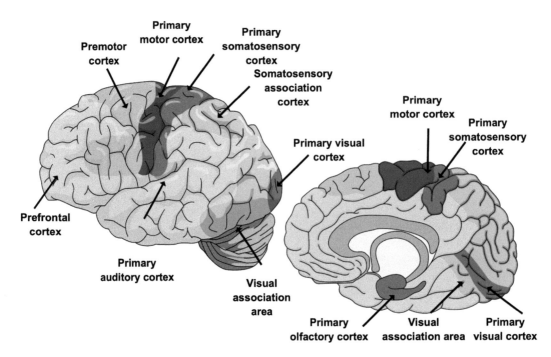

Fig. 17.12 Functional areas of the cerebral cortex

In general, the frontal lobe is involved in diverse behavioral functions of cognition and emotions including executive or decision-making (Tables 17.1 and 17.2). The precentral gyrus is known as the primary motor cortex, which controls the mechanical actions of movement. Notice that the primary motor cortex of one hemisphere controls movement on the contralateral side of the body, as 90% of motor axons cross the midline in the lower brainstem and upper cervical spinal cord. The premotor areas, which are important for motor decisions and movement planning, are adjacent to the primary motor cortex, anteriorly. The inferior frontal gyrus contains Broca's area, in the left hemisphere (side of dominance) in most people, and is essential for the articulation of speech. One should note that much of the frontal lobe is an association cortex. The prefrontal association cortex, located in the most anterior portion of the frontal lobe, is important in thought, cognition, and emotions [10]. The medial frontal cortex, sometimes called the medial prefrontal area, is important in arousal and motivation. The cingulate gyrus, medial frontal lobe, and most of the orbital gyri are primarily emotional processing association areas [10].

The primary somatosensory cortex, which is located in the postcentral gyrus of the parietal lobe, mediates our sensory perceptions of touch, pain, and limb position. The remaining portion of the parietal lobe constitutes the parietal association cortices, including the superior and inferior

Table 17.2 Functional neuroanatomy

	Location	Function
Limbic system	Cingulate and parahippocampal gyri, hippocampal formation, amygdaloid nucleus, mammillary bodies, and the anterior thalamic nucleus	Involved in the control of emotion, behavior, and drive also appears to be important to memory
Anterior cingulate	Anterior aspect of the cingulate gyrus	Important in attention and volitional control of cognitive and motor functions. Mirrors frontal lobe functions
Posterior cingulate	Posterior aspect of the cingulate gyrus	Plays an integrative role in visuospatial processing and memory
Primary motor cortex	Precentral gyrus	Participates in controlling the mechanical actions of movement
Premotor areas	Anteriorly to the primary motor cortex	Important for motor decision making and movement planning
Prefrontal association cortex	Most anterior portion of the frontal lobe	Important in thought, cognition, and emotions
Medial prefrontal area	Medial frontal cortex	Important in arousal and motivation
Primary somatosensory cortex	Postcentral gyrus	Mediates our perceptions of touch, pain, and limb positioning
Parietal association cortex	Superior and inferior parietal lobules	Processes and integrates somatic and sensory information
Primary visual cortex	In the walls and depths of the calcarine fissure	Important in the initial stages of visual processing and awareness of visual stimulus
Visual association cortex	Surrounding the primary visual cortex	Plays a role in visual stimulus analysis, including the perception of the shape and color of objects
Primary auditory cortex	Superior temporal gyrus on the gyri of Heschl	Perception and localization of sounds
Broca's area	Inferior frontal gyrus (in most people in the left hemisphere)	Articulation of speech
Wernicke's area	Superior temporal gyrus (in most people in the left hemisphere)	Specialized for speech, including spoken and written language comprehension

parietal lobules. The superior parietal lobule is a higher-order somatosensory area, for higher-level processing of somatic and other sensory information. The inferior parietal lobule integrates diverse sensory information for processes such as perception, language, mathematical reasoning, and visuospatial cognition [10].

The occipital lobe has a more singular function, subserving vision. The primary visual cortex, located in the walls and depths of the calcarine fissure on the medial brain surface, performs the initial stages of visual processing, including the awareness of visual stimulus. The surrounding higher-order visual areas are the visual association cortices, which perform visual stimuli analyses, such as the perception of shapes and colors [10].

The temporal lobe mediates a variety of sensory processes as well as that of memory and emotions. The primary auditory cortex works with surrounding areas in the superior temporal gyrus as well as regions in the lateral and the superior temporal sulci, and the auditory association cortex, for the perception and localization of sounds. Wernicke's area, in the superior temporal gyrus and, in most people, in the left hemisphere (the side of dominance), is specialized for speech, and mediates spoken and written language comprehension. The primary olfactory cortex is located on the medial aspect of the temporal lobe, in the uncus, and connects directly to the limbic system. The middle temporal gyrus, particularly the portion close to the occipital lobe, is essential for the perception of visual motion, while the inferior temporal gyrus mediates the perception of visual form and color [10].

The insular cortex plays a role in the processing and integration of taste, visceral and pain sensation, and vestibular functions [10].

Note that the posterior association area is where visual, auditory, and somatosensory association areas meet, and the anterior association area includes the prefrontal cortex.

Vasculature of the Brain and Vascular Disease

Brain function is critically dependent on an uninterrupted supply of oxygenated blood. The major vessels of the brain include the cortical branches of the anterior, middle, and posterior cerebral arteries (Fig. 17.13). The three major cerebral artery territories fit together like a "jigsaw puzzle", as they supply the hemispheres. Areas of confluence between two territories are known as "watershed areas" and are particularly vulnerable to hypoperfusion.

The anterior cerebral arteries (ACA) supply most of the medial hemispheric surface, except for the occipital lobe. The ACA cortical branches supply the anterior two-thirds of the medial hemispheres and convexity, and the penetrating branches supply the medial basal ganglia, corpus callous genu, and anterior limb of internal capsule. The middle cerebral arteries (MCA) typically supply most of the lateral and superior surface of the brain, except for the convexity, inferior temporal gyrus, and the anterior tip of the temporal lobe (although this may vary). Its penetrating branches, the medial lenticulostriate arteries supply the medial basal ganglia, caudate nucleus, and internal capsule, while the lateral lenticulostriate arteries supply the lateral putamen, caudate nucleus, and external capsule. The posterior cerebral arteries (PCA) supply the occipital poles and most of the undersurface of the temporal lobe except for its tip, which is usually supplied by MCA. Their penetrating branches supply the midbrain, thalami, posterior limb of the internal capsule and optic tract. The ventricular/choroidal branches supply the choroid plexus of the third/lateral ventricles, parts of the thalami, the posterior commissure, and the cerebral peduncles. The splenial branches supply the posterior body and splenium of the corpus callosum [19].

It is advisable to recall the possibility of vascular contribution to cognitive impairment when analyzing brain images in the context of neurodegeneration, as it implies a spectrum of age-related vascular pathologies, including not only stroke, but microinfarcts, microhemorrhages, leukoaraiosis, and cerebral amyloid angiopathy [20]. The presence of comorbidities and coexisting diseases, such as macro- and microvascular changes, must be taken into consideration, particularly when uncertain or atypical image patterns do not definitively fit to one of the known neurodegenerative diseases [21].

VASCULAR TERRITORIES OF THE BRAIN

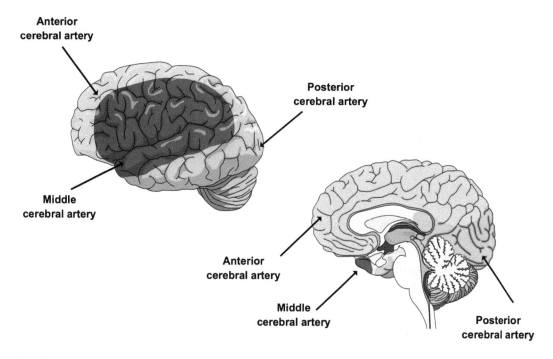

Fig. 17.13   Vascular territories of the brain

Molecular Imaging Radiotracers Approved for Clinical Use: Normal Physiology, Age Variants, Best Practices, and Artifacts

Normal Physiology

Knowledge of specific radiotracer biodistribution and normal variability is fundamental for the recognition of characteristic patterns of abnormalities and to perform adequate scan interpretation. Diagnostic accuracy can be improved with multimodality images, which combine SPECT and PET with CT or MRI, to better describe functional and spatial/structural information, and the addition of semiquantitative analyses may provide further benefit. However, these multimodal/multi-informational approaches can also introduce potential sources of interference and artifacts, which should be recognized to avoid potential misdiagnoses.

This section will describe the physiologic distribution of most of the readily available brain imaging radiopharmaceuticals, including perfusion/metabolism, protein deposition (Amyloid

and Tau) and nigrostriatal dopaminergic pathway integrity, as well as factors that can affect image quality and create potential artifacts.

Metabolic and Perfusion Radiotracers
Normal Physiologic Distribution

Current knowledge indicates that a variety of neurodegenerative disorders have global and focal effects on neuronal activity, which usually result in alterations of brain metabolism and perfusion. Glucose is the major source of energy for the brain, which does not have substantial storage capacity, and thus requires a continuous supply from plasma to maintain activity. Decreased neuronal activity due to neurodegenerative processes can be detected directly or indirectly by either glucose metabolic and perfusion imaging, since regional neuronal activity and blood flow are tightly coupled with normal brain autoregulation. At present, metabolic tracers are widely available for PET, but only perfusion tracers are available for SPECT imaging. Perfusion SPECT can be applied in dementia workup and presents similar pathologic findings as metabolic PET; however PET imaging is usually more accurate due to a combination of factors including a higher spatial resolution, sensitivity, improved attenuation correction, and nature of available tracers, as well as limitations to SPECT quantification.

The most widely used SPECT perfusion tracers are 99mTc-labeled compounds ethyl-cysteine-dimer (ECD) and hexamethyl-propylene-amine-oxime (HMPAO). They possess very similar kinetic properties in normal brain tissue, but have differences in "in vitro" stability, uptake mechanisms, cerebral distributions, and dosimetry [22]. They are lipophilic compounds which penetrate an intact blood-brain barrier by simple diffusion and subsequently remain in brain tissue due to conversion into hydrophilic compounds [23].

In a normal cerebral perfusion SPECT scan (Image 17.1), there is up to a fourfold higher radiotracer uptake in cortical gray matter relative to white matter. Activity is also high in the subcortical gray matter, such as the basal ganglia, and is highest in the cerebellum. Typically, the activity is evenly distributed between the lobes of the brain with mostly left/right symmetry. There are differences in the perfusion patterns between 99mTc-HMPAO and 99mTc-ECD, which is likely due to variation in the mechanisms responsible for their cerebral accumulation [24]. Images with 99mTc-ECD seem to reflect metabolic activity more closely than those with 99mTc-HMPAO [24]. In the HMPAO-SPECT images, relatively high activity can be observed in the basal ganglia and cerebellum, while in ECD-SPECT images, high activity can be observed in the medial aspect of the occipital lobe [24]. Note that the variation in visual cortex activity may also be due to tracer uptake with open or closed eyes. When comparing the perfusion SPECT images to 18F-fluorodeoxyglucose (FDG) PET images, the most prominent difference related to radiotracer distribution is the higher uptake in the cerebellum.

The PET radiotracer, FDG, is a glucose analog and hence the prime metabolic marker for neuronal activity. Regional consumption of FDG reflects the demand of energy at rest and during brain activation. With respect to pathological processes, FDG uptake reflexes glucose consumption at the synapses. The tracer crosses the blood-brain barrier via the glucose transporter and is enzymatically altered in brain tissue by hexokinase-mediated phosphorylation, resulting in the substrate, FDG-6-phosphate, which cannot be further utilized for glycolic metabolism, and remains trapped in the cell. In addition, FDG brain uptake depends not only on neuronal activity, but also can reflect the consumption of glucose by the astrocytes in support of neuronal function, transport mediated by the glucose transporter 1 (GLUT1) across the blood-brain barrier, and possibly pathological inflammatory conditions such as microglial activation [25]. Interestingly, when cortical projection neurons are affected by diseases such as stroke, epilepsy, and neurodegeneration, not only the primary lesion shows decreased FDG uptake, but also synapses in remote areas connected to the primary lesion can show decreased uptake [21].

In normal subjects, brain FDG uptake is usually symmetrical, but slight differences can be observed among different brain regions (Image 17.2). The most intense FDG uptake occurs in the primary visual cortex and posterior cingulate as well as the frontal eye fields. Uptake is usually higher in the frontal, parietal, and occipital areas than in temporal cortex. Metabolic activity is usually lower in medial temporal cortex, including hippocampal areas, than in neocortical regions [26]. The subcortical putamen, caudate nucleus, and thalamus have relatively moderate uptake. With a lower prevalence, generally below 10%, slight asymmetries in FDG uptake can be observed in the Wernicke area, the frontal eye fields, and the angular gyrus [26]. The white matter is relatively photopenic.

Normal Physiologic Distribution of Radiotracers for Protein Deposition (Amyloid and Tau)

Aberrant intracellular or extracellular deposition of self-aggregating misfolded proteins is a common finding in primary neurodegenerative disorders. These abnormal proteinaceous deposits are characteristic disease features, which can provide information about the molecular pathogenesis of a neurodegenerative disorder. Over the past 20 years, the amyloid cascade hypothesis has guided most research of Alzheimer's disease (AD) suggesting that beta amyloid (Aβ) is the

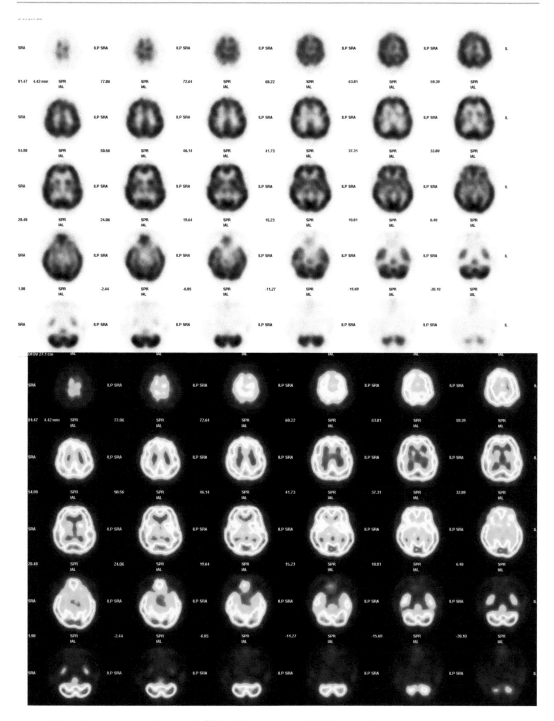

Image 17.1 The normal distribution of a ^{99m}Tc-ECD perfusion SPECT in a healthy control is displayed in axial plane

initial trigger of the disease and precedes pathological tau as well as symptom onset, by decades. However evidence indicates that tau deposition is more associated with neurodegeneration and cognitive decline [27].

The first PET tracer for imaging Aβ plaques was developed at the University of Pittsburg and was called 11C-Pittsburg Compound B (11C-PIB), but the short half-life of the C^{11} isotope presented limitations for widespread clinical use.

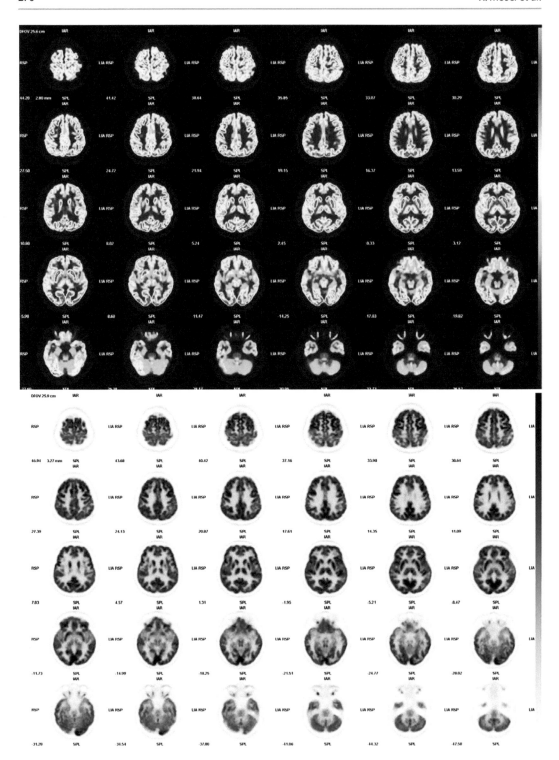

Image 17.2 The normal distribution of an 18F-FDG-PET in a healthy control is displayed in axial plane

Subsequently, 18F-labeled tracers were developed and are now commercially available, with 18F-florbetapir, 18F-flutemetamol, and 18F-florbetaben approved for clinical imaging (Images 17.3, 17.4, and 17.5). It is important to remember that although these radiotracers share a common imaging target and present similar imaging characteristics, they differ in tracer

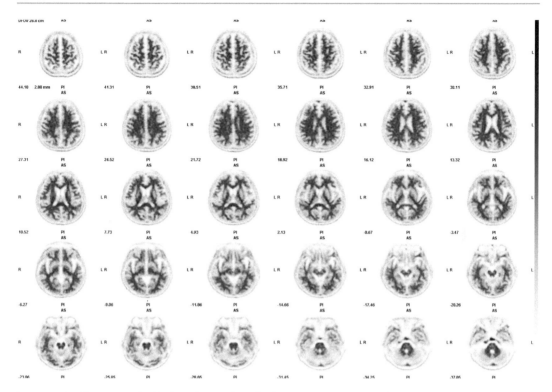

Image 17.3 The normal distribution of a negative 18F-florbetapir PET in a healthy control is displayed in the axial plane

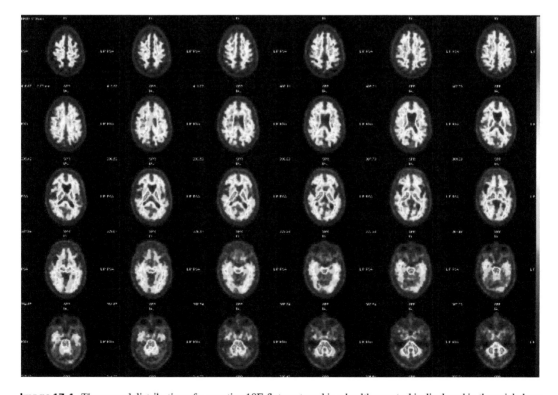

Image 17.4 The normal distribution of a negative 18F-flutemetamol in a healthy control is displayed in the axial plane

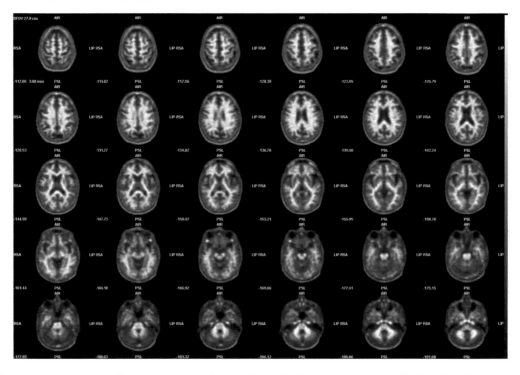

Image 17.5 The normal distribution of a negative 18F-florbetaben in a healthy control is displayed in axial plane

kinetics, specific binding ratios, and optimal imaging parameters, and have specific recommendations for injected dose, time from injection to imaging, and scan duration [28].

Normal amyloid tracer biodistribution for a negative Amyloid-PET scan shows nonspecific white matter uptake and little or no binding in the gray matter, resulting in a very clear gray to white matter contrast. The uptake pattern resembles a blueprint of typical white matter anatomy, with numerous concave arboreal ramifications that do not reach the cortical ribbon. A clear, wide, irregular gap between the cerebral hemispheres is usually visible. The gray matter uptake intensity observed in the cerebellar cortex is less than that usually seen in the normal cerebral cortical regions due to closer proximity of white matter structures to the gray matter. Note that the amount of normal white matter uptake varies with the radiotracer used.

Research advances, particularly in the field of AD, have motivated investigations on the role of tau pathology in neurodegenerative disease. Several neurodegenerative diseases are characterized by tau aggregates, which can vary by disease in either morphological or ultrastructural conformations. Accumulating evidence suggests a closer association between the density and neocortical spread of neurofibrillary tangles (NFTs) measured by Tau-PET with neurodegeneration and cognitive decline in AD in comparison to that of Amyloid-PET [29, 30], despite the apparent presence of amyloid pathology prior to tau accumulation [31].

However, the development of Tau-PET tracers has been challenging, with limitations due to the intracellular target location, a relatively low target expression, and a high concentration of competing off-target binding sites [32]. Recently, the Tau-PET tracer, 18F-flortaucipir (previously known as AV-1451), with high affinity to paired helical filaments and insoluble neurofibrillary tangles, was approved by the United States Food and Drug Administration (FDA) for clinical use [33]. The tracer retention pattern corresponds well with Braak staging of neurofibrillary tau pathology. However, 18F-flortaucipir PET imaging faces challenges with off-target binding, especially in the basal ganglia, and has a higher affinity to "AD-like" tau aggregates in comparison to other neurodegenerative tauopathies. Novel "second-generation" Tau-PET tracers have somewhat overcome these shortcomings with respect to the known off-target binding sites, and in principle, may translate into a higher

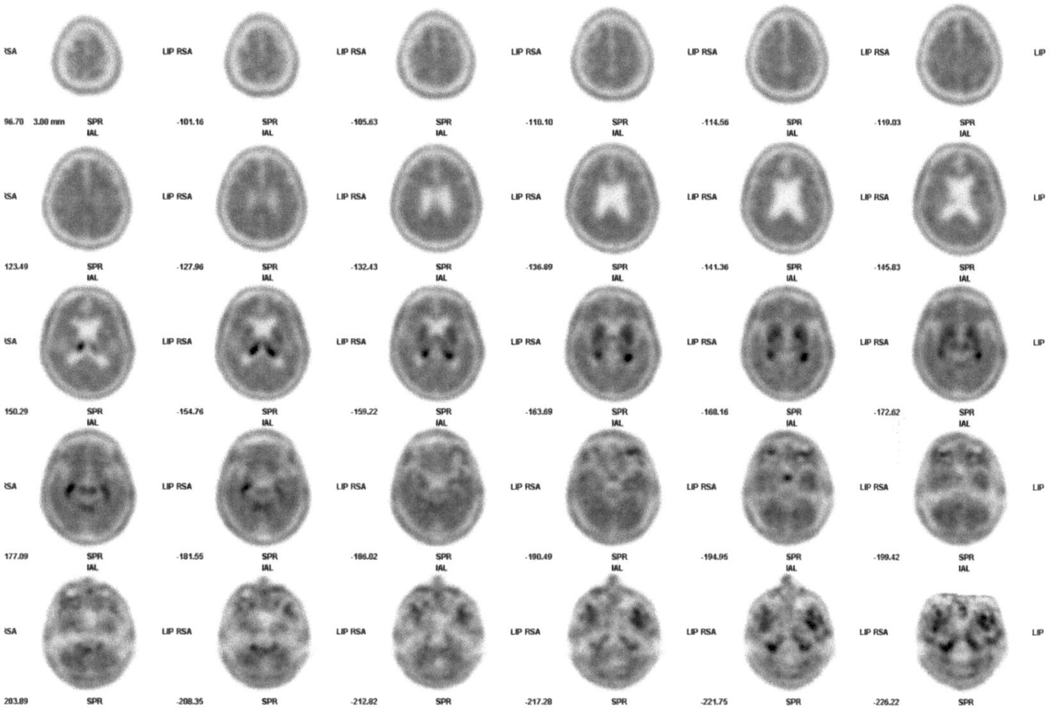

Image 17.6 The normal distribution of 18F-flortaucipir in a healthy control (72 yo male Aβ−, MMSE 28) is displayed in axial plane. Images show no significant tracer uptake in cortical region with "off-target" binding in basal ganglia and thalamus, and in the choroid plexus

sensitivity for the detection of early secondary and primary tauopathies [34].

In cognitively normal young individuals, 18F-flortaucipir PET shows little focal radiotracer retention besides the off-target binding in the brainstem, striatum, and retina [35] (Image 17.6). Second-generation tracers show significantly less off-target binding, as seen with 18F-PI-2620 (Image 17.7). Knowledge of radiotracer off-target binding is fundamental for an accurate interpretation of a Tau-PET scan (Image 17.8). Note that in elderly individuals with normal cognition, an age-related increase in radiotracer retention following the anatomically specific patterns of neocortical susceptibility to tau deposition is expected [32].

The Normal Physiologic Distribution of Tracers for Nigrostriatal Dopaminergic Pathway Integrity (18F-Fluorodopa PET and DAT-SPECT)

Dopaminergic function, presynaptic and postsynaptic, can be assessed through molecular imaging. However, in clinical practice, the most widely available tracers bind to presynaptic dopamine nerve terminals, with specific targets of dopamine synthesis, 18F-Fluorodopa PET (18F-DOPA-PET), as well as the dopamine transporter, DAT-SPECT agents.

From a pathophysiological viewpoint, dopaminergic neurodegeneration as detected by 18F-DOPA-PET tends to be less than that seen with DAT-SPECT. However, with regard to imaging, both tracers can diagnose presynaptic dopaminergic deficits with excellent sensitivity and specificity, in early stages of Parkinson's disease (PD) [36]. PET provides a higher spatial resolution than SPECT and is better for quantification, but SPECT is more affordable and more readily available in clinical practice. DAT-SPECT with 123I–ioflupane (DaT scan) is mainly used in Europe and the US, while Asia and South America primarily use the 99mTc-labeled tropane derivative (99mTc-TRODAT-1) for SPECT imaging. These tracers provide a measure of neuronal integrity by binding to sites on the presynaptic dopamine neuron, with highest density in the striatum.

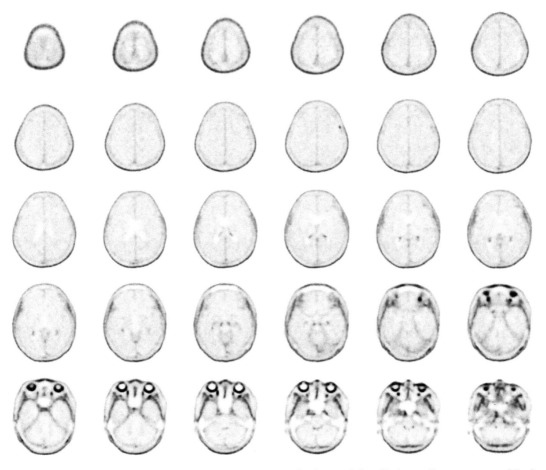

Image 17.7 The normal distribution of 18F-PI2620 in a healthy control (74 yo male Aβ−, MMSE 30) is displayed in axial plane. The images show no significant tracer uptake in cortical region and "off-target" binding in sub- stantia nigra and choroid plexus. (Image courtesy of Prof Villemagne and Rowe, University of Melbourne, Australia)

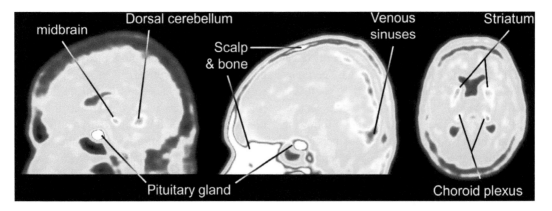

Image 17.8 Areas of frequent 18F-flortaucipir off-target binding. (This image is a derivate from Sonni I, Lesman Segev OH, Baker SL, et al. Evaluation of a visual interpre- tation method for tau-PET with 18F-flortaucipir. *Alzheimers Dement (Amst)*. 2020;12(1):e12133. Published 2020 Nov 28. doi:10.1002/dad2.12133, with permission from: John Wiley & Sons, Inc)

In normal subjects, the striatal uptake is homogeneous and symmetrical, although a mild asymmetry may be present in normal controls. The normal striata are comma-shaped structures, with symmetric well-delineated borders (Image 17.9).

With 18F-DOPA-PET the local maximum striatal uptake is normally in the putamen, while in DAT-SPECT, uptake appears more evenly distributed (Images 17.10, 17.11, and 17.12). Despite the higher spatial resolution with PET, extrastriatal uptake due to monoaminergic inner-

vation is low and usually undetectable. In cases where nigrostriatal degeneration is present, catecholaminergic (locus coeruleus) and dopaminergic (substantia nigra) nuclei may become more visible, exhibiting a kind of a "Mickey Mouse" shape in the midbrain, due to a global reduction of striatal uptake [37].

Aging Effects on Imaging

Normal aging is associated with brain weight reduction, cortical atrophy, and altered white mat-

NORMAL STRIATUM

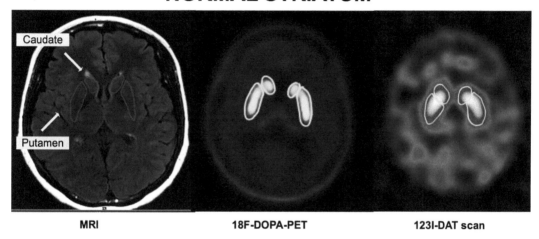

Image 17.9 Normal striatum in the axial plane is demonstrated in MRI (left), 18F-DOPA-PET (middle), and 123I-DAT-SPECT (right)

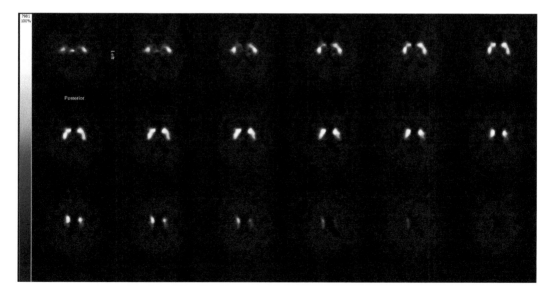

Image 17.10 The normal distribution of 123I–ioflupane SPECT is displayed in axial plane

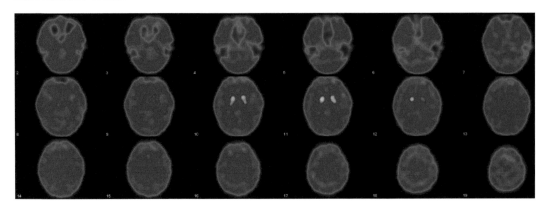

Image 17.11 The normal distribution of 99mTc-TRODAT-1 SPECT is displayed in axial plane

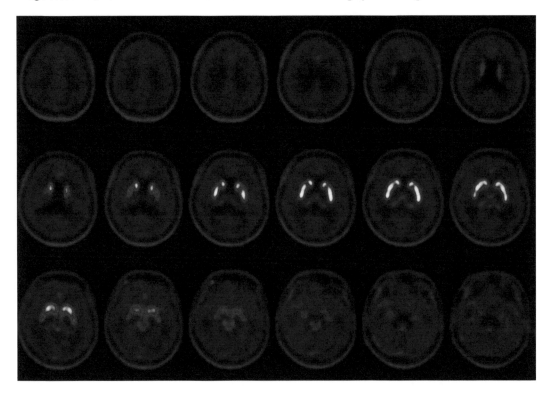

Image 17.12 The normal distribution of 18F-FDOPA-PET is displayed in axial plane

ter, as well as molecular and functional changes. Knowledge of the expected normal aging variability is essential for adequate study interpretation.

Tracers for Metabolism and Perfusion

Generally, the aging process is characterized by a progressive loss of brain volume, as indicated by prominent sulci and fissures, and is accompanied by varying degrees of hypoperfusion/hypometabolism in cortical and subcortical gray matter. Decreased cerebral glucose metabolism has been predominately reported in the frontal, cingulate, and temporal lobes with normal aging [38]. Age-related glucose hypometabolism seems to predominate in the medial frontal regions with brain atrophy in the lateral frontal and parietal regions, and parallel changes of both volume and glucose metabolism in the anterior cingulate gyrus [38] (Image 17.13). Imaging of cortical glucose metabolism is particularly altered when cortical thickness is further decreased. A common interpretation error occurs in the superior aspects of the parietal cortex, which can appear to have diminished intensity in older patients, leading to a

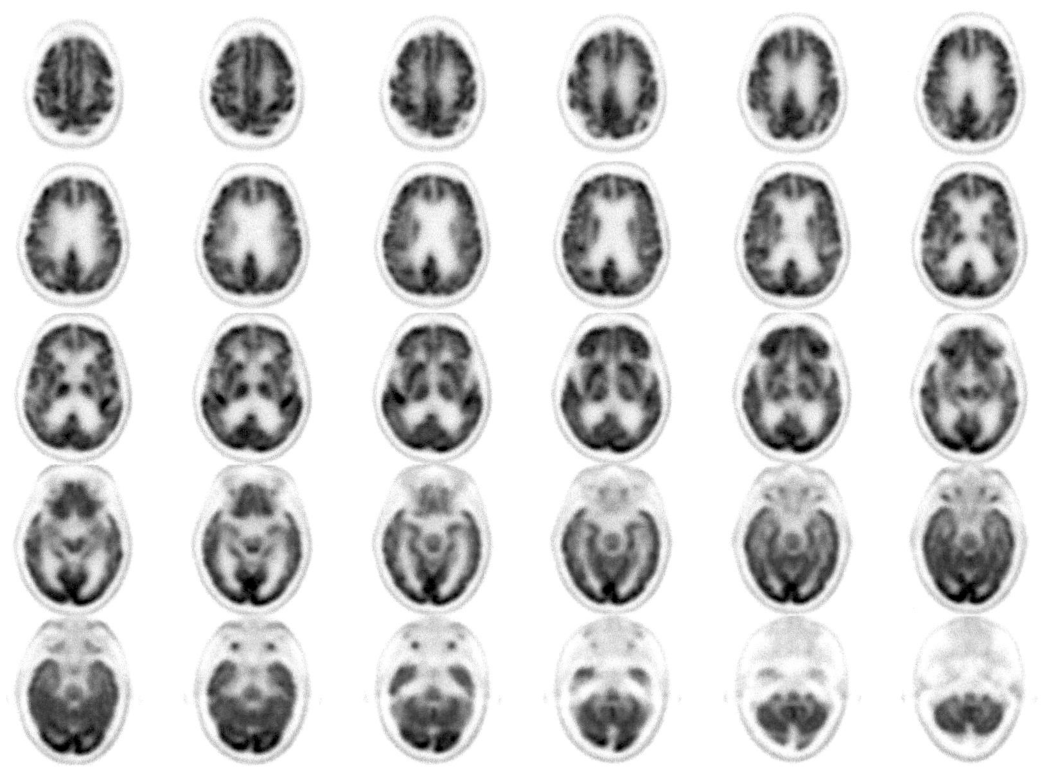

Image 17.13 The 18F-FDG transaxial images reveal the evident sulcal widening within each hemisphere in aging cortical atrophy. Generalized atrophy can be assessed at the level of the lateral ventricles by examining the inter-hemispheric fissure, and at the level of the third ventricle by examining the separation between the left and right sides of the thalamus, differently from young healthy subjects, where left and right cerebral hemispheres, as well as left and right thalami, are in close apposition to each other

description of biparietal hypometabolism (Images 17.14 and 17.15). These changes, if not carefully analyzed, can be a confounding factor in the distinction between a normal case and one with subtle disease, particularly in cases of equivocal cognitive impairment [26]. In fact, if carefully analyzed, isolated superior biparietal hypometabolism should not be interpreted as Alzheimer's disease, which characteristically affects the inferior parietal cortex prior to the more superior portion of the cortex. This pattern of superior biparietal hypometabolism occurs when atrophy-driven sulcal widening affects the external face of the cortical ribbon. The resultant partial volume effect can be readily confirmed by examining the corresponding sagittal views. The metabolism of the cerebellum also tends to increase with normal aging, which can be appreciated visually, not only as a relative intensity caused by global hypometabolism of the cortex, but also reflects an actual increased rate of glucose utilization by the cerebellum in absolute terms in elderly subjects [39].

Tracers of Protein Deposition

In amyloid imaging, an atrophied brain may lead to false-positive results due to an overestimation of radiotracer uptake in the thinned cortex, which can be based on the spillover activity from the white matter uptake (Image 17.16). However, in cases of severe atrophy, false-negative results due to an inability to differentiate the thin ribbon of amyloid-positive cortex from the adjacent white matter uptake can also occur, which can erroneously resemble the typical appearance of nonspecific white matter uptake in a healthy control subject [6]. The uncertainty related to the location or edge of the gray matter on the amyloid-PET scan can be decreased with co-registration to CT or MRI.

In Tau-PET imaging, age-related increased radiotracer retention in the midbrain, caudate,

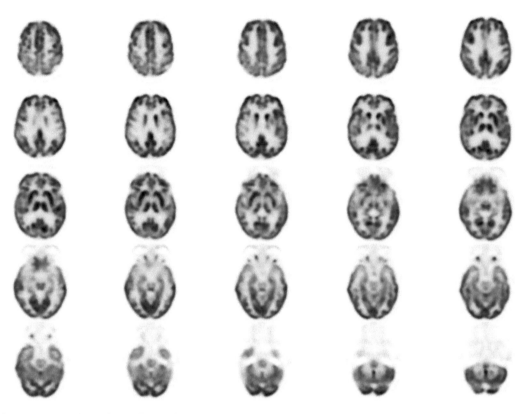

Image 17.14 18F-FDG-PET images in axial view demonstrating relatively low uptake in the superior part of parietal lobe due to sulcal widening caused by atrophy leading to partial volume effect

Image 17.15 CT, PET, and PET/CT co-registered images of the patient on Image 7.14. Note the more prominent cortical atrophy in the superior aspects of the parietal cortex leading to an impression of hypometabolism, which can be readily confirmed by examining the corresponding sagittal views. Mildly decreased FDG uptake of isolated superior parietal lobes is less likely to represent Alzheimer's disease which characteristically affects inferior parietal cortex before involving more superior portion of the neocortex

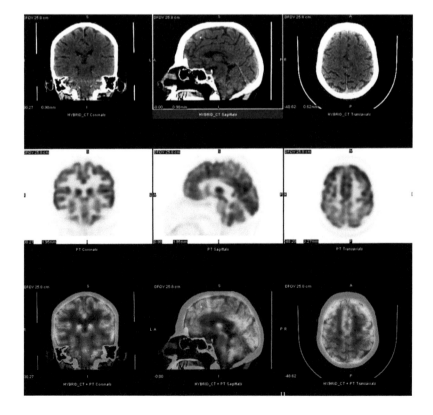

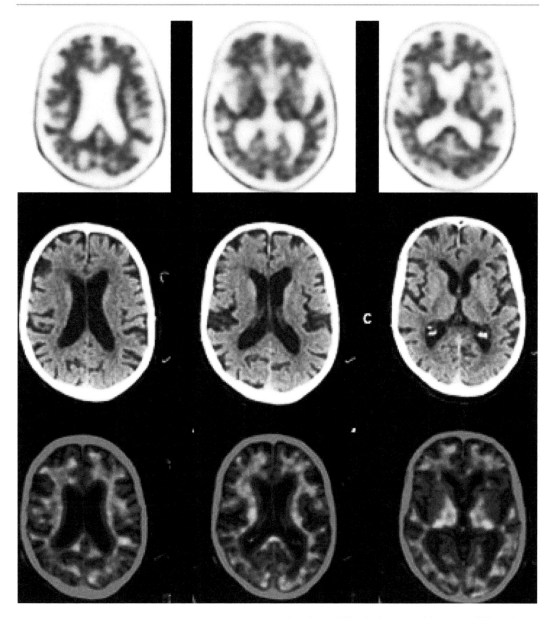

Image 17.16 18F-florbetapir transaxial images in an elderly patient with significant cortical atrophy, particularly in the left temporal cortex. Cortical atrophy may lead to misinterpreting the amyloid-PET images as false positive due to difficulty in gray–white matter differentiation. Review of the anatomical images is mandatory to prevent such pitfall

putamen, pallidum, and thalamus, which follows anatomically specific patterns of neocortical susceptibility to tau deposition, can be observed in elderly individuals with normal cognition [32]. Tau pathology is almost universally present in aging and may appear first in temporal lobe allocortex/medial temporal lobe (MTL). The pathology remains mostly confined to these regions with moderate spread into the neocortical temporal lobe, and minor infiltration into other neocortical areas such as the ventral frontal cortex [35]. The spread of tau outside of the MTL, to the lateral and inferior temporal, and other neocortical regions has been associated with increased Aβ pathology, which suggests that Aβ aggregation may play a facilitating role in the AD pathological cascade [35] (Image 17.17).

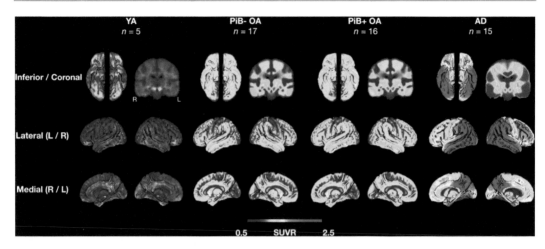

Image 17.17 Tau deposition in young healthy adults, normal aging adults, and AD patients. Surface projections and coronal slices are presented for young healthy adults (YA), older adults (OA) split into PiB- and PiB+ subgroups for illustration, and AD patients. Differences between cognitively healthy participants and young controls were primarily localized in inferior and lateral temporal subregions, while patient vs. young control differences extended into other temporal as well as parietal and frontal cortical regions. (Reprinted with permission from [Elsevier]: [**Neuron**] (Schöll, Michael et al. "PET Imaging of Tau Deposition in the Aging Human Brain." *Neuron* vol. 89,5 (2016): 971–982. doi:10.1016/j. neuron.2016.01.028))

Tracers of Nigrostriatal Dopaminergic Pathway Integrity

Age-related central atrophy may also alter the tracer binding, location, or appearance of the striatal structures. In fact, multicenter initiatives have demonstrated that normal aging is associated with a dopaminergic tracer signal reduction of about 5.5–6% per decade [40, 41] (Image 17.18). Normal 18F-DOPA striatal uptake seems less dependent on age than that seen with the DAT-SPECT tracers. Special attention should be taken particularly when performing semiquantitative analyses, as there is no universal age-dependent cutoff for determining normal versus abnormal. Ideally, each institution should establish their own reference values using a healthy control group or, when not feasible, have the procedure calibrated to a normal subject database [37]. Correlation with CT and MRI may be of fundamental importance to better delineate structural atrophy and identify anatomic lesions.

Best Practices and Factors That Affect Image Appearance

With brain imaging, it is important to remember that, in addition to adequate study acquisition and processing, the correct image interpretation depends on adequate patient preparation. In general, one should avoid any factors which may interfere with normal radiopharmaceutical distribution. Such important aspects include the withholding of potentially interfering medications and adequate control of environmental variables. For example, FDG-PET and perfusion SPECT require a resting condition before the injection and during the tracer uptake phase, as specific stimulation can generate brain activation, in specific regions as well as in remote cortical and subcortical areas. In addition, hyperglycemia can reduce whole brain FDG uptake (Image 17.19), with some evidence suggesting a more prominent reduction in the posterior parieto-occipital cortices, which may affect study accuracy when evaluating patients suspected of AD [42]. With dopaminergic tracers, a significant pitfall is the need for the pre-administration of carbidopa to block the peripheral uptake of 18F-DOPA and to improve tracer availability in the striatum. There is also a significant list of medications and drugs, which can interfere with DAT uptake (Image 17.20).

Of note, patients with neurologic deficits may require special care or even sedation, which should be performed with caution to avoid inter-

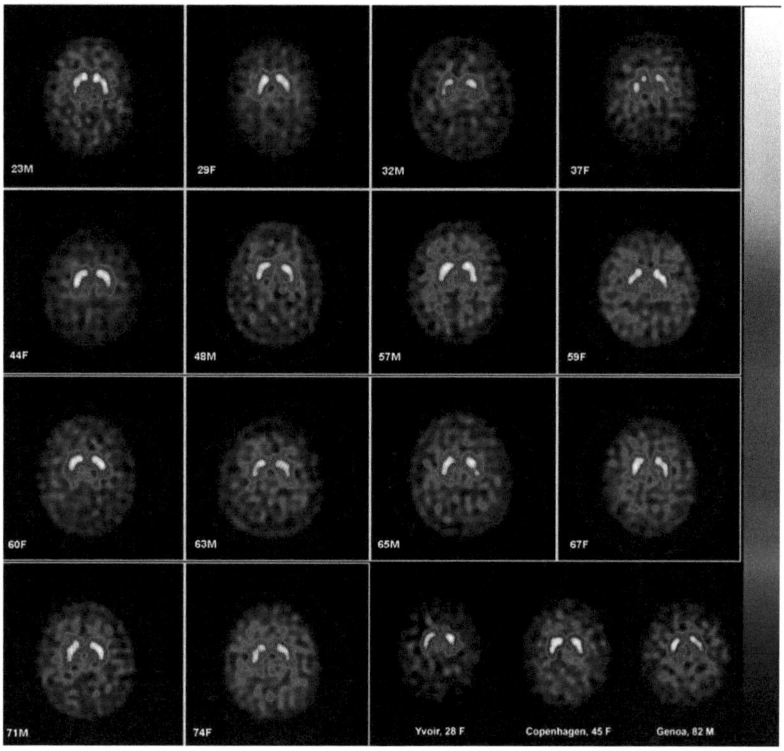

Image 17.18 Representative 123I-FP-CIT DAT-SPECT images of healthy controls of different ages, which show age-related decline in striatal uptake, with the average decline of approximately 5.5% per decade. (Reprinted by permission from **Springer Nature**: **European Journal of Nuclear Medicine**: (European multicentre database of healthy controls for [123I] FP-CIT SPECT (ENC-DAT): age-related effects, gender differences and evaluation of different methods of analysis, Andrea Varrone et al), (2013) Eur J Nucl Med Mol Imaging. 2013 Jan;40(2):213–27. doi: 10.1007/s00259-012-2276-8. Epub 2012 Nov 16. PMID: 23160999)

ference with normal radiotracer distribution. For further information, it is advisable to check brain imaging guidelines of the major international societies of nuclear medicine, namely the Society of Nuclear Medicine and Molecular Imaging (SNMMI) and the European Association of Nuclear Medicine (EANM), for more details regarding patient preparation, precautions, image acquisition, dosimetry, and image processing [22, 25, 28, 37, 43].

Technical Artifacts

An important first step for reading an imaging study is to assess the technical quality (Table 17.3). In brain imaging the most common artifacts are related to motion. Notably in elderly patients with cognitive disorders, motion may occur for a variety of reasons, particularly due to a lack of attention or from concomitant movement disorders. Motion-related artifacts may cause blurred activity over brain structures and inaccuracies in quantification. Misregistration between the functional and anatomical images can lead to inaccurate attenuation correction and generate false areas of increased or decreased activity. These circumstances can potentially result in misdiagnoses (Images 17.21 and 17.22). Fortunately, recent advances in artificial intelligence (AI) algorithms have promise to minimize motion-related artifacts by decreasing the image acquisition times as well as correcting for motion.

Another important issue for brain imaging is correct patient positioning, as a change in head orientation can make the proper identification of anatomical structures challenging, as well as in the evaluation of symmetry. This is particu-

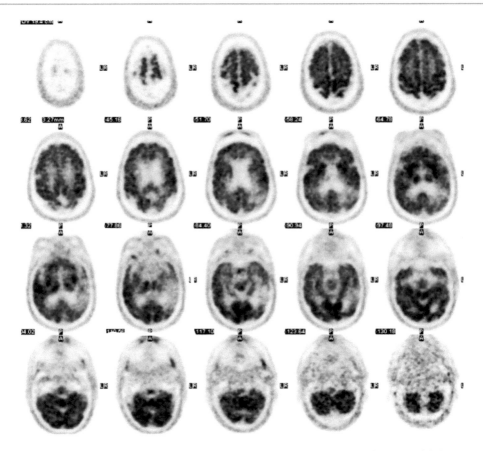

Image 17.19 Hyperglycemia reduces 18F-FDG uptake and degrades image quality as shown in axial views. Note the generalized decreased uptake in bilateral cerebral cortices and poor visualization of sulci and gyri

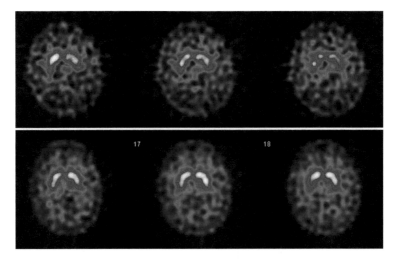

Image 17.20 A 64-year-old man with tremors had the initial Dopamine transporter single-photon emission computerized tomography (SPECT) imaging (DaTscan) showing abnormally patchy striatal tracer distribution (top row). The patient was not instructed to stop methylphenidate before the examination. A repeat DaTscan, 25 days later with drug discontinuation, showed normal striatal features (bottom row). (Reprinted by permission from [**Elsevier**]: [Mayo Clinic Proceedings] [False-Positive DaTscan Features With Methylphenidate and Phentermine Therapy, Kenneth N. Huynh, Ba D. Nguyen, November 2018, © 2018 Mayo Foundation for Medical Education and Research DOI: https://doi.org/10.1016/j.mayocp.2018.09.012)

Table 17.3 Common technical artifacts

Related to	Findings
Motion	Blurred activity/inaccuracies in quantification
Function/anatomy image misregistration	Incorrect attenuation correction with areas of increased or diminished activity due to over/under correction
Misalignment in patient positioning	Difficulty in identification of anatomic structures and evaluation of symmetry
Processing	Inadequate filtering can degrade image resolution
Scaling	False impression of global reduced uptake when structures with higher activity are included in the processing field

larly important when analyzing DAT-SPECT and 18F-DOPA-PET, as positioning artifacts can lead to misinterpretation of the results, which may suggest striatal denervation (Image 17.23). For quality assurance, the inspection of brain symmetry can be done on the transaxial view with respect to in-plane rotation, which can confirm that the structures are symmetric in appearance. If the visual inspection reveals asymmetric placement, image reorientation can generally be performed, since most facilities obtain brain images by three-dimensional (3D) acquisition. In patients with limited neck mobility, the image resolution may be suboptimal

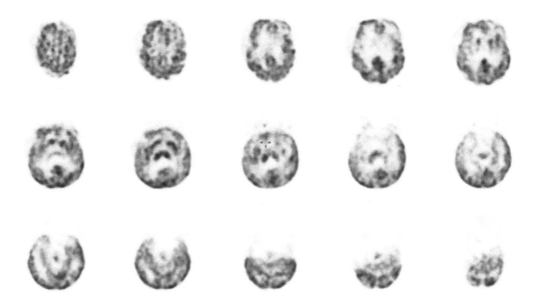

Image 17.21 18F-FDG axial plane showing blurred images due to head movement during PET imaging acquisition

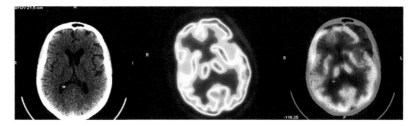

Image 17.22 Axial views of 18F-FDG-PET showing hypometabolism in right frontal and temporal lobes due to incorrect attenuation correction artifact caused by patient head motion between the acquisition of CT and PET images

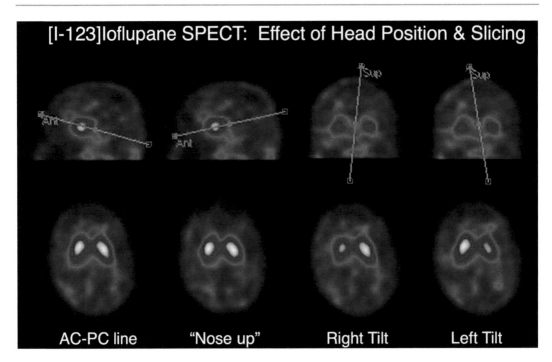

Image 17.23 123I-Ioflupane images. The axial images show asymmetry of the caudate and putamen due to effect of non-ideal head positioning, which may lead to a false-positive scan interpretation

when the head is not centered in the scanner field of view [44].

Correct image processing is also fundamental for optimal image quality. Additional considerations with respect to technical quality include smoothing, which should be applied to reduce noise without degrading the image resolution.

Scaling artifacts may occur if structures outside the brain with high tracer uptake are included within the processing field. This can lead to a false reduction in global uptake, as demonstrated by the inclusion of the salivary glands on DAT-SPECT (Image 17.24). When inspecting images, in addition to errors from the above-mentioned sources, attenuation correction errors should also be suspected when deeper structures in the brain appear washed out, indicating a greater degree of photon attenuation before reaching the scanner detectors.

Automated voxel-based statistical analysis software has been proven to reduce interob-

server variation, can be used for the training of novice readers, and can improve the accuracy of study interpretation [45]. In addition, such software can be used to investigate the relationship between metabolic changes and abnormal protein deposition, as well as the anatomical basis for such alterations, and includes the ability to compare an individual patient to a normal control database. Two-dimensional and three-dimensional semiquantitative methods have also been utilized as an adjunct to visual assessment of striatal binding in the analysis of nigrostriatal dopaminergic pathway integrity, with intra- and inter-operator variabilities dependent on the degree of operator intervention. When utilizing these methods, one should consider the possibility of errors and artifacts, such that the findings should always be confirmed by a visual read of the images (Images 17.25 and 17.26).

IMAGES NORMALIZED TO SALIVARY GLANDS

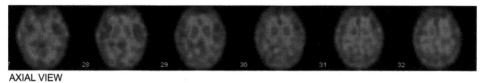

AXIAL VIEW

IMAGES CORRECTLY NORMALIZED

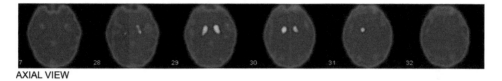

AXIAL VIEW

CORONAL
VIEW

99mTc-TRODAT

Image 17.24 Scaling artifact in 99mTc- TRODAT-1 SPECT images. The first image row shows diffuse striatal uptake reduction due to scaling artifact related to the inclusion of the salivary glands in the processing field. The second and third image rows show normal striatal uptake after image reprocessing in axial and coronal planes, respectively

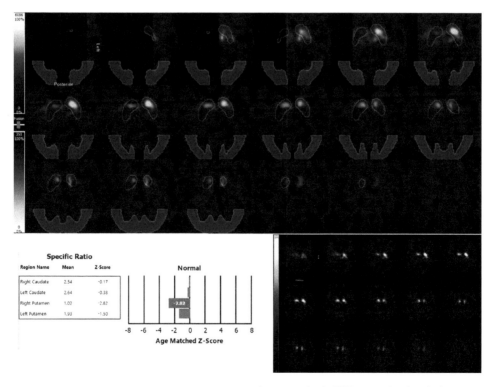

Region Name	Mean	Z-Score
Right Caudate	2.54	-0.17
Left Caudate	2.64	-0.38
Right Putamen	1.02	-2.82
Left Putamen	1.93	-1.50

Specific Ratio

Normal

-8 -6 -4 -2 0 2 4 6 8
Age Matched Z-Score

Image 17.25 Artifact caused by semiquantitative software processing. The axial images visually show a clearly abnormal scan. However, the striatum is not fully scanned with some small parts of the ventral striatum missing, which is a common problem in routine practice in older patients. Consequently, the VOIs cannot be placed adequately, and in fact are placed partly outside the brain, which induces artificially high uptake ratios (reconstruction and quantification within BRASS). (Image courtesy from Dr. J. Booij, Academic Medical Center, University of Amsterdam)

3D-SSP

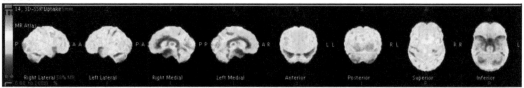

Z-SCORE MAP

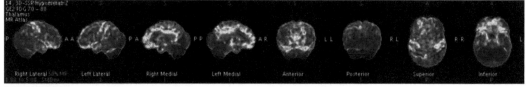

AXIAL VIEW

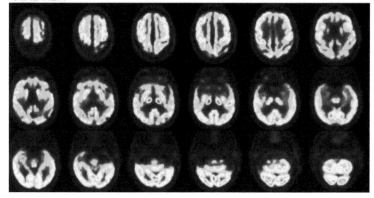

18F-FDG

Image 17.26 Another example of artifact caused by semiquantitative software processing using semiquantitative (3D-SSP) technique. In this case, the voxel semiquantitative analysis artifacts due to significant cortical atrophy are observed, particularly in medial frontal lobes

Image Interpretation and Reporting

Image interpretation should begin with a global appreciation of the images. In fact, brain images are better analyzed on a computer screen, rather than on printed image files, because intensity thresholds can be adjusted and pixel displays optimized. A display view with multiple slices provides a good general overview of the whole brain radiotracer distribution, despite the necessity of scrolling through the images.

Caution should be used in the selection of contrast levels and with background subtraction, as artifacts can be created by inappropriate thresholding. Usually, analysis of brain molecular images is performed using color and black-white linear scales, although certain 18F-labeled amyloid tracers require interpretation using a specific color scale, according to manufacturer's guidelines (Images 17.3, 17.4, and 17.5). In general, a gray scale is good for identifying hot areas, while the color scale is better for identifying areas of reduced activity. A continuous color scale is important to create the maximal diagnostic advantage by spreading the gradations over the entire scale. In fact, noncontinuous color scales may be confusing or misleading if abrupt color changes occur.

An adjunct analysis of molecular images with structural images, such as CT or MR, is beneficial, if not fundamental. Areas of missing or deformed tissue may indicate cerebrovascular insults (Image 17.27), posttraumatic, postsurgical, or other disease-related changes. The relative expansion of white matter and/or ventricular spaces may represent hydrocephalus (Image 17.28), while asymmetries can be secondary to

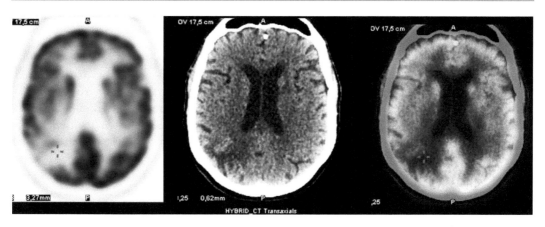

Image 17.27 18F-FDG in cerebrovascular insult. Hypometabolism in area of brain gliosis due to vascular insult is shown in the right parietal lobe

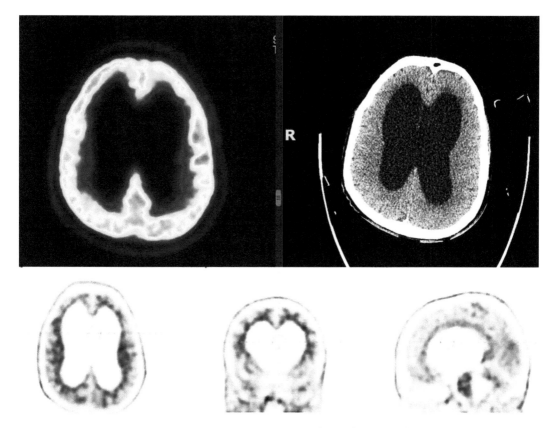

Image 17.28 Hydrocephalus. The 18F-FDG-PET image demonstrates generalized thinning of bilateral cerebral cortices, which is corresponding to the marked dilatation of the ventricular system on the CT images. The cortical uptake is usually preserved, except in the vicinity of the ventricles, most likely from partial volume effect. The higher FDG uptake at the high convexity, including central region can also be seen

mass effects or tumors. As previously mentioned, atrophy can be a pitfall for imaging interpretation, particularly in severe cases, where anatomical verification is necessary for the correct delineation between gray and white matter, as well as for the identification of areas of reduced uptake due to partial volume effects. Ideally molecular imaging and anatomical diagnostic studies should be acquired simultaneously, but nondiagnostic anatomical studies can be co-registered with diagnostic CT or MR through commercial software. Visual side by side correlation has important limitations particularly when assessing small abnormalities or structures.

The accurate interpretation of brain images is not as simple as the identification of a hot or cold spot, such as in cancer diagnosis, in that it may require the evaluation of uptake in a particular structure relative to other brain regions. It can be difficult to determine which imaging findings are significant, and ultimately, an understanding of the normal range for a particular image will lead to better recognition of abnormalities or patterns of abnormalities for a final or differential diagnosis. In this manner, semiquantitative or automated voxel-based statistical algorithms, in addition to axial, sagittal, and coronal views, can provide standardized, objective, and quantitative validation of observed changes in neurodegenerative disorders. With automated voxel-based statistical analysis, a large amount of information is condensed into a few hemispheric surface maps on which the regional statistical deviation from the age-matched "normal" database can be overlaid [1]. The surface rendered displays of the study data and the deviation from the normal range allow a sampling of the brain volume, without the extensive neuroanatomic expertise needed for the quantification process itself.

FDG-PET and Perfusion SPECT Image Interpretation

The most common indications for FDG-PET and perfusion SPECT in neurodegenerative diseases are for the differential diagnosis of dementing disorders and relatively early stages of neurodegeneration, particularly when an MRI and CT are negative for structural causes [21]. An accurate interpretation of these studies requires recognition of typical metabolic patterns caused by different types of dementia (Table 17.4). In addition to recognizing the patterns of decreased metabo-

lism or perfusion found with a particular type of neurodegenerative disease, to avoid a misdiagnosis, it is also important to recognize and identify the areas or structures, which are typically spared. Whenever a pattern is atypical or associated with other nonexpected abnormalities, the possibility of an alternative etiology or an association with other pathologies should always be considered and will increase the uncertainty of the diagnosis. The presence of comorbidities such as cerebrovascular disease or mixed Alzheimer's disease and dementia with Lewy bodies (DLB) may confound the interpretation of a brain imaging study. In addition to mixed or overlapping pathologic conditions, dementia syndromes may also exhibit atypical manifestations [46]. It is particularly important to remember that in later stages of neurodegenerative disorders, altered metabolism/perfusion becomes more widespread, and overlapping disorders may converge, in part due to the complex interconnectivity of the neuronal regions involved. Presently, there is no clinical indication for repeat FDG-PET scans to monitor disease progression or to evaluate treatment response in dementia patients, but in cases of equivocal and/or nondiagnostic imaging findings at early disease stages, further evaluation in 6–12 months may be helpful in patients with progressive cognitive decline [46]. Additionally, atypical FDG-PET findings can be further evaluated with the use of disease-specific imaging or fluid biomarkers for a more precise assessment of the causal pathologic processes in dementing disorders.

In imaging analysis, a visual interpretation is a vital component. When assessing global cortical metabolism or perfusion, it is critically important to use internal reference structures to identify relative abnormalities, which can be challenging for physicians who are not familiar with brain PET or SPECT images. In this manner, computer-assisted analysis can improve the learning curve of novice readers, as discussed in Chap. 13. Although several software packages for semiquantitative analysis of brain images are available (SPM, Mimvista, Cortex ID, PMOD, etc.) most of the following case examples were processed using the freely available software

Table 17.4 FDG-PET and disease-related imaging findings

Disease	Image findings
Alzheimer's disease	Decreased uptake in the posterior cingulate gyri, precuneus, posterior temporal and parietal association cortices, and may involve the frontal/prefrontal association cortices in severe cases Sparing of the sensorimotor cortex and relatively preserved metabolism in the visual and anterior cingulate cortices, basal ganglia, thalamus, and posterior fossa
Dementia with Lewy body	Decreased uptake in the temporoparietal and occipital lobe involving the associative and primary visual cortex Relatively preserved uptake in the posterior cingulate cortex (cingulate island sign)
Behavioral-variant FTD (bvFTD)	Decreased uptake in the frontal and anterior temporal lobes, and often involves caudate nucleus
Semantic-variant PPA (svPPA) or semantic dementia (SD)	Asymmetric decreased uptake in anterior temporal lobe, with the left temporal lobe often more severely affected than the right Decreased uptake may involve the inferior frontal lobe
Nonfluent (agrammatic)-variant PPA (nfvPPA)	Decreased uptake predominantly in the left lateral posterior frontal cortex, superior medial frontal cortex, and insula
Logopenic-variant PPA (lvPPA)	Decreased uptake in the lateral temporal cortex and inferior parietal lobule, often more severe in the left hemisphere The right parietotemporal cortices can be spared, in contrast to typical AD
Progressive supranuclear palsy (PSP)	Focally decreased uptake in the midbrain, as well as more diffuse decrease in the medial frontal and anterior cingulate cortices. Decreased uptake in the caudate and thalamus
Corticobasal degeneration (CBD)	Asymmetric decreased uptake in the frontoparietal regions without sparing of the sensorimotor cortex, basal ganglia, and thalamus Often asymmetric relative to the clinical symptoms
Multiple system atrophy	Decreased uptake in the striatum, frontal, prefrontal, and temporal cortices, brainstem and cerebellum, with more pronounced in the putamen and lenticular nuclei in Parkinsonian type (MSA-P), and more pronounced in brainstem and cerebellum in cerebellar type (MSA-C)
Vascular dementia (VAD)	Decreased uptake in the brain cortices with focal cortical pattern related to the affected vascular territory, and often involve deep gray nuclei, cerebellum, primary cortexes, middle temporal gyrus, and anterior cingulate cortex

[21, 46, 64–66]

3D-SSP to improve diagnostic accuracy. This semi-quantitative statistical mapping technique using a normal database for brain PET was developed in 1995[47]. Similar approaches are now available on clinical commercial workstations.

In the following sections, we will describe the structured process to identify abnormalities on an FDG-PET scan, which is also applicable to perfusion SPECT. NEUROSTAT/3D-SSP processing has been applied to improve diagnostic accuracy.

Example Case 1

A 64-year-old male patient, hypertensive, with progressive cognitive decline over 3 years, behavioral changes, and a positive family history for dementia. Investigation of AD × FTD. CDR: 2.

The FDG-PET images in the axial plane are shown (Images 17.29 and 17.30).

Visual Interpretation

A display of the transaxial images permits an initial global analysis of the brain, allowing an appreciation of the metabolic activity in specific regions relative to the other brain structures. One should remember when evaluating neurodegenerative diseases that it is important to identify spatial patterns of altered metabolism, as well as the degree of such alterations, i.e., mild, moderate, or severe.

In this patient, one can observe signs of cortical atrophy with a widening of the fissures, nota-

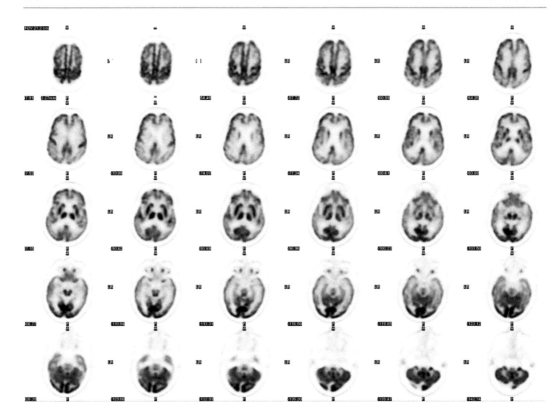

Image 17.29 18F-FDG transaxial views black and white

Image 17.30 18F-FDG transaxial views color scale

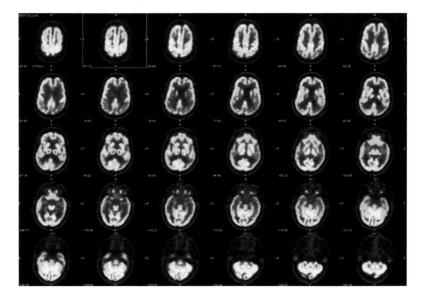

bly the interhemispheric and peri-sylvian. Normal metabolic activity can be appreciated in the sub-cortical structures, including the putamen and caudate nucleus, and thalamus bilaterally (Image 17.31). The sensorimotor cortex appears to have a more intense and conspicuous uptake relative to

the parietal and the frontal cortices. However, with careful analysis, one can appreciate that the sensorimotor cortex has slightly reduced metabolic activity relative to the striatum, which is a normal finding. The sensorimotor cortex appears to have increased uptake compared to the parietal and frontal cortices because the activity in that region is preserved in contrast to the metabolic reduction of the adjacent parietal and frontal association cortices (Image 17.32). Please note that this patient was imaged with relatively high "nose-up" head position, and the primary sensorimotor cortex appears to be located more posteriorly than those seen in a usual head position.

Visually one can appreciate that the reduction in uptake of the parietal cortex is more pronounced than in the frontal cortex, with a slight

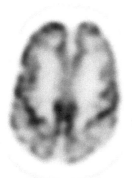

Image 17.31 Normal uptake in striatum and thalamus

asymmetry of the involvement in the frontal lobes, where the left side is slightly more affected than the right (Image 17.33).

In this patient, hypometabolism can be also observed in the posterior cingulate and precuneus, which can be better appreciated in the sagittal view (Image 17.34). One should remember that in normal individuals, the posterior cingulate is a region with very high baseline metabolic activity compared to other brain regions. In the workup of dementia patients, this region should be carefully evaluated, in particular the posterior cingulate, due to its early involvement in AD pathology [48].

The images also indicate a slightly higher metabolic activity in visual cortex relative to the occipital association cortex, which is a normal finding when the tracer injection and uptake occur with the patient's eyes open in a dimly lit room. The occipital lobes do not exhibit hypometabolism; however, a reduction is seen bilaterally in the temporal cortex when compared with the occipital cortex (Image 17.35). A good way to identify metabolic or perfusion abnormalities in the temporal lobe is to look for activity in the transitional region between the occipital and the temporal lobes, which should be unremarkable in a normal scan. A marked difference in uptake as observed in this patient, with decreased uptake in the temporal lobe compared to the occipital lobe, should be interpreted as a reduction in temporal lobe metabolism. In order to avoid misinterpretation, one

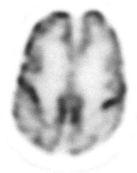

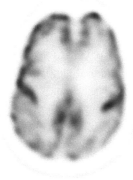

Image 17.32 Normal sensorimotor cortex uptake, with severe reduction in parietal uptake. Frontal lobes uptake reduction is less intense than in parietal lobes

Image 17.33 Uptake reduction in the parietal cortex more pronounced than in frontal cortex

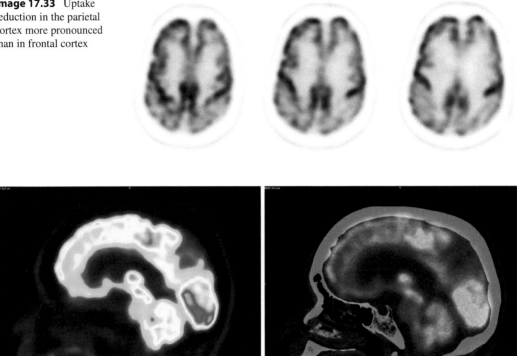

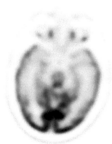

Image 17.34 Reduced uptake in posterior cingulate and precuneus

Image 17.35 Slightly higher uptake in visual cortex relative to the occipital association cortex and reduced uptake in temporal lobes

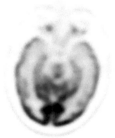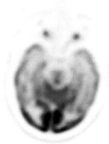

should note that, under normal conditions, activity is slightly lower in the medial temporal cortex, including in the hippocampal areas than in the lateral temporal areas.

In this patient, the metabolic activity in the cerebellum is preserved, as well as in the previously noted sensorimotor cortices and striata (Image 17.36). It is worth emphasizing that, when analyzing brain images, a diagnosis of specific neurodegenerative disease pattern not only includes the identification of spatial patterns for altered metabolism, but also involves the recognition of certain regions, not affected by the pathology, which are relatively spared.

Semi-quantitative Analysis

Voxel-based analytical approach based on freely available software (3D-SSP) (Image 17.37).

The top row shows the metabolic activity provided by a surface rendered map of the brain image, while the second row provides a surface rendered statistical "z-score" map of the regional deviation compared to the "normal" database, which has been superimposed on to a template MRI. Usually, when analyzing a z-score map, regions of blue/green or higher on the color scale (Z-score >1.5) should be regarded as likely abnormal, but the distribution as well as the severity of the hypometabolism should be used for the diagnosis [47]. The patient's semiquantitative analysis shows severe hypometabolism in the posterior cingulate gyri, precuneus, posterior temporal and parietal lobes (colored red), with moderate to severe hypometabolism in the frontal lobes (colored in yellow/red), and slightly worse on the left side.

Impression

This case illustrates AD (early-onset) with hypometabolism involving the posterior cingulate gyri, precuneus, and posterior temporal and parietal association cortices, and extending to the frontal/prefrontal association cortices as well. A key image finding, which indicates the diagnosis of AD and not FTD in this patient, and in nearly all cases of advanced AD, is that the posterior cingulate gyrus is preferentially involved (see greater hypometabolism in the 3D-SSP z-score map), with a pattern of more severe posterior temporoparietal lobe hypometabolism when compared to

the frontal lobes. Another key feature for the diagnosis of AD is the sparing of the sensorimotor cortex, which appears more conspicuous when contrasted with the adjacent hypometabolism, as well as relatively preserved metabolism in the visual and anterior cingulate cortices, basal ganglia, thalamus, and posterior fossa [46].

Early-onset Alzheimer's disease (EOAD), which affects patients under the age of 65 years, usually represents a challenge for diagnosis. It is frequently associated with an atypical clinical presentation, and usually has a more rapid progression, more generalized cognitive deficits, and is accompanied by greater cortical atrophy and hypometabolism compared to late-onset patients (LOAD) of a similar disease stage [49]. For a similar clinical severity, literature involving FDG-PET has indicated the presence of more extensive and severe hypometabolism in EOAD compared with LOAD, which is preferentially located in the posterior areas, particularly in the

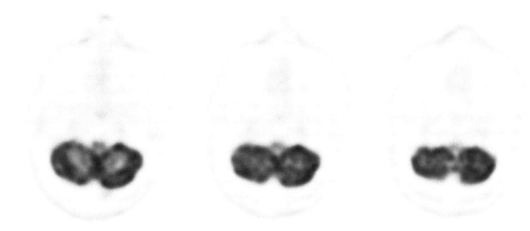

Image 17.36 Normal cerebellar uptake

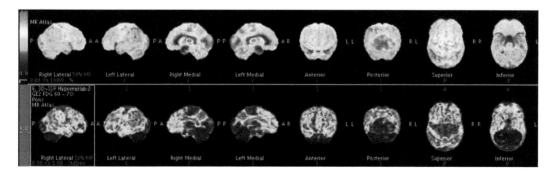

Image 17.37 Semiquantitative analysis: 3D-SSP. Top row: Surface rendered data. Bottom row: rendered z-score

parietal and temporal lobes. In addition, there are greater abnormalities in the frontal lobe and the subcortical structures such as basal ganglia and thalamus. As the disease progresses, the pattern of involvement in brain regions becomes relatively uniform over time [49].

Amyloid-PET Interpretation

The use of Amyloid-PET is usually indicated: (1) when a patient has objectively confirmed cognitive impairment of uncertain cause after a comprehensive evaluation by a dementia expert, where the differential diagnosis includes AD dementia, and (2) when knowledge of the presence or absence of Aβ pathology is expected to increase diagnostic certainty or alter patient management [28]. In most cases, the patients are likely to have persistent or progressive unexplained MCI, a core clinical criteria for possible AD with an unclear clinical presentation (either an atypical clinical course or an etiologically mixed presentation), or the patient has progressive dementia, but with atypical early age of onset (usually <65 years) [28]. Note that, in accordance with the appropriate use criteria for Amyloid-PET, which was developed by a Task Force from the SNMMI and the Alzheimer's Association, Amyloid-PET is not recommended: (1) for patients with core clinical criteria for probable Alzheimer's disease and a typical age of onset; (2) to determine dementia severity, based on an isolated positive family history of dementia or the presence of the APOE-4 genotype; (3) in patients with a cognitive complaint unconfirmed by clinical examination; (4) in lieu of genotyping for suspected autosomal mutation carriers; and (5) in asymptomatic individuals or for nonmedical usage (e.g., legal interest, insurance coverage, or employment screening) [50].

When interpreting an Amyloid-PET, physicians should be aware of the prevalence of amyloid positivity in normal older individuals, which may not be related or relevant to the presenting symptoms. The estimates for age-specific posi-

tivity rates in population studies are around <5% between 50 and 60 years old, 10% in 60–70, 25% in 70–80, and >50% in 80–90 years [50]. Another caveat is that a positive amyloid scan can occur with pathologies other than AD. For example, amyloid is found in 50–70% of patients with DLB, but not in patients with frontotemporal dementia (FTD) [51]. Indeed, amyloid pathology can coexist with other diseases. Notably, a variable degree of AD pathology can be found in patients with vascular dementia. In this manner, the appropriateness of Amyloid-PET requires knowledge of all relevant findings, which include a clinical evaluation, laboratory tests, and imaging findings to weight the relevance of each component [50].

An amyloid-PET interpretation and report comprises a qualitative binary algorithm, to assess the study as positive or negative for Aβ amyloid plaque deposition. Tracer-specific training for image interpretation is provided by the manufacturers, and users are recommended to take appropriate training prior to clinical interpretation. The criteria for positivity and negativity are slightly different across available tracers (18F-florbetapir, 18F-flutemetamol, or 18F-florbetaben). Familiarity with brain anatomy is critical. Semiquantitative techniques may be helpful [28].

In a positive scan, a significant amount of Aβ amyloid deposition is seen in the gray matter. The visual analysis requires optimized evaluation of the gray–white matter differentiation, with an adequate image size display. A gray scale display is generally preferred for 18F-florbetaben and 18F-florbetapir, but a specific color scale is also recommended for 18F-flutemetamol. The images are normally analyzed in the transaxial orientation, but a corresponding display of coronal and sagittal planes may be used to better define the uptake localization. One must take care to have the correct brain orientation, because if it is slightly oblique, uptake in white matter can be mistaken for cortical binding [51].

The following example case gives a general instruction for how to identify abnormalities on an amyloid-PET scan.

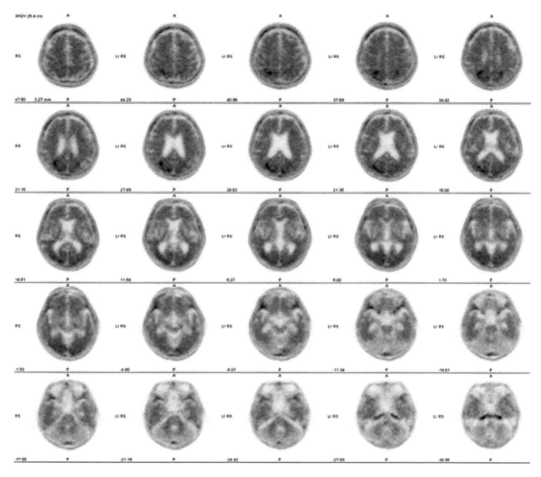

Image 17.38   18F-florbetapir amyloid-PET images in axial plane

Example Case 2

A 77-year-old female who presented with atypical cognitive impairment, possibly representing AD. The 18F-florbetapir Amyloid-PET images in axial plane are shown (Image 17.38).

Visual Interpretation

An initial review of the transaxial images gives a global impression of the brain, from the bottom to the top, and allows an initial confirmation of normal gray–white matter differentiation in the cerebellum, with a clear delineation of the gray and white matter. Note that the cerebellar cortex is expected to be mostly free of Aβ deposition, even in subjects with cerebral cortical amyloid disease. Nonspecific uptake in the pons and cerebellar peduncle can be used as a reference intensity for image display across subjects.

The next step is to examine all cerebral cortical and subcortical regions, to screen for abnormal gray matter radiotracer uptake. Specific attention should be paid to the lateral temporal, frontal, posterior cingulate, precuneus, and parietal cortices, where most distinct radiotracer accumulation occurs in Aβ-positive subjects. The image shows significant amounts of gray matter Aβ deposition in all of the previously described areas. Note the presence of striatal radiotracer uptake as well. Striatal binding can be an elucidating finding for positivity in subjects with major cortical atrophy, where the distinction between a thin ribbon of amyloid-positive cortex from adjacent white matter may not be clear [28].

In this patient, a blurred distinction of the gray to white matter junction can be observed. In contrast, negative scans have nonspecific white matter uptake with little to no binding in the gray matter, and resemble an image of white matter distribution. In fact, a key feature for distinguishing Aβ-positive from Aβ-negative scans is the loss of gray to white matter contrast, with radiotracer uptake extending to the edge of the cerebral cortex and forming a smooth, regular boundary. One can appreciate the sharp cortical margin of uptake in this patient, rather than the white matter sulcal pattern typical of a negative scan. The gap between the two hemispheres is ill defined, appearing as a thin, regular line, as opposed to a clear, wide, irregular gap between the cerebral hemispheres seen in a negative scan. The abnormal radiotracer uptake observed is symmetric, affecting both right and left lobar structures. Areas of increased uptake compared to the white matter can be appreciated in the parietal lobes of this case.

Quantification/Semi-quantitative Analysis

Voxel-based analytical approach using 3D-SSP (Images 17.39 and 17.40).

The cerebellum is generally used as a reference region for visual and semiquantitative interpretation, due to an absence of cerebellar cortex Aβ deposition, even in subjects with cerebral cortical amyloid disease. Under circumstances in which there may be plaque in the cerebellum, the pons should be used as the reference region. The radiotracer package insert usually provides specific guidelines on the number of affected cortical regions required for a diagnosis of a positive scan [28]. In this example, the 3D-SSP Z-score map shows generalized higher amyloid deposition as compared to the normal population in all cortical

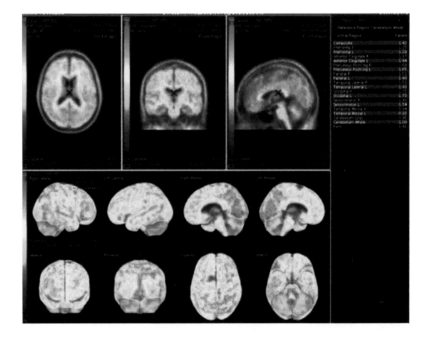

Image 17.39 18F-florbetapir amyloid-PET semiquantitative analysis (3D-SSP)

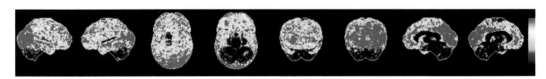

Image 17.40 18F-florbetapir amyloid-PET semiquantitative analysis (3D-SSP) Z-score map

regions, particularly the precuneus, and posterior cingulate, as well as in the occipital, parietal, lateral temporal, and prefrontal cortices. The global cortical SUVR using the whole cerebellum as a reference region is 1.42, which is higher than the suggested cutoff (>1.1, Amyvid leaflet [52]). Note that there are cases where an intermediate or indeterminate uptake pattern may be encountered.

Impression

This case illustrates significant deposition of Aβ amyloid in the brain (a positive scan).

It is critically important to recall that a positive scan is not indicative of AD by itself. Positive findings can occur in non-AD forms of dementia, other neurologic diseases, in older subjects without cognitive impairment, and can coexist with other pathologies. However, a negative scan does not exclude the presence of a non-AD dementing illness. In fact, a negative scan indicates that the patient is unlikely to have AD at the time of imaging, or in case of patients presenting with MCI, that progression to AD dementia is unlikely [28].

Tau-PET Interpretation

As a new modality, the clinical applications for Tau-PET are still under development [30]. Tau-PET with 18F-flortaucipir was recently approved by the FDA for the clinical setting, enabling the noninvasive detection of in vivo tau deposition, in suspected cases of AD. However, 18F-flortaucipir PET has not been recommended for the clinical evaluation of other tauopathies, such as Traumatic Encephalopathy Syndrome (TES), which is the clinical manifestation of pathologically defined Chronic Traumatic Encephalopathy (CTE). Flortaucipir also shows some limitations in the early detection of AD [33, 53]. Recently, second-generation Tau-PET tracers have been shown to be sensitive to both primary and secondary tauopathies, but further clinical studies are required to judge their utility in a clinical context [54, 55].

Currently, several groups are developing appropriate use criteria for tau-PET. One example of the appropriate use criteria for Tau-PET

with 18F-flortaucipir [32] indicates its use in the following clinical scenarios: (1) when the cause of cognitive impairment remains uncertain after a comprehensive clinical evaluation by an expert; (2) the disease history and routine examination cannot confirm the definitive diagnosis of AD; (3) there is a need to differentiate AD from other neurodegenerative tauopathies; and (4) there is a need to determine the extent of the tau deposition in AD.

When interpreting a Tau-PET scan, the physician should keep in mind the assessment of the density and distribution of the NFTs in the brain, and that a positive scan, by itself, does not establish a definitive diagnosis of AD. Presently, a positive scan should be interpreted in combination with positive amyloid biomarkers (cerebrospinal fluid or Amyloid-PET) and clinical information supportive of an AD diagnosis. Additionally, a positive 18F-flortaucipir PET result does not exclude the coexistence of other neurodegenerative disorders such as FTLD.

Visual reading has only been standardized for 18F-flortaucipir PET and, similar to Amyloid-PET, the interpretation comprises a qualitative binary algorithm, to assess the study as positive or negative. A negative scan typically shows no increased neocortical tracer retention or shows increased tracer retention isolated to the mesial temporal, anterolateral temporal, or frontal regions only. A positive scan typically shows widespread tracer uptake with bilateral neocortical deposition in the posterolateral temporal, occipital, parietal and precuneus, medial prefrontal and cingulate, and lateral prefrontal regions [33].

While interpreting a scan in the context of AD, the reader should be attentive if the pattern of tau distribution is coherent with what is typically observed within the AD spectrum. Note that in subjects with mild cognitive impairment and AD, uptake seems to spread from the mesial temporal lobes to iso-cortical areas, which is consistent with the Braak and Braak staging of neurofibrillary tau pathology. The NFT pathology begins in the transentorhinal cortex before spreading to the medial and inferior temporal lobes, the parietal-occipital regions, and the rest of the neocortex [31].

In a recent paper, Sonni et al. [56] described four patterns of 18F-Flortaucipir distribution, which can assist the reader to better align the observed imaging findings regarding positivity of the scan with the likelihood of being associated with AD as follows:

- Pattern I (negative scan): absence of 18F-Flortaucipir signal in any brain area.
- Pattern II (mild temporal binding only): mild to moderate increase of 18F-Flortaucipir signal, limited to the medial temporal cortex and fusiform gyrus (probably consistent with early Braak stage tau pathology, which may be seen in older individuals with or without cognitive decline).
- Pattern III (AD-like binding): 18F-Flortaucipir distribution not restricted to the medial temporal/fusiform area, but extending to the lateral temporal, parietal, or frontal cortices (consistent with the neuropathological distribution of tau in an advanced Braak stage/$\geq$ IV).
- Pattern IV (non-AD-like): atypical signal distribution, not following the expected Braak distribution of NFTs (consistent with non-AD syndromes).

A caveat with Tau-PET is that several features can make the image analysis more challenging. Contrary to amyloid imaging, where white matter predominant off-target binding is a consistent feature across Aβ-radiotracers, with tau tracers, the presence of off-target binding can be highly variable across individuals, both in terms of severity and location. Indeed, high variation in signal intensity between patients, differing regional distributions, and a mild-to-moderate signal observed in non-AD-associated conditions can complicate the interpretation [56]. In the mesial temporal regions, potential bleed-in from off-target binding in the choroid plexus and atrophy-associated partial volume effects may represent additional challenges for visual interpretation.

Moreover, the reader should be aware of the limited sensitivity of 18F-flortaucipir for the detection of early-stage tau pathology. When positive, the scan indicates the presence of widely distributed tau neuropathology in neocortical areas (B3: Braak stages V/VI, with NFTs widely distributed throughout the neocortex), but a negative scan does not rule out the presence of minor tau pathology (B0 and B1: no NFTs and Braak stage I/II with NFTs predominantly in the entorhinal cortex and closely related areas, respectively), (B2: Braak stages III/IV, with abundant NFTs in the hippocampus and amygdala, and some extension into the association cortices) or amyloid pathology. In these cases, an additional evaluation to confirm the absence of AD pathology may be necessary. Indeed, patients with a negative Tau-PET, but worsening in cognitive function, may require a subsequent imaging to detect progression to a B3 level of tau pathology [33].

The following sections give general instructions for how to identify abnormalities on a Tau-PET scan.

Example Case 3

A 60-year-old male who presented progressive symptoms of cognitive impairment with initial diagnosis of suspected AD. The 18F-Flortaucipir PET images in axial plane are shown (Images 17.41 and 17.42).

Visual Interpretation

While analyzing the images, the goal is to identify and locate areas of tracer activity in the neocortex, which are greater than the background activity, as well as to verify that the location is coherent with patterns observed for the AD spectrum. The inferior portion of the cerebellum should be used as a reference region for no binding, with care taken to exclude the superior portion, since 18F-flortaucipir retention may be observed in the superior portion of cerebellar gray matter [32]. Color scales may be used according to the reader's preference, but for optimal display, it is advisable to adjust a color scale for a rapid transition between two distinct colors.

The initial review of the transaxial images should give an overall global assessment of the

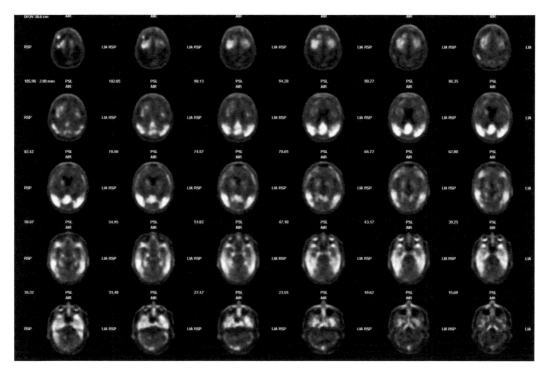

Image 17.41   18F-Flortaucipir PET images in transaxial views (black and white)

Image 17.42   18F-Flortaucipir PET images in transaxial views (color scale)

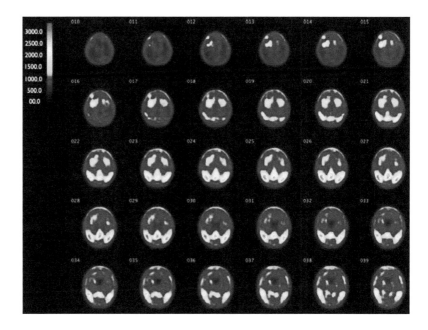

brain, with particular attention to the lobar anatomy, sites of increased uptake, and "off-target" binding. Sagittal and coronal images (not shown) should be analyzed as well, to adjust the orientation for head tilt. A sagittal slice just off the midline should be used to align the inferior frontal and inferior occipital poles in the horizontal plane.

It is advisable to begin the inspection with the temporal lobes, followed by the occipital, parietal, and frontal lobes bilaterally. Note that the temporal lobe should be subdivided into quadrants: anterolateral temporal (ALT), anterior mesial temporal (AMT), posterolateral temporal (PLT), and posterior mesial temporal (PMT) for the evaluation. This detailed description is fundamental, as increased neocortical activity in the mesial temporal, anterolateral temporal, and/or frontal regions, when isolated, may represent a negative study. In contrast, a positive scan shows increased neocortical activity in the posterolateral temporal, occipital, or parietal/precuneus regions, with or without frontal activity [57].

In this example, the image shows bilateral increased neocortical activity in the mesial temporal, posterolateral temporal cortices, as well as in the parietal/precuneus and posterior cingulate regions. Focal and continuous uptake in the midfrontal regions, which is greater in the right hemisphere, can be observed. There is also mild "off-target" binding in the striata and choroid plexus.

The increased neocortical activity in the posterolateral temporal, and parietal/precuneus and posterior cingulate regions with frontal involvement is determinant for study positivity, but not the mesial temporal lobe activity. It is also important to remember when interpreting a study that neocortical activity in either hemisphere, not just bilateral involvement, can contribute to the identification of a positive pattern. Isolated or noncontiguous foci should be evaluated with caution.

Quantification/Semi-quantitative Analysis

Voxelwise semiquantitative analysis with SPM software (Image 17.43).

Currently there is no automated, voxelwise, quantitative or semiquantitative analysis software commercially approved for clinical applications with 18F-Flortaucipir in suspected AD. As used clinically in a broad sense, standardized uptake value ratios (SUVRs) can be applied for quantification, as indicated below, using the inferior cerebellum as a reference region.

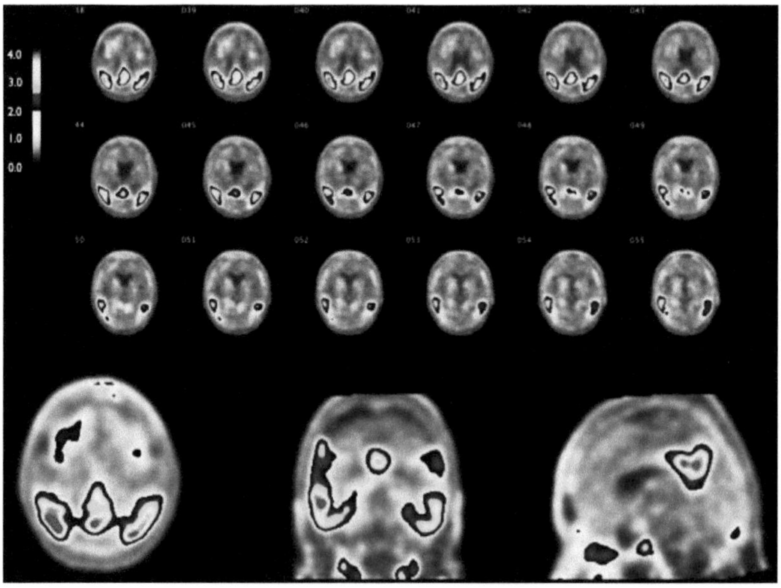

Image 17.43 Voxelwise semiquantitative analysis with SPM software

In this patient, the voxelwise analysis relative to the cerebellar gray matter demonstrates areas of significant increase of 18F-flortaucipir deposition in the precuneus, and posterior cingulate gyrus, as well as the medial and lateral temporal cortices bilaterally, with a small degree of deposition in the right frontal cortex.

Impression

This case illustrates a typical pattern of tau pathology in AD, most dominant in regions summarized as B3 (i.e., Braak V/VI), and indicative of widely distributed tau neuropathology, which represents the determination of a positive scan.

DAT-SPECT and 18F-DOPA-PET Interpretation

The most common indication for presynaptic dopaminergic imaging, DAT-SPECT agents and 18F-Fluorodopa PET is the differential diagnosis between neurodegenerative parkinsonian syndromes and non-dopamine deficiency etiologies of parkinsonism. Notably, patients become symptomatic after a significant number of striatal projections originating from the substantia nigra have degenerated. In this manner molecular imaging studies may be particularly useful for patients with atypical syndromes, overlapping symptoms, unsatisfying response to therapy, or in early/mildly symptomatic stages of disease, which can demonstrate a high negative predictive value.

In accordance with EANM practice guidelines/SNMMI procedure standards for dopaminergic imaging in parkinsonian syndromes 1.0 [37], presynaptic dopaminergic imaging is particularly indicated: (1) to support the differential diagnosis between essential tremor and neurodegenerative parkinsonian syndromes, (2) to help distinguish between DLB and other dementias, particularly for differentiation from AD, (3) to support the differential diagnosis between parkinsonism due to presynaptic degenerative dopamine deficiency from other forms of parkinsonism, which include the differentiation of idiopathic Parkinson's disease (IPD), and from drug-induced, psychogenic, or vascular parkinsonism, and (4) to detect early presynaptic parkinsonian syndromes.

One should be aware that presynaptic dopaminergic imaging cannot clearly distinguish IPD and DLB from progressive supranuclear palsy (PSP), cortical basal degeneration (CBD), or the putaminal variant of multisystem atrophy (MSA) (Table 17.5). In fact, what does distinguish atypical parkinsonism from all forms of multisystem Lewy body disease (MLBD), which includes PD, is a lack of peripheral post-ganglionic autonomic neuropathy and, in such cases, cardiac MIBG imaging may be of use. Another presynaptic dopaminergic imaging limitation is the characterization of subjects who clinically appear to have parkinsonism, but do not have decreased striatal DAT signal, known as "scans without evidence for dopaminergic deficit" (SWEDD) [58]. However, new evidence suggests that SWEDD subjects are unlikely to have IPD [59].

When interpreting a DAT-SPECT or 18F-DOPA-PET scan using the transaxial plane, the reader should check if the striata appears as normal, comma-shaped structures with symmetric, well-delineated borders, while taking into consideration the patient's age and morphological information provided by other imaging modalities, such as CT or MR. In abnormal scans, the striatum has reduced intensity on one or both sides, with a change in shape, which can present as an oval or circle. Visual assessment is usually sufficient for the evaluation of striatal left/right symmetry and striatal subregions, particularly for experienced readers; however semi-quantitative analysis may be applied to improve accuracy, most notably in complex or borderline cases. The most applied semi-quantitative analysis uses the specific binding ratio (SBR), calculated as the striatal target-to-background ratio (usually the occipital cortex), which can be obtained manually or using software.

In cases with an abnormal striatal appearance, the reader should verify that the head alignment is correct, to exclude the possibility of artifactual left-right asymmetry. Anatomical lesions or conditions, which could alter the tracer binding, location, or shape of the striatal structures should

Table 17.5 DAT-SPECT and DOPA-PET disease expected imaging findings

Disease	Image findings
Idiopathic Parkinson's disease (IPD)	A "*dot shape*" is typical from the earliest stages of disease. The putamen (in particular the posterior part) of the most affected hemisphere is more severely affected than the caudate nucleus; the putamen of the less affected hemisphere tends to be involved early (often before the caudate nucleus of the most affected side)
Essential tremor	Normal uptake
Psychogenic parkinsonism	Normal uptake
Drug-induced parkinsonism	Normal uptake
Alzheimer's disease	Normal uptake
Vascular parkinsonism	Normal or only slightly diminished uptake except when an infarct directly involves a striatal structure
Dementia with Lewy body	Reduced uptake substantially overlapping IPD features[a]
Multiple system atrophy	Reduced uptake, often overlapping IPD features (uptake reduction tends to be more symmetric as compared to IPD)
Progressive supranuclear palsy	Reduced uptake, often overlapping IPD features (uptake reduction tends to be more symmetric and to involve the caudate nucleus earlier in disease course as compared to IPD)
Corticobasal degeneration	Reduced uptake, overlapping IPD features (uptake reduction sometimes more asymmetric as compared to IPD and often involving both the putamen and caudate head)
Frontotemporal dementia	Reduced uptake in 30–60% of patients with sporadic FTD (usually less pronounced than in IPD)

Adapted from Morbelli S et al. EANM practice guideline/SNMMI procedure standard for dopaminergic imaging in Parkinsonian syndromes 1.0. Eur J Nucl Med Mol Imaging. 2020 Jul;47(8):1885–1912. doi: 10.1007 s00259-020-04817-8. Epub 2020 May 9. PMID: 32388612; PMCID: PMC7300075
[a]Around 10% of patients with pathologic proven DLB show a normal DAT-SPECT at the time of the clinical diagnosis, possibly becoming abnormal after 1.5–2 years

be considered as well. In these situations, anatomical correlation from multimodal images (e.g., SPECT/CT, PET/CT, or PET/MR) or previous imaging studies should be performed. The level of striatal activity should always be compared with the background activity, to check for normalization errors.

A DAT-SPECT or 18F-DOPA-PET imaging interpretation and report comprises a qualitative binary algorithm, to assess if a presynaptic dopaminergic deficit is present or absent.

The following sections give general instructions for how to identify abnormalities on an 18F-DOPA-PET scan.

Example Case 4

A 45-year-old female with a history of two years of progressive left upper extremity clumsiness when performing activities like getting dressed or peeling fruit, and mild tremor. She has no previous history of rapid eye movement (REM) sleep behavior disorder, constipation, or reduction of smell. The neurological examination evidenced an UPDRS III score of 21 and a Hoehn-Yahr score of 1. She does not show abnormalities in any of the blood test analysis performed, as well as in the brain and cervical MRI scans.

The 18F-Fluorodopa PET images in an axial plane are shown (Image 17.44).

Visual Interpretation

The axial slices show moderate contrast between the striatal and the cortical uptake. The uptake in the striatum is clearly asymmetric and more conspicuously decreased on the right side. Note that the decrease is more pronounced in the putamen than in the caudate, particularly in the posterior part.

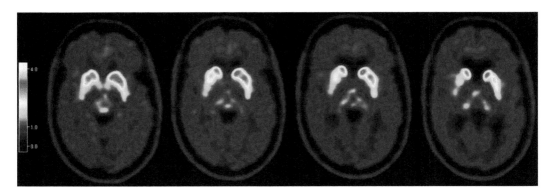

Image 17.44 18F-Fluorodopa PET images in in transaxial views

Quantification/Semi-quantitative Analysis

Voxelwise, semi-quantitative analysis based on *syngo*.via MI Neurology software (Image 17.45).

In this case, the original PET study was spatially normalized to a standard template. The semiquantitative analysis was performed by calculating the ratio between the activity in the striata in reference to the occipital cortex (area with the lowest brain activity), using predefined volumes of interest of the different regions of the striatum (caudate, anterior putamen and posterior putamen) as well as the occipital cortex. One should note that an abnormal finding can be observed in both striata, which is more marked on the right side, and particularly more prominent in the putamen (Z-Score below 2 standard deviations).

Impression

In conjunction, the appearance of the images and the semiquantitative values obtained indicate that a presynaptic dopaminergic deficit is present, as manifested by the abnormal brain distribution and metabolism of FDOPA, which is most notable with the asymmetrical denervation (right higher than left) and rostrocaudal gradient. This finding indicates that the etiology of the parkinsonian syndrome in this patient is related to degeneration of the substantia nigra, which supports the clinical diagnosis of neurodegenerative parkinsonism.

Brain Molecular Image Reporting

In general, an adequate study report must contain: (1) the patient's clinical information and indication for the scan; (2) comparison/prior imaging exams; (3) the imaging technique employed; (4) a description of the findings; and (5) the impression.

Table 17.6 provides formats for the essential findings, description, interpretation, and conclusions as recommended by specific guidelines [25, 28, 32, 37, 60].

While reporting an FDG-PET or perfusion SPECT brain imaging study, the conclusion should state the diagnosis based on the findings of a characteristic disease pattern, while taking into consideration the clinical presentation. Whenever the findings represent an uncharacteristic disease pattern, statements to explain why a specific diagnostic entity could not be determined should be included. When appropriate, a differential diagnosis should be provided as well as a suggestion for follow-up or additional studies to better clarify/confirm the suspected diagnosis [25, 60].

In Amyloid-PET and Tau-PET studies, the impression should clearly state if the scan is positive or negative. For inconclusive studies, the potential reasons such as low count rate, head motion during imaging, unexpected focal lesions, cortical atrophy, or other issues should be described [28, 32].

In dopaminergic imaging with DAT-SPECT and 18F-DOPA-PET, the impression should state

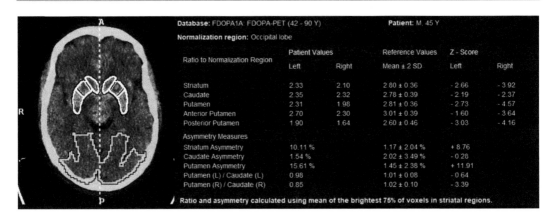

Image 17.45 Voxelwise, Semi-quantitative analysis based on *syngo*.via MI Neurology software

Table 17.6 Specific report contents

	FDG-PET/Perfusion SPECT	Amyloid-PET	Tau-PET	DAT-SPECT/18F-DOPA-PET
Findings description	• Abnormalities: – Location – Extent – Symmetry/asymmetry – Reference to a normal database (when performing quantification)	• Uptake in cerebellum • Degree and location of cerebral atrophy • Loss of gray–white matter differentiation • Areas of pathological uptake • Uptake above white matter	• Pathological uptake • Affected areas	• Striatal binding compared to background • Abnormalities: – Location – Intensity of reduction – Significant asymmetry
Interpretation/conclusion	• Characteristic disease pattern • Noncharacteristic disease pattern (provide differential diagnosis)	• Positive (significant Aβ deposition) • Negative (no evidence of significant Aβ deposition) • Indeterminate[a]	• Positive (increased/abnormal neocortical tracer retention) • Negative (no neocortical tracer retention) • Indeterminate[a]	• Presynaptic dopaminergic deficit present • Presynaptic dopaminergic deficit absent

Data taken from [22, 25, 27, 31, 36, 42, 57]

[a] In case of an indeterminate result, state possible reasons

if a presynaptic dopaminergic deficit is present or absent. A more comprehensive diagnostic comment can be included depending on the imaging findings or on the availability of previous studies. Similarly, follow-up or additional studies can be recommended to clarify or confirm the suspected diagnosis [37].

Clinical Case Reporting

Case 1 (Courtesy of Professor Kazunari Ishii)

Kazunari Ishii

Indication/Clinical Information

A 70-year-old male patient with a family-anecdotal description of several years of forgetfulness. At the time of presentation, he could not remember the minute by minute conversation, and kept repeating the same questions. He was aware of his forgetfulness.

Scan Interpretation

(Images. 17.46, 17.47, and 17.48).

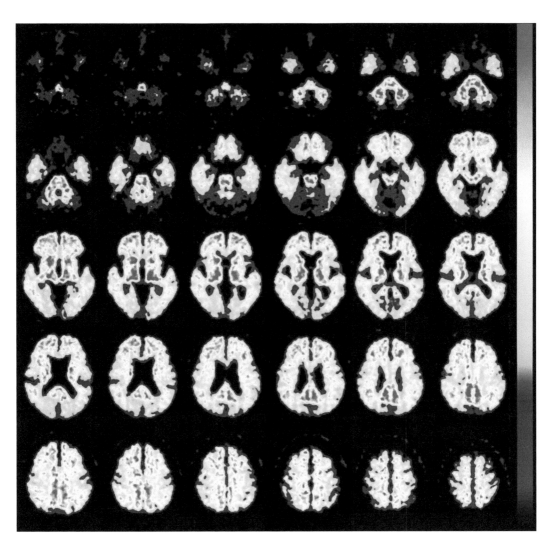

Image 17.46 The Amyloid-PET scan with 18F-flutemetamol shows severe bilateral frontal and posterior cingulate/precuneus cortical radiotracer deposition with a loss of gray–white matter contrast. There is also bilateral striatal deposition and slight deposition in parietotemporal regions, which indicates a significant amount of cerebral Aβ deposition (a positive scan)

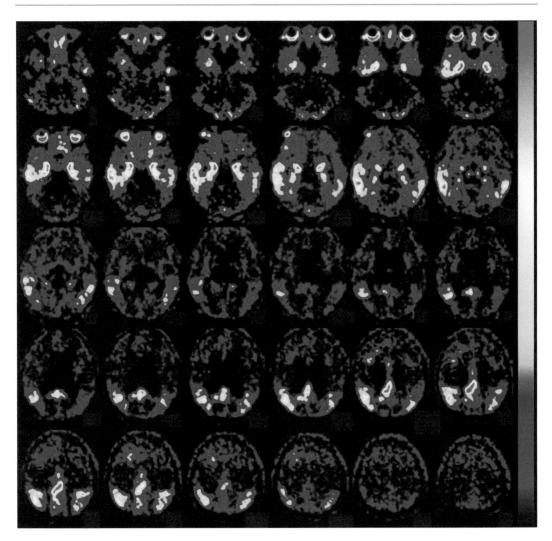

Image 17.47 The Tau-PET scan with 18F-MK6240 shows bilateral medial and lateral temporal, posterior cingulate/precuneus, and parietal cortical radiotracer uptake, which indicates a significant amount of cerebral tau deposition (a positive scan)

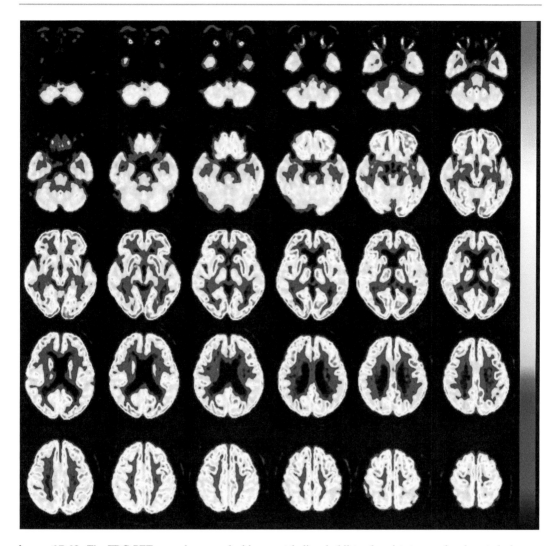

Image 17.48 The FDG-PET scan shows marked hypometabolism in bilateral parietotemporal and posterior/precuneus cortices, demonstrating the typical hypometabolic pattern of Alzheimer's disease

Teaching Points

This patient represents a traditional classic demonstration of A + T + N+ case with a typical case of AD clinical presentation where the neuropathological changes of Aβ deposition, tau deposition, and neurodegeneration were evaluated with Amyloid-PET, Tau-PET, and 18F-FDG-PET imaging.

Note that the diagnostic patterns of AD with PET imaging include increased tracer accumulation in the parietotemporal, frontal, and posterior/precuneus cortices on the Amyloid and Tau-PET images, and decreased accumulation (hypometabolism) in the parietotemporal, frontal, and posterior/precuneus cortices on the FDG-PET scan.

Case 2 (Courtesy of Professor Kazunari Ishii)

Kazunari Ishii

Indication/Clinical Information

A 78-year-old male patient with a history of memory decline for 2–3 years. According to his family, his emotional state has manifested with increased anger. No movement impairment was observed.

Scan Interpretation

(Images. 17.49, 17.50, and 17.51).

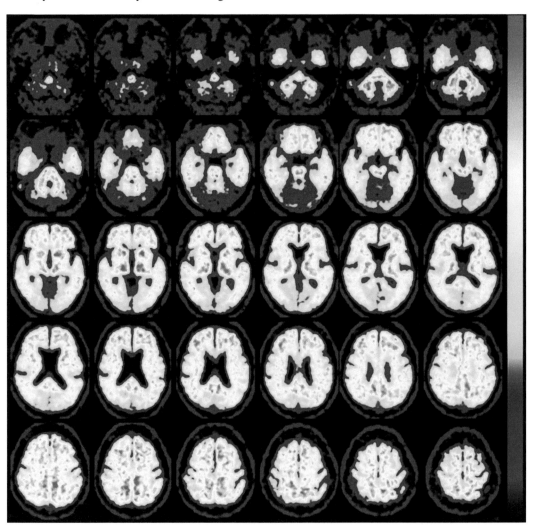

Image 17.49 The Amyloid-PET scan with 18F-flutemetamol shows frontal and parietotemporal cortical radiotracer deposition, with loss of gray–white matter contrast, and high deposition in the striatal and posterior cingulate/precuneus regions. These findings indicate a significant amount of cerebral Aβ deposition (a positive scan)

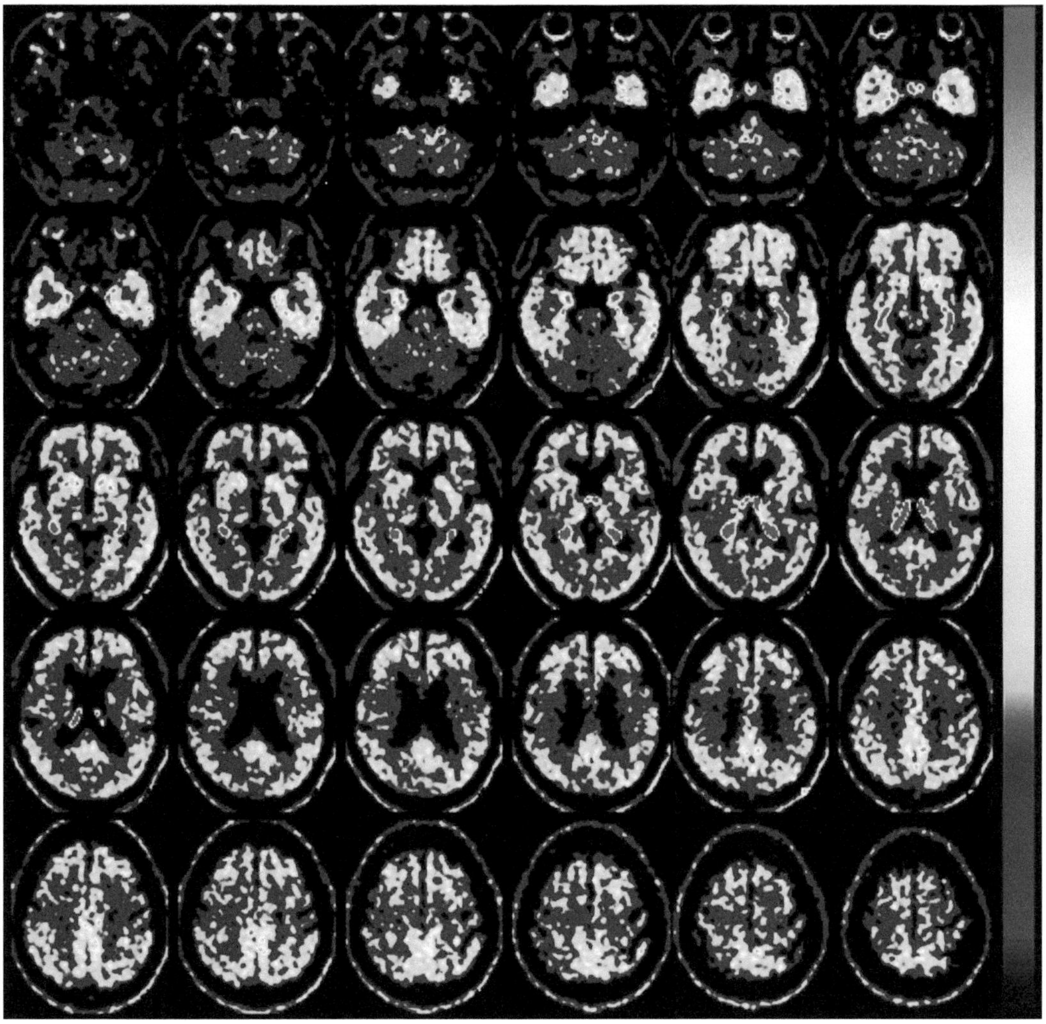

Image 17.50 The Tau-PET scan with 18F-PM-PBB3 shows increased radiotracer uptake in the bilateral lateral temporal, frontal, posterior cingulate/precuneus, and parietal cortices, as well as the amygdala. These findings indicate a significant amount of cerebral tau deposition (a positive scan). Note that PM-PBB3 has a strong affinity for the choroid plexus, which is considered off-target binding

Teaching Points

In this patient, the FDG-PET shows an atypical metabolic pattern, with frontal dominant hypometabolism, which favors a diagnosis of FTD; however the slightly decreased parietal and posterior cingulate metabolism may indicate the presence of AD pathology as well. Note that in some circumstances, FDG-PET may not differentiate the frontal variant of AD (fvAD) from the behavioral variant of FTD (bvFTD) very well or alternatively two pathologies, AD and FTLD, can coexist in the same patient, especially in elderly ones.

The fvAD is quite uncommon when compared to other subtypes of AD. Usually the memory decline tends to develop earlier and is more severe than in FTD, and the clinical presentation may be confounded with bvFTD. Usually, amyloid deposition is not observed in bvFTD, where the pathological condition mostly derives from intracellular aggregates of tau protein or TAR DNA-binding

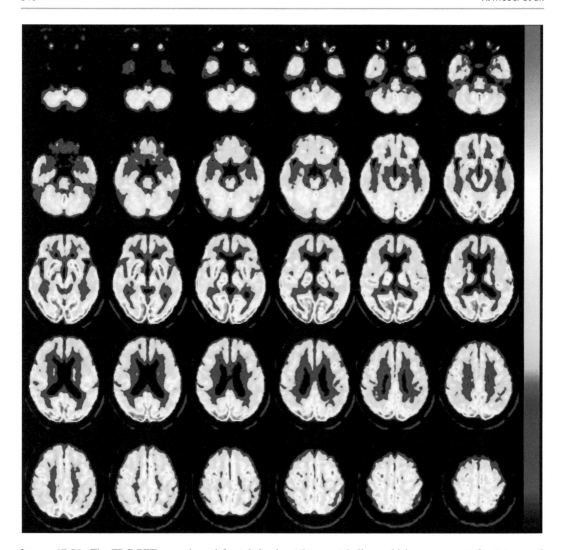

Image 17.51 The FDG-PET scan showed frontal dominant hypometabolism, which may suggest frontotemporal lobar degeneration (FTLD). Bilateral parietal and posterior cingulate metabolism is slightly decreased

protein 43 and, less frequently, from intracellular fused in sarcoma inclusions [61].

In this patient, the additional Amyloid and Tau-PET scans verified the presence of AD pathology, favoring the diagnosis of fvAD, but the Tau-positive findings are not specific to Tau isoforms seen in AD versus FTLD. Therefore, leaving the possibility of bvAD vs FTLD despite the use of 3 different molecular imaging methods.

Case 3 (Courtesy of Professor Kazunari Ishii)

Kazunari Ishii

Indication/Clinical Information

A 62-year-old male patient who had been aware of his forgetfulness for some time. Recently, he was unable to recognize people's faces. He had been suffering from sleep apnea syndrome for 2 years.

He indicated that a month prior, he saw his deceased father-in-law painting a picture. He did not have parkinsonism or any neurological symptoms.

Scan Interpretation

(Images. 17.52, 17.53, and 17.54).

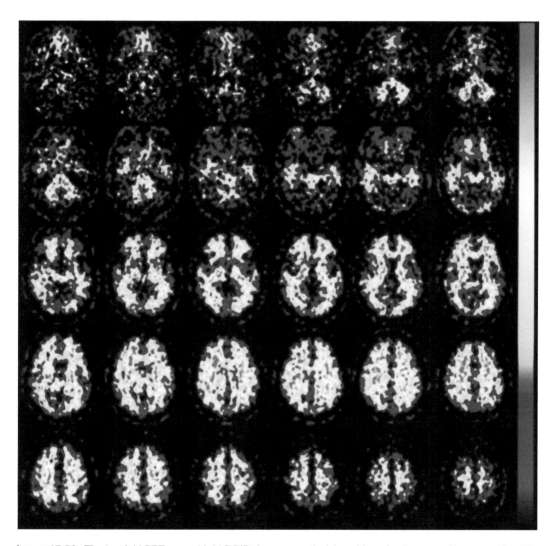

Image 17.52 The Amyloid-PET scan with 11C-PiB shows no cortical deposition of radiotracer with nonspecific white matter accumulation. These findings indicate no to very slight cerebral Aβ deposition (a negative scan)

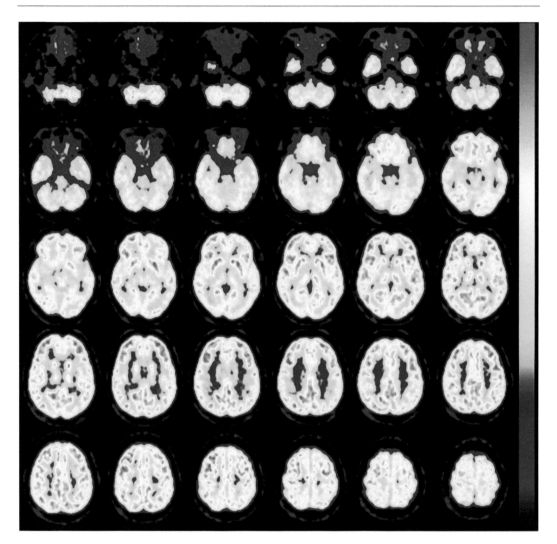

Image 17.53 The FDG-PET scan demonstrates marked hypometabolism in the bilateral parietotemporal, precuneus, and occipital cortices with primary visual cortex involvement. However, the relatively preserved metabolism in the middle cingulate cortex shows a slight "cingulate island sign" (CIS)

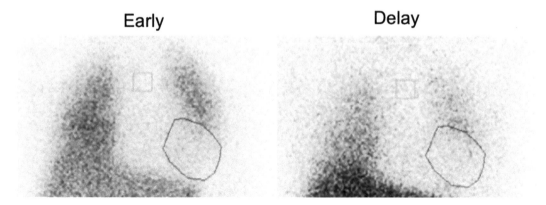

Image 17.54 The 123I-metaiodobenzylguanidine (MIBG) myocardial scintigraphy shows no myocardial uptake in the early or delayed phase, with an increased washout ratio

Teaching Points

This patient's FDG-PET scan shows hypometabolism in the occipital cortices, in addition to the bilateral parietotemporal and precuneus, supporting a diagnosis of DLB. Note that decreased uptake in the visual association cortex can also be seen in AD, and that decreased uptake in the primary visual cortex, as observed in this patient, can more accurately differentiate DLB from AD. The presence of the "cingulate island" sign also indicates the possibility of DLB, as the disease typically does not involve metabolic impairment of the posterior cingulate cortex.

Up to a half of clinically diagnosed DLB cases were negative for amyloid deposition, even though there is hypometabolism in parietotemporal cortices [62]. DAT-SPECT imaging and 123I-MIBG myocardial scintigraphy can help to differentiate DLB from AD. MIBG myocardial scintigraphy shows low uptake of MIBG in the Lewy body-related disorders, including Parkinson's disease, DLB, pure autonomic failure, and rapid eye movement sleep behavior disorder (RBD). The differentiation of DLB versus AD is critical for symptomatic drug treatments involving neuroleptics, which can cause severe adverse reactions in DLB [21].

Case 4 (Courtesy of Professor Min-Kai Chen)

Ming-Kai Chen

Indication/Clinical Information

A 79-year-old male presented with progressive visuospatial and visuoperceptual dysfunction, as well as short-term memory decline for approximately 8 years. In the past 4 years, he developed auditory and visual hallucinations, which occurred on a daily basis. He had no tremors or sleep disturbances, but his wife mentioned slowed movements of insidious onset. The neuropsychological testing was suggestive of DLB with some features of AD. The MRI was mostly unremarkable, with minor white matter microvascular changes.

Scan Interpretation

(Images. 17.55, 17.56, and 17.57).

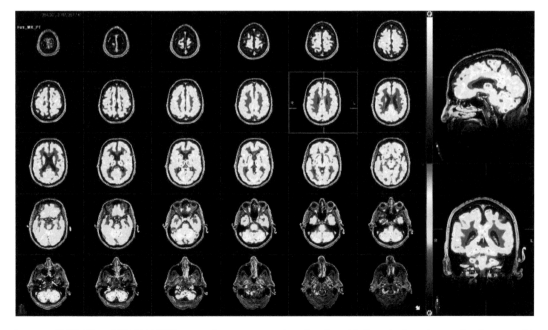

Image 17.55 The 18F-FDG-PET scan demonstrates hypometabolism in the right temporal lobe, bilateral parietal lobes, precuneus, and occipital lobes. Note that there is reduced metabolism in the primary visual cortex with relative sparing of the posterior cingulate cortex, indicating the CIS. These findings are suggestive of DLB

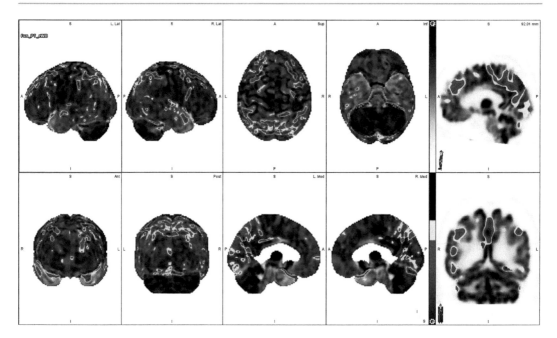

Image 17.56 The 3D-SSP images of the F-18-FDG-PET scan reveal significant hypometabolism in the right temporal lobe, bilateral parietal lobes, precuneus, and occipital lobes as compared to the normal database, which supports the findings by the visual assessment

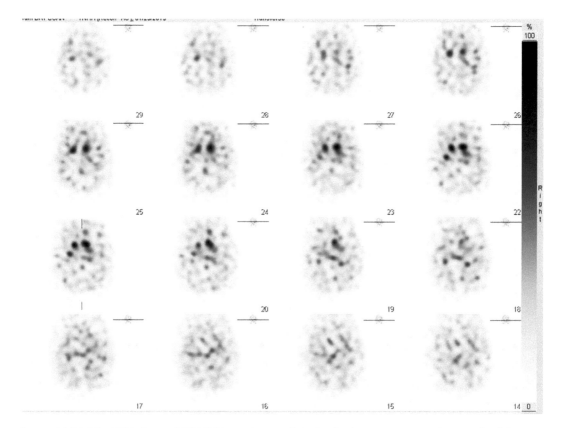

Image 17.57 The 123I-ioflupane SPECT/CT scan shows significantly reduced DaT scan uptake in the right and left striata, with more extensive involvement in the putamen. Striatal reductions are more prominent on the right, compared to the left. These findings are consistent with a pre-synaptic dopaminergic deficit of a parkinsonian syndrome

Teaching Points

Posterior cortical atrophy, considered the most common atypical presentation of Alzheimer disease (PCA-AD), has some clinical overlap with DLB, presenting with visual hallucinations and rapid eye movement sleep behavior disorder (RBD).

Notably both pathologies, DLB and PCA-AD, are associated with 18F-FDG-PET hypometabolism predominantly in the occipital and temporoparietal cortices. The relative preservation of posterior cingulate indicating CIS typically described in favor of DLB should be analyzed with caution. It is important to recall that posterior cingulate hypometabolism is not a reliable sign of the presence of Alzheimer's disease when dealing with atypical clinical presentations. In fact, the CIS can also be observed in PCA as well as DLB, although it is often asymmetric [63].

In this patient, the abnormal DAT scan is indicative of DLB, as AD has limited disruption of the dopaminergic system. Additionally, the patient cerebrospinal fluid biomarkers essentially excluded AD.

Case 5

Indication/Clinical Information

A 73-year-old female patient (8 years of education) presented with progressive multiple domain cognitive impairment of 3–4 years duration. According to her relatives, she had some difficulty in expressing herself or finding the appropriate words, but she was able to repeat sentences. She was well oriented but expressed some memory deficits (forgetful of some conversation details). She remained autonomous for daily living activities. The mini-mental state examination (MMSE) was 18 out of 30, and the neuropsychological assessment showed a mild multiple domain cognitive impairment with predominant involvement of language (mixed aphasia) and executive functions with no relevant neuropsychiatry symptoms.

Scan Interpretation

(Images. 17.58, 17.59, 17.60, and 17.61).

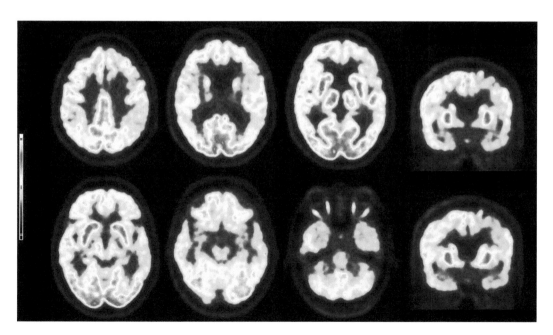

Image 17.58 The axial 18F-FDG-PET image indicates frontal and temporoparietal hypometabolism, more marked in the left hemisphere. Interestingly, the left inferoposterior frontal and anterior temporal cortices exhibit clear hypometabolism

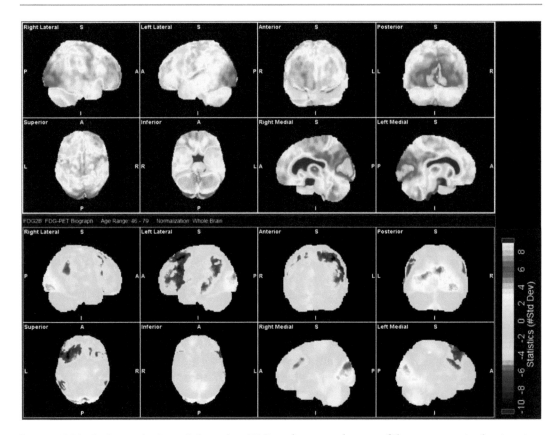

Image 17.59 Surface projections of the patient FDG-PET scan (upper row) and statistical surface projection maps after comparison to a normal database adjusted to the patient's age (lower row) are shown. There is significant hypometabolism in frontal and temporoparietal regions, which are more prominent in the left hemisphere, shown as a decrease of the z-score greater than two standard deviations (blue color in the lower row). These images clearly depict a pattern of dominant frontal hypometabolism, characteristic of FTLD. One should also note the absence of posterior cingulate hypometabolism

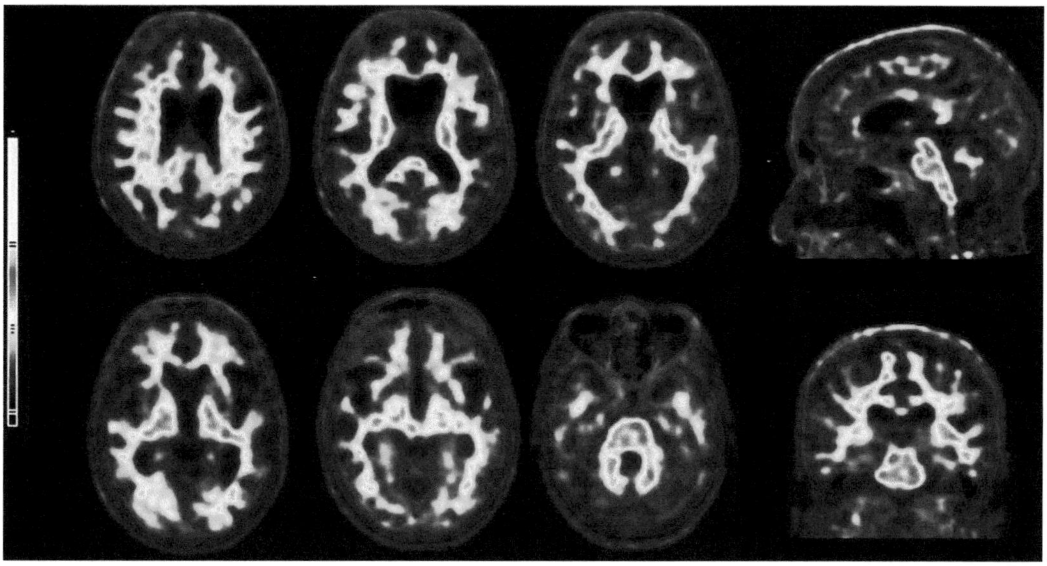

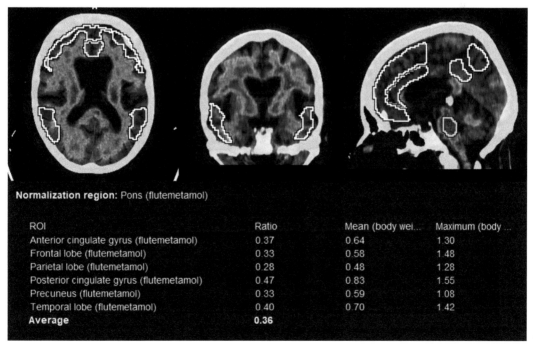

Image 17.60 The amyloid-PET scan with 18F-flutemetamol indicates a high contrast of white matter without uptake in the frontal, parietotemporal, and posterior cingulate/precuneus cortices, or in the striata. This is a clear example of a negative amyloid-PET scan, which indicates absence or lack of cerebral Aβ deposition. In other words, the presence of Alzheimer's pathology can be ruled out

Normalization region: Pons (flutemetamol)

ROI	Ratio	Mean (body wei...	Maximum (body ...
Anterior cingulate gyrus (flutemetamol)	0.37	0.64	1.30
Frontal lobe (flutemetamol)	0.33	0.58	1.48
Parietal lobe (flutemetamol)	0.28	0.48	1.28
Posterior cingulate gyrus (flutemetamol)	0.47	0.83	1.55
Precuneus (flutemetamol)	0.33	0.59	1.08
Temporal lobe (flutemetamol)	0.40	0.70	1.42
Average	**0.36**		

Image 17.61 Semiquantitative analysis of 18F-Flutemetamol PET images is shown. The global standard uptake value ratio (SUVR) was calculated by dividing the SUV in different cortical areas (volumes of interest) using the pons as a reference region. In this case the global SUVR was 0.36 (positive values are equal or higher than 0.6)

Teaching Points

In this case, the FDG-PET indicates a large region of frontal hypometabolism, with temporo-parietal involvement. Therefore, based exclusively on this pattern it may be difficult to completely exclude AD, as some variants exhibit language as the predominant symptom (logopenic aphasia). The additional amyloid-PET scan verified the absence of AD pathology and supported the etiology of frontotemporal lobe degeneration. Nevertheless, the FDG scan shows a clearly left dominant involvement with more marked inferoposterior frontal and anterior temporal (including temporal pole) hypometabolism. This pattern is highly consistent with primary progressive aphasia and specifically the non-fluent variant of primary progressive aphasia. Interestingly, an FDG-PET scan forms part of the current diagnostic criteria in support of a diagnosis of primary progressive aphasias.

Conclusion

Molecular imaging possesses the unique ability to image and quantify brain function "in vivo"; however image interpretation can be challenging and requires specific training. Here, we have provided a broad overview of molecular brain imaging, from the fundamentals, which include an overview of structural and functional brain anatomy, to a review of most of the clinically available radiotracers. We have outlined the common causes of artifacts and other factors which can interfere with accurate image interpretation. We hope this information will help readers improve their understanding of how to interpret and report different imaging studies in the clinical evaluation of neurodegenerative disorders. Lastly, we have included illustrative cases with typical and atypical presentations of different pathologies. Our hope is that the knowledge acquired through this chapter will encourage the development and expansion of molecular brain imaging in clinical practice.

Acknowledgments The authors would like to thank Drs. Kazunari Ishii (Kindai University, Japan), Ming-Kai Chen (Yale University, USA), Chakmeedaj Sethanandha (Mahidol University, Thailand), Jan Booij (University of Amsterdam, Holland), and Victor Villemagne (University of Melbourne, Australia) for contributing the images and cases for this chapter.

Appendix

MR Atlas

The images presented are from a healthy middle-aged male subject, acquired on a GE SIGNA Pioneer 3.0T MRI scanner. Each page contains images in axial plane from top-to-bottom, demonstrating the structures whose recognition is essential in the interpretation of a molecular imaging scan.

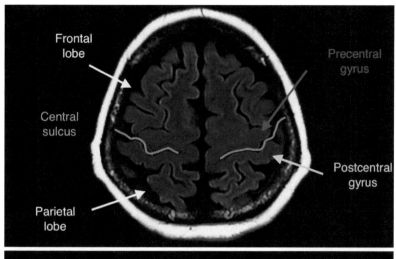

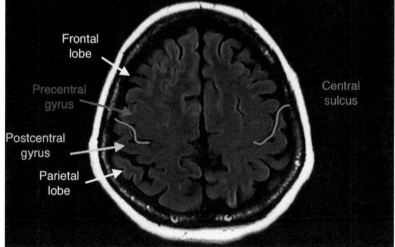

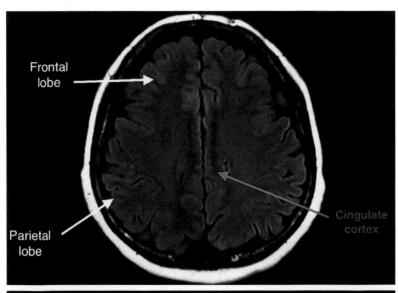

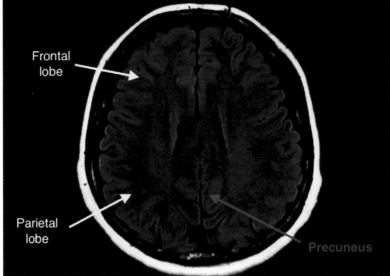

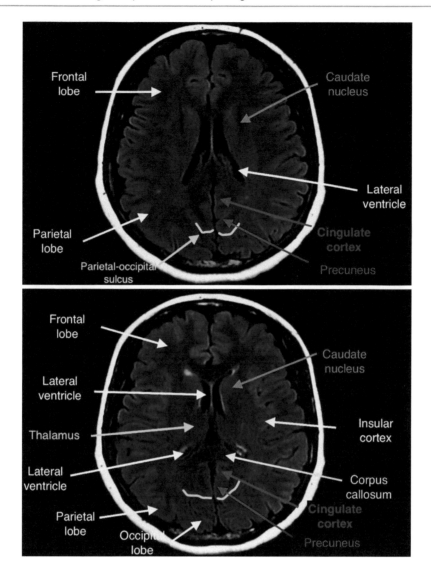

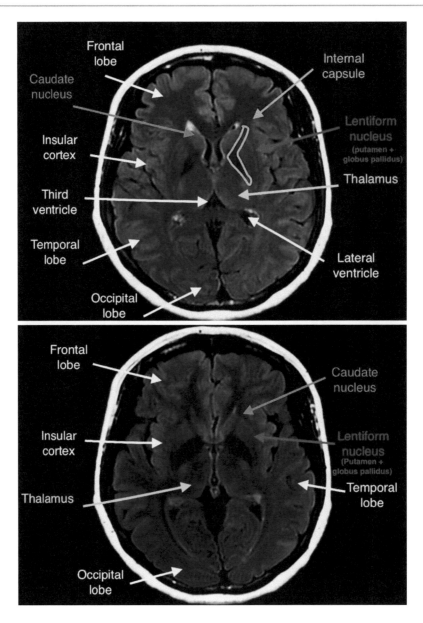

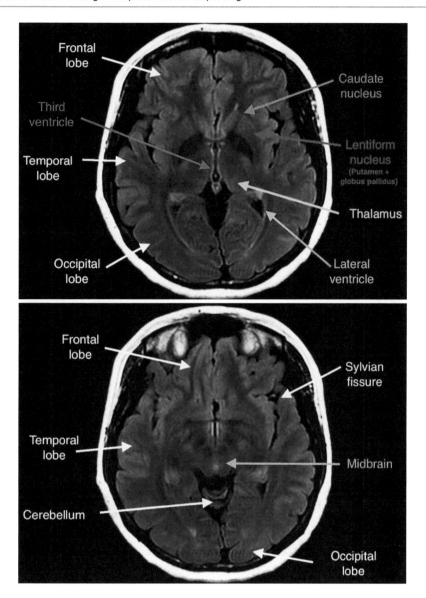

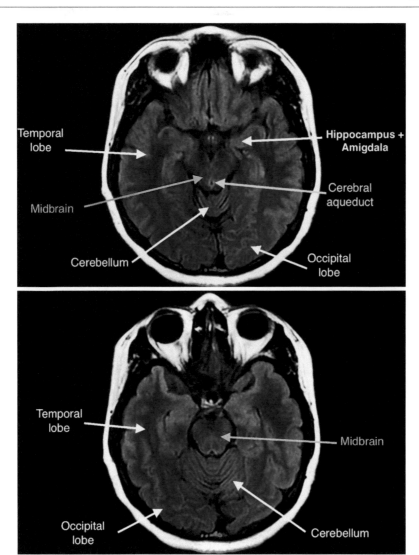

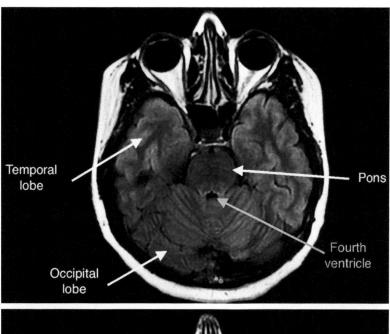

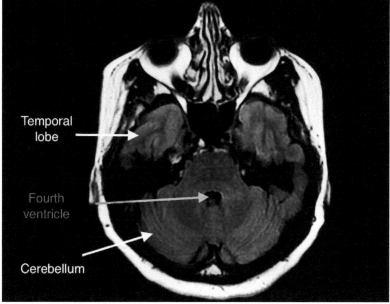

FDG Atlas

The images presented are from a healthy cognitively normal middle-aged female subject, acquired on a PET/CT (Discovery PET/CT scanner). The PET images were co-registered to the patient's MR acquired in a 3T MR system (Ingenia, Philips Medical system). Each page contains images in axial plane from top-to-bottom, demonstrating the structures whose recognition is essential in the interpretation of a molecular imaging scan.

Images courtesy from Dr. Chakmeedaj Sethanandha, Faculty of Medicine Siriraj Hospital, Mahidol University, Bangkok, Thailand.

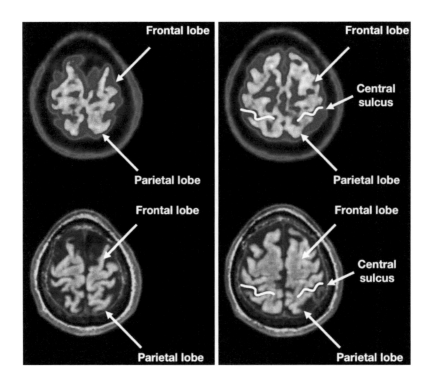

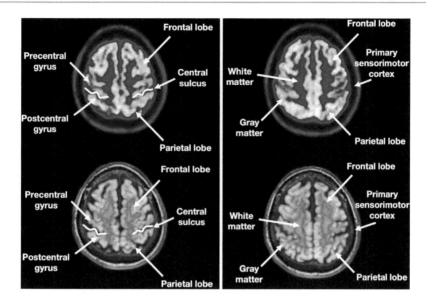

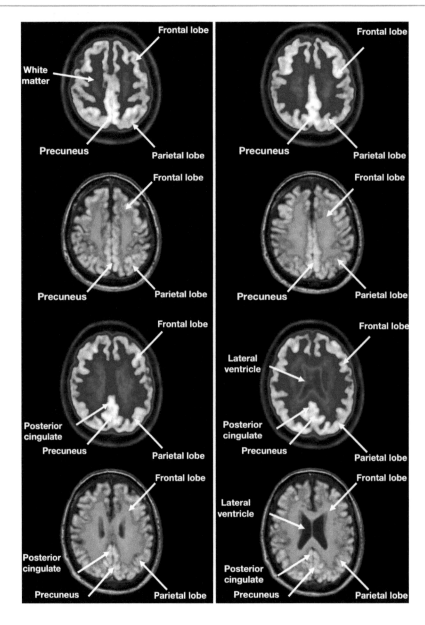

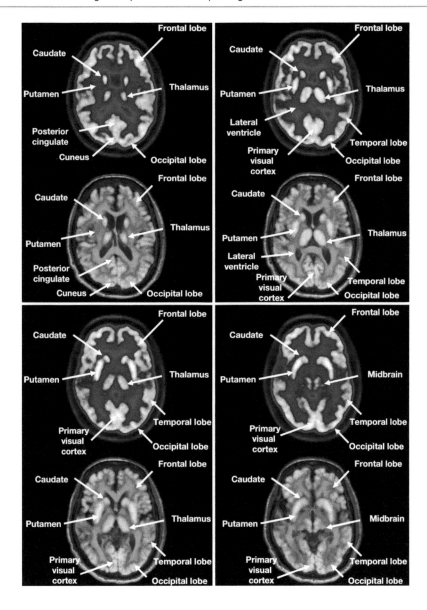

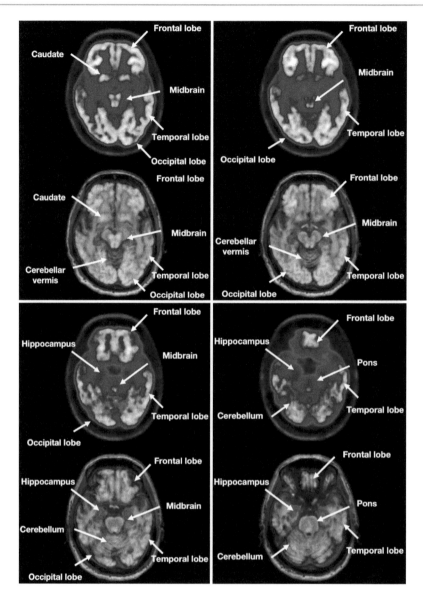

References

1. Jenkinson M, Chappell M. Introduction to neuroimaging analysis. In: Oxford neuroimaging primers. 1st ed. Oxford: Oxford University Press; 2018.

2. Haines DE, et al. Neuroanatomy in clinical context: an atlas of structures, sections, systems, and syndromes. 9th ed. Philadelphia: Wolters Kluwer Health; 2015.

3. Hendelman W. Atlas of functional neuroanatomy. 3rd ed. Boca Raton: CRC Press; 2015.

4. Lee TC, et al. Netter's correlative imaging: neuroanatomy. Netter clinical science. Philadelphia, PA: Elsevier Saunders; 2015.

5. Berger W, Berger J. Neuroanatomy. Case closed! Boca Raton: CRC Press; 2017.

6. Agarwal N, Port JD. Neuroimaging: anatomy meets function. 1st ed. Cham: Springer International Publishing; 2018.

7. Splittgerber R, Lippincott W, Wilkins. Snell's clinical neuroanatomy. 8th ed. Philadelphia: Wolters Kluwer; 2018. p. xxvi, 527 pages: illustrations (black and white, and colour).

8. Waxman SG, Waxman SG. Clinical neuroanatomy. In: McGraw-Hill's AccessNeurology. 29th ed. New York: McGraw-Hill Education LLC; 2020.

9. Berkowitz AL. Clinical neurology and neuroanatomy: a localization-based approach. In: Berkowitz A, editor. Neurology collection. 1st ed. New York, NY: McGraw-Hill Education LLC; 2017.

10. Martin JH, Martin JH. Neuroanatomy: text and atlas. In: McGraw-Hill's access neurology. 5th ed. New York: McGraw-Hill Education LLC; 2021.

11. Bui T, Das JM. Neuroanatomy, cerebral hemisphere. In: StatPearls, StatPearls Publishing Copyright © 2021. Treasure Island, FL: StatPearls Publishing LLC; 2021.

12. Talairach J, Tournoux P. Co-planar stereotaxic atlas of the human brain: 3-dimensional proportional system: an approach to medical cerebral imaging. Stuttgart/New York: Thieme Thieme Medical; 1988. p. viii, 122 p. : ill. (chiefly col.)

13. Brock DG, Mancall EL, Gray H. Gray's Clinical neuroanatomy: the anatomic basis for clinical neuroscience (Clinical neuroanatomy). W B Saunders Company; 2011.

14. Jacobson S, et al. Neuroanatomy for the neuroscientist. Cham: Springer; 2018.

15. Van Heertum RL, Tikofsky RS, Ichise M. Functional cerebral SPECT and PET imaging. 4th ed. Philadelphia, PA: Lippincott Williams & Wilkins; 2010. p. xvi, 458 pages: illustrations (some color)

16. Anand KS, Dhikav V. Hippocampus in health and disease: an overview. Ann Indian Acad Neurol. 2012;15(4):239–46.

17. Vanderah TW, Gould DJ, Ebscohost. Nolte's the human brain: an introduction to its functional anat-

omy. In: ClinicalKey. 7th ed. Philadelphia, PA: Elsevier; 2016.

18. Kenhub. Cerebral cortex. March 14, 2022. https://www.kenhub.com/en/library/anatomy/cerebral-cortex.

19. Osborn AG. Diagnostic and surgical imaging anatomy: brain, head & neck, spine. London: Amirsys; 2006. 227pages : illustrations (some colour)

20. Toth P, et al. Functional vascular contributions to cognitive impairment and dementia: mechanisms and consequences of cerebral autoregulatory dysfunction, endothelial impairment, and neurovascular uncoupling in aging. Am J Physiol Heart Circ Physiol. 2017;312(1):H1–H20.

21. Minoshima S, et al. Brain [F-18]FDG PET for clinical dementia workup: differential diagnosis of Alzheimer's disease and other types of dementing disorders. Semin Nucl Med. 2021;51(3):230–40.

22. Kapucu OL, et al. EANM procedure guideline for brain perfusion SPECT using 99mTc-labelled radiopharmaceuticals, version 2. Eur J Nucl Med Mol Imaging. 2009;36(12):2093–102.

23. Kung HF, Kung MP, Choi SR. Radiopharmaceuticals for single-photon emission computed tomography brain imaging. Semin Nucl Med. 2003;33(1):2–13.

24. Koyama M, et al. SPECT imaging of normal subjects with technetium-99m-HMPAO and technetium-99m-ECD. J Nucl Med. 1997;38(4):587–92.

25. Guedj E, et al. EANM procedure guidelines for brain PET imaging using [(18)F]FDG, version 3. Eur J Nucl Med Mol Imaging. 2022;49(2):632–51.

26. Berti V, Mosconi L, Pupi A. Brain: normal variations and benign findings in fluorodeoxyglucose-PET/computed tomography imaging. PET Clin. 2014;9(2):129–40.

27. Saroja SR, et al. Differential expression of tau species and the association with cognitive decline and synaptic loss in Alzheimer's disease. Alzheimers Dement. 2022;18(9):1602–15.

28. Minoshima S, et al. SNMMI procedure standard/EANM practice guideline for amyloid PET imaging of the brain 1.0. J Nucl Med. 2016;57(8):1316–22.

29. Bischof GN, et al. Impact of tau and amyloid burden on glucose metabolism in Alzheimer's disease. Ann Clin Transl Neurol. 2016;3(12):934–9.

30. Bejanin A, et al. Tau pathology and neurodegeneration contribute to cognitive impairment in Alzheimer's disease. Brain. 2017;140(12):3286–300.

31. Ricci M, et al. Tau biomarkers in dementia: positron emission tomography radiopharmaceuticals in tauopathy assessment and future perspective. Int J Mol Sci. 2021;22(23)

32. Tian M, et al. International consensus on the use of tau PET imaging agent (18)F-flortaucipir in Alzheimer's disease. Eur J Nucl Med Mol Imaging. 2022;49(3):895–904.

33. Mattay VS, et al. Brain tau imaging: Food and Drug Administration approval of (18)F-flortaucipir injection. J Nucl Med. 2020;61(10):1411–2.

34. Bischof GN, et al. Clinical validity of second-generation tau PET tracers as biomarkers for Alzheimer's disease in the context of a structured 5-phase development framework. Eur J Nucl Med Mol Imaging. 2021;48(7):2110–20.

35. Scholl M, et al. PET imaging of tau deposition in the aging human brain. Neuron. 2016;89(5):971–82.

36. Eshuis SA, et al. Comparison of FP-CIT SPECT with F-DOPA PET in patients with de novo and advanced Parkinson's disease. Eur J Nucl Med Mol Imaging. 2006;33(2):200–9.

37. Morbelli S, et al. EANM practice guideline/SNMMI procedure standard for dopaminergic imaging in Parkinsonian syndromes 1.0. Eur J Nucl Med Mol Imaging. 2020;47(8):1885–912.

38. Zhang K, et al. PET imaging of neural activity, beta-amyloid, and tau in normal brain aging. Eur J Nucl Med Mol Imaging. 2021;48(12):3859–71.

39. Silverman D, Silverman D. PET in the evaluation of Alzheimer's disease and related disorders. 1st ed. New York: Springer; 2009.

40. Varrone A, et al. European multicentre database of healthy controls for [123I]FP-CIT SPECT (ENC-DAT): age-related effects, gender differences and evaluation of different methods of analysis. Eur J Nucl Med Mol Imaging. 2013;40(2):213–27.

41. Parkinson Progression Marker Initiative. The Parkinson Progression Marker Initiative (PPMI). Prog Neurobiol. 2011;95(4):629–35.

42. Burns CM, et al. Higher serum glucose levels are associated with cerebral hypometabolism in Alzheimer regions. Neurology. 2013;80(17):1557–64.

43. Juni JE, et al. Procedure guideline for brain perfusion SPECT using (99m)Tc radiopharmaceuticals 3.0. J Nucl Med Technol. 2009;37(3):191–5.

44. Salmon E, Bernard Ir C, Hustinx R. Pitfalls and limitations of PET/CT in brain imaging. Semin Nucl Med. 2015;45(6):541–51.

45. Kim J, et al. Usefulness of 3-dimensional stereotactic surface projection FDG PET images for the diagnosis of dementia. Medicine (Baltimore). 2016;95(49):e5622.

46. Brown RK, et al. Brain PET in suspected dementia: patterns of altered FDG metabolism. Radiographics. 2014;34(3):684–701.

47. Minoshima S, et al. A diagnostic approach in Alzheimer's disease using three-dimensional stereotactic surface projections of fluorine-18-FDG PET. J Nucl Med. 1995;36(7):1238–48.

48. Minoshima S, et al. Metabolic reduction in the posterior cingulate cortex in very early Alzheimer's disease. Ann Neurol. 1997;42(1):85–94.

49. Kim EJ, et al. Glucose metabolism in early onset versus late onset Alzheimer's disease: an SPM analysis of 120 patients. Brain. 2005;128(Pt 8):1790–801.

50. Johnson KA, et al. Appropriate use criteria for amyloid PET: a report of the Amyloid Imaging Task Force, the Society of Nuclear Medicine and Molecular Imaging, and the Alzheimer's Association. J Nucl Med. 2013;54(3):476–90.

51. Rowe CC, Villemagne VL. Brain amyloid imaging. J Nucl Med. 2011;52(11):1733–40.
52. Amyvid (florbetapir F 18 Injection) Leaflet. 2012. https://www.accessdata.fda.gov/drugsatfda_docs/label/2012/202008s000lbl.pdf.
53. Jie C, et al. Tauvid: the first FDA-approved PET tracer for imaging tau pathology in Alzheimer's disease. Pharmaceuticals (Basel). 2021;14(2)
54. Brendel M, et al. Assessment of 18F-PI-2620 as a biomarker in progressive supranuclear palsy. JAMA Neurol. 2020;77(11):1408–19.
55. Mueller A, et al. Tau PET imaging with (18)F-PI-2620 in patients with Alzheimer disease and healthy controls: a first-in-humans study. J Nucl Med. 2020;61(6):911–9.
56. Sonni I, et al. Evaluation of a visual interpretation method for tau-PET with (18)F-flortaucipir. Alzheimers Dement (Amst). 2020;12(1):e12133.
57. Eli Lilly and Company. TAUVID TM (flortaucipir F 18 injection) Leaflet. 2020. https://pi.lilly.com/us/tauvid-uspi.pdf.
58. Langston JW, Wiley JC, Tagliati M. Optimizing Parkinson's disease diagnosis: the role of a dual nuclear imaging algorithm. NPJ Parkinsons Dis. 2018;4:5.
59. Marek K, et al. Longitudinal follow-up of SWEDD subjects in the PRECEPT study. Neurology. 2014;82(20):1791–7.
60. Waxman AD, Lewis DH, Herscovitch P, Minoshima S, Ichise M, Drzezga AE, Devous MD, Mountz JM. Society of Nuclear Medicine procedure guideline for FDG PET brain imaging 1.0; 2009.
61. Li CH, et al. Frontal variant of Alzheimer's disease with asymmetric presentation mimicking frontotemporal dementia: case report and literature review. Brain Behav. 2020;10(3):e01548.
62. Ossenkoppele R, et al. Prevalence of amyloid PET positivity in dementia syndromes: a meta-analysis. JAMA. 2015;313(19):1939–49.
63. Whitwell JL, et al. (18)F-FDG PET in posterior cortical atrophy and dementia with Lewy bodies. J Nucl Med. 2017;58(4):632–8.
64. Minoshima S, Cross D, Thientunyakit T, Foster NL, Drzezga A. 18F-FDG PET imaging in neurodegenerative dementing disorders: insights into subtype classification, emerging disease categories, and mixed dementia with copathologies. J Nucl Med. 2022;63(Suppl 1):2S–12S.
65. Chandran V, Stoessl AJ. Imaging in multiple system atrophy. Neurol Clin Neurosci. 2014;2:178–87. https://doi.org/10.1111/ncn3.125.
66. Shivamurthy VKN, Tahari AK, Marcus C, Subramaniam RM. Brain FDG PET and the diagnosis of dementia. Am J Roentgenol. 2015;204(1):W76–85.

Index